Controversies
in Oncology

Controversies
in Oncology

Edited by

Peter H. Wiernik, M.D.
Professor of Medicine
University of Maryland School of Medicine
Director, Baltimore Cancer Research Center
Baltimore, Maryland

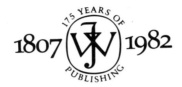

A WILEY MEDICAL PUBLICATION
JOHN WILEY & SONS / **New York • Chichester • Brisbane • Toronto**

Library of Congress Cataloging in Publication Data
Main entry under title:

Controversies in oncology.

(A Wiley medical publication)
Includes index.
1. Cancer—Treatment.   I. Wiernik, Peter H.
II. Series. [DNLM: 1. Neoplasms—Drug therapy.
QZ 266 C7645]
RC270.8.C67   616.99'406   81-11420
ISBN 0-471-05925-0   AACR2

Printed in the United States of America

10 9 8 7 6 5 4 3 2 1

To Roberta, and Julie, Lisa, and Peter

To Roberta, and Julie, Lisa, and Peter

Contributors

Joseph Aisner, M.D.
Associate Professor of Medicine
University of Maryland Hospital
Head, Clinical Oncology Branch
Baltimore Cancer Research Center
Baltimore, Maryland

Robert S. Benjamin, M.D.
Associate Professor of Medicine
University of Texas Cancer Center
Chief, Section of Clinical Pharmacology
Department of Developmental Therapeutics
M.D. Anderson Hospital and Tumor Institute
Houston, Texas

Daniel E. Bergsagel, M.D.
Professor of Medicine
University of Toronto
Chief of Medicine
Princess Margaret Hospital
Toronto, Canada

Clara D. Bloomfield, M.D.
Professor of Medicine
University of Minnesota School of Medicine
Director, Masonic Leukemia Treatment Center
Minneapolis, Minnesota

Fernando Cabanillas, M.D.
Associate Professor of Medicine
University of Texas Cancer Center
Associate Internist
Department of Developmental Therapeutics
M.D. Anderson Hospital and Tumor Institute
Houston, Texas

Florence Chu, M.D.
Chairman and Attending Radiation Therapist
Department of Radiotherapy
Memorial Sloan-Kettering Center
New York, New York

James D. Cox, M.D.
Professor of Radiology
Department of Radiation Therapy
Medical College of Wisconsin
Milwaukee, Wisconsin

Isaac Djerassi, M.D.
Director of Hematology-Oncology
Fitzgerald Mercy Division
Mercy Catholic Medical Center
Darby, Pennsylvania

John R. Durant, M.D.
Professor of Medicine
University of Alabama Medical Center
Director, Comprehensive Cancer Center
Birmingham, Alabama

John C. Fletcher, Ph.D.
Assistant for Bioethics
Clinical Center
National Institutes of Health
Bethesda, Maryland

Emil Freireich, M.D.
Ruth Harriet Aimsworth
Professor of Developmental Therapeutics
University of Texas Cancer Center
Head, Department of Developmental Therapeutics
Adult Division
M.D. Anderson Hospital and Tumor Institute
Houston, Texas

Arvin S. Glicksman, M.D.
Chairman, Department of Radiation-Oncology
Rhode Island Hospital
Providence, Rhode Island

Philip H. Gutin, M.D.
Assistant Professor in Residence
Department of Neurosurgery
University of California
San Francisco, California

Daniel Hollard, M.D.
Professor and Chairman
Department of Blood Diseases
University Hospital of Grenoble
Grenoble, France

Diana Lake-Lewin, M.D.
Associate Attending Physician
Division of Hematology-Oncology
St. Michaels Medical Center
Newark, New Jersey

Monique Laurent, Ph.D
Commissariat à l'Energie Atomique
Centre d'Etudes Nucléaires de Grenoble
Laboratoire d'Hématologie
Grenoble, France

Burton J. Lee, M.D.
Attending Physician
Memorial Sloan-Kettering Center
New York, New York

Arthur C. Louie, M.D.
Research Fellow
Department of Medicine
Division of Oncology
Stanford University
Stanford, California

Kenneth B. McCredie, M.D.
Professor of Medicine
University of Texas Cancer Center
Chief, Leukemia Service
Department of Developmental Therapeutics
M.D. Anderson Hospital and Tumor Institute
Houston, Texas

Keith Mills, M.D.
Director of Hematology-Oncology
Fitzgerald Mercy Division
Mercy Catholic Medical Center
Darby, Pennsylvania

Franco M. Muggia, M.D.
Professor of Medicine
Director, Division of Oncology
New York University Medical Center
New York, New York

Jane E. Myers, B.S.
Research Assistant
Memorial Sloan-Kettering Cancer Center
New York, New York

Henry G. Ohanissian, M.D.
Hematology-Oncology
Mercy Catholic Medical Center
Philadelphia, Pennsylvania

Santiago Pavlovsky, M.D.
Chairman
Grupo Argentino De Tratamiento De La Leucemia Aguda
Buenos Aires, Argentina

Philip A. Pizzo, M.D.
Head, Infectious Disease Section
Pediatric Oncology Branch
National Cancer Institute
National Institutes of Health
Bethesda, Maryland

Carol S. Portlock, M.D.
Associate Professor of Medicine
Section of Medical Oncology
Yale University School of Medicine
New Haven, Connecticut

Douglas Pritchard, M.D.
Consultant, Department of Orthopedics
Mayo Clinic
Rochester, Minnesota

Saul A. Rosenberg, M.D.
Professor of Medicine & Radiology
Chief, Division of Oncology
Stanford University Medical Center
Stanford, California

Marcel Rozencweig, M.D.
Head, Investigational Drug Section
Department of Chemotherapy
Service de Médecine et Laboratoire d'investigation
Clinique H.J. Tagnon
Institute Jules Bordet
Centre des Tumeurs de l'universitaire
Libre de Bruxelles
Brussells, Belgium

Charles A. Schiffer, M.D.
Associate Professor of Medicine
University of Maryland Hospital
Head, Cell Component Therapy Section
Baltimore Cancer Research Center
Baltimore, Maryland

Stephen C. Schimpff, M.D.
Professor of Medicine
University of Maryland Hospital
Head, Section of Infection of Microbiological Research
Baltimore Cancer Research Center
Baltimore, Maryland

Nathan Schnaper, M.D.
Professor of Psychiatry
University of Maryland Hospital
Head, Psychiatric Section
Baltimore Cancer Research Center
Baltimore, Maryland

Lucius F. Sinks, M.D.
Professor of Adolescence Oncology
Chief, Adolescence Oncology
Vincent T. Lombardi Cancer Research Center
Georgetown University Medical Center
Washington, D.C.

Jean Jacques Sotto, M.D.
Assistant Professor of Hematology
Department of Hematology and Oncology
Service d'Hématologie
Center Hospitalier et Universitaire
  de Grenoble
La Tronche, France

Jung Sun Kim, M.D.
Associate Professor
Department of Pediatrics
Jefferson University Medical School
Associate Director
Research Hematology and Oncology
Mercy Catholic Medical Center
Philadelphia, Pennsylvania

Peter H. Wiernik, M.D.
Professor of Medicine
University of Maryland School of Medicine
Director, Baltimore Cancer Research Center
Baltimore, Maryland

Shiao Y. Woo, M.D.
Assistant Professor
Department of Pediatrics
Division of Pediatric and
    Adolescent Hematology-Oncology
Vincent T. Lombardi Cancer Research Center
Georgetown University Medical Center
Washington, D.C.

Preface

Oncology is a rapidly advancing field on all fronts. Only a third of a century has passed since the first demonstration that drugs could favorably affect the course of a malignant disease, and only a couple of decades have passed since the first proof of cure of advanced disease with radiotherapy (Hodgkin's disease) or chemotherapy (choriocarcinoma and childhood acute lymphocytic leukemia) was obtained. For the most part, progress in cancer treatment has been steady and unfaltering. On rare occasions, however, premature conclusions led us down the wrong path and cost us all precious time in achieving our ultimate goal of effective therapy for most patients with cancer.

The purpose of this volume is to point out that certain important conclusions drawn by some from present-day studies are not universally subscribed to. It is hoped that the information collected here will stimulate others to perform studies that will lead to the ultimate resolution of the issues discussed.

I wish to express my sincere gratitude to the authors who contributed their expertise to this effort and to Mr. Robert Hurley, Medical Editor, John Wiley & Sons, Inc., whose advice and patience are equally appreciated.

Peter H. Wiernik

Contents

PART 3   SUPPORTIVE CARE   221

Controversies
in Oncology

Part 1

HEMATOLOGIC MALIGNANCIES

1

Combined Modality Treatment of Early Stage Hodgkin's Disease

Peter H. Wiernik

Some important aspects of the management of patients with Hodgkin's disease are still controversial and they often lead to debate that fails to generate a consensus on the issues. The accumulation of new data from several sources in recent years that bear on the proper staging and treatment of patients with Hodgkin's disease may shed light on some of these issues that are so important to our patients.

A number of studies have indicated that a combined modality approach to some patients with Hodgkin's disease confined to lymph nodes offers them the best chance of cure. However, Portlock and coworkers (1) have argued that the overall survival of groups of patients so treated is not enhanced by such aggressive treatment because "salvage" chemotherapy for patients who are radiation failures results in the cure of a significant fraction of such patients. The data represented in Figure 1, however, suggest that the long-term results of "salvage" chemotherapy may not be as impressive as the short-term results. Others (2) have reached similar conclusions.

Proponents of the radiotherapy alone approach to all patients with Hodgkin's disease confined to lymph nodes also argue that the frequency of acute leukemia in patients with Hodgkin's disease is greatest in those who receive combined modality therapy. Close examination of relevant data, however, demonstrates that the incidence of acute leukemia is greatest in patients who are initially treated with extended field radiotherapy, relapse, and then receive "salvage" combination chemotherapy. Nevertheless, the incidence of acute leukemia in patients who are intensively treated for Hodgkin's disease serves as a signal that the long-term complications of such treatment may dictate that the entire approach to Hodgkin's disease treatment be reexamined. Some pilot data have demonstrated the potential of combination chemotherapy alone for the successful induction of complete remission in early Hodgkin's disease. Although

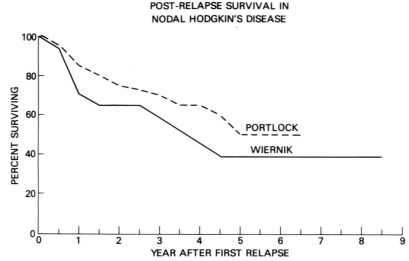

Figure 1. The Stanford (Portlock) and Baltimore Cancer Research Center (Wiernik) data concerning postrelapse survival for early-stage Hodgkin's disease treated initially with radiotherapy alone.

chemotherapy alone may be associated with more acute toxicity than radiotherapy, the chronic complications of radiotherapy may be greater. Chemotherapy alone for localized Hodgkin's disease is, of course, investigational, and the observation of a sufficient number of patients so treated for, perhaps, a decade will be necessary before the relative merit of this approach to a standard one can be fully evaluated.

The purpose of this chapter is to discuss some of these issues critically and to make recommendations based on available data for the treatment of patients with Hodgkin's disease apparently confined to lymph nodes.

THE COMBINED MODALITY APPROACH

Two major and similar early studies comparing radiotherapy alone with radiotherapy and chemotherapy for Hodgkin's disease confined to lymph nodes have yielded similar results. Both demonstrated a statistically significant improvement in continuous disease-free survival after combined modality treatment compared with radiotherapy alone (3,4), and, in both studies, total survival was also better in that treatment group; but the differences were not significant for some stages of disease. The lack of statistical significance to the overall survival differences between the two treatment groups has led the Stanford group to recommend radiotherapy alone for patients with early stage Hodgkin's disease, as discussed by Dr. Portlock in this volume. They recommend withholding combination chemotherapy until the patient relapses after initial radiotherapy treatment, and they justify that approach with three major arguments. First, that approach obviously spares the majority of patients chemotherapy because the majority of patients do not relapse after radiotherapy alone. Furthermore, as mentioned above, post relapse, or "salvage" chemotherapy, is said to be eminently successful (1)—so successful that the total survival of patients treated initially only with radiotherapy compared with that of patients treated initially with combined modality therapy is not statistically significantly different. Last, acute leukemia occurs with greater frequency in Hodgkin's disease patients who have been treated with the combined modality approach compared with those treated with radiotherapy alone. These arguments have led many oncologists to conclude that initial combined modality treatment is not in the best interest of the patient with early stage Hodgkin's disease.

Before examining these issues in detail, it seems appropriate to update the results of our own study of 74 evaluable patients that began 10 years ago and was closed to accrual of new patients in January 1974. Earlier evaluations of this study have been published (4,5).

OVERALL RESULTS

Figure 2 demonstrates a statistically significant advantage for stage IA, IB, IIA, and IIB patients treated with the combined modality approach with respect to disease-free survival compared with patients treated with extended field radiotherapy only. However, Figure 3 indicates that total survival, although better for the combined modality group, is not statistically significantly different between the treatment groups. Figure 4 illustrates two important points. The first is that, as was noted for stage I and II patients, stage IIIA patients also have a highly statistically significantly better disease-free survival when treated with radio-

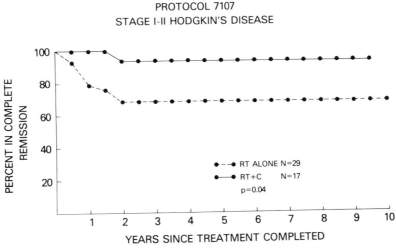

Figure 2. Complete remission duration curves for stage I and II patients treated with extended field radiotherapy alone or followed by six courses of MOPP chemotherapy. Patients were first entered on this study of the Baltimore Cancer Research Center in 1971 (see text for details).

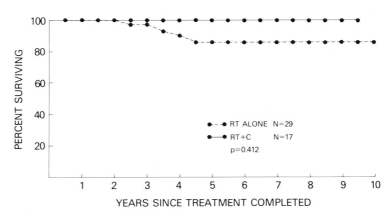

Figure 3. Survival curves for the patients in Figure 1.

therapy and chemotherapy compared with patients treated with radiotherapy only. Second, late relapses occur in Hodgkin's disease, and any final meaningful evaluation of a study such as this one must be made many years after the last patient has been entered on study. Figure 5 demonstrates that the overall survival advantage for patients with stage IIIA disease that is afforded by combined modality treatment is statistically significant compared with that of total nodal radiotherapy alone.

In an effort to identify stage IIA patients with a high probability of relapse, an exhaustive analysis of pretreatment characteristics of each patient was made and correlated with outcome. This analysis identified patients with E stage of

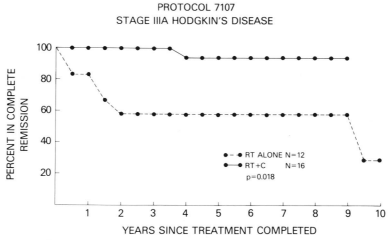

Figure 4. Complete remission duration curves for patients with stage IIIA entered on the same study depicted in Figures 1 and 2.

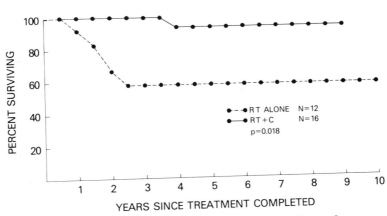

PROTOCOL 7107
STAGE IIIA HODGKIN'S DISEASE

Figure 5. Survival curves for the patients in Figure 3.

the lung as a small group of patients (15% of all patients entered in that study) with a significantly poorer disease-free and overall survival compared with patients of the same stage without E disease when radiotherapy alone was the treatment (4). No such differences were noted between the two groups if combined modality treatment was used (4). This observation stimulated us to look retrospectively at a larger group of patients who were treated by us (6). In that review of 102 patients, which included the 74 patients described above, 18 had E stage of the lung. The E stage patients had again significantly poorer disease-free and overall survival compared with patients of the same stage without E stage disease when treated with radiotherapy alone. Again, these differences between E stage and other patients were not evident when therapy was radiotherapy followed by six courses of MOPP. The majority of the relapses in E stage patients were regional recurrences in the lung parenchyma after radiotherapy alone (7). We also noted that almost 80% of the relapsed patients had E stage disease in association with very large mediastinal masses (7). We concluded from these observations that early stage Hodgkin's disease patients with very large mediastinal masses often had direct pulmonary extension of disease from these masses, and patients with such masses had significantly higher relapse and death rates compared with other patients of similar stages when treated with radiotherapy alone. Treatment with radiotherapy followed by MOPP eliminated these differences (4,6,7).

Since our observations on patients with large mediastinal masses and E stage of the lung were published, others (8–12) have reported similar results after radiotherapy, and others have reported improved results after combined modality treatment (13,14). These data have led some to conclude recently that the failure of radiation to control mediastinal Hodgkin's disease is the major therapeutic problem remaining in patients without symptoms (15).

The relationship discussed above between local control with radiotherapy and size of the mediastinal mass parallels observations made in other malignant diseases. A definite relationship between tumor size and radiation dose required for local control has been established for breast cancer and squamous cell carcinoma of the head and neck (16–20), as pointed out by Thar et al. (9). The problem in Hodgkin's disease is that higher than standard mantle irradiation doses in a patient with a large mediastinal mass are not possible unless significant cardiopulmonary damage to the patient is deemed acceptable. In fact, upper mantle irradiation to the usual field at the usual dose in such a patient may cause more cardiopulmonary toxicity than previously appreciated. A small fraction of patients who receive irradiation to the entire cardiac silhouette develop radiation-related pericarditis that usually spontaneously resolves. It may, however, occasionally become chronic and constrictive and require pericardiectomy (21). In addition, an occasional young patient developing myocardial infarction after mediastinal irradiation for Hodgkin's disease has been reported. Coronary artery intimal proliferation consistent with radiation damage has been associated with coronary artery occlusion in some such cases (22). Systematic examination of hearts from young people dying of lymphoma has revealed a previously unappreciated incidence of coronary artery narrowing and fibrous thickening of the mural and valvular endocardium in patients previously heavily irradiated to the mediastinum (23). More important, perhaps, is the fact that asymptomatic pericardial effusion, restrictive cardiomyopathy, and systolic left ventricular dysfunction can be demonstrated many years after mediastinal irradiation for Hodgkin's disease in enough patients to cause one group of investigators to conclude that lifelong cardiologic follow-up for all such patients is indicated (24).

Most Hodgkin's disease patients who received irradiation to large mediastinal masses have some permanent evidence of minimal to moderate pulmonary fibrosis demonstrable on chest x-ray films. Few patients, it is true, have clinically significant pulmonary dysfunction after such treatment. However, long-term studies of such patients have not been reported until recently. Do Pico et al. (25) reported significant declines in diffusing capacity for carbon monoxide, vital capacity, and inspiratory capacity usually occurring in the year following upper mantle irradiation. These changes were transient and not clinically important in most cases, but in some they were severe and even, rarely, fatal.

My conclusion from these data is that mantle irradiation should not be intensified in field or dose for the patient with a large mediastinal mass. The only alternative compatible with cure of Hodgkin's disease is to augment the radiation treatment with adjuvant chemotherapy. Dr. Portlock expresses a different view in her chapter in this volume. She would prefer to deliver local "boost" therapy up to a total dose of 5,000 rad to involved regions in patients with massive mediastinal disease and to irradiate the whole ipsilateral lung with a dose of 1,500 to 1,650 rad in four to five weeks in patients with pulmonary hilar involvement. These recommendations are made even though the Stanford group has recently also reported that large mediastinal mass patients have poorer disease-free ($P = .007$) and overall ($P = .10$) survival when treated with radiotherapy alone compared with patients with small mediastinal masses or none at all (26). It is interesting to note that, although the Stanford group observed inferior disease-free survival for patients with E stage disease treated with radiotherapy alone compared with patients without E stage disease similarly treated, the difference was not significant (27). These data are only quantitatively different from our data quoted above, not qualitatively. Dr. Portlock ascribes the difference to the fact that our radiation technique did not permit tumoricidal doses to all areas of known or suspected pulmonary disease. This is not the case (see Fig. 6).

My interpretation of the results of the Stanford and Baltimore studies is that they are not very different: the more mediastinal and contiguous pulmonary disease, the less likely radiotherapy alone is to cure the patient, and the more likely is adjuvant MOPP therapy to affect disease-free and overall survival favorably.

It is also possible to identify a subgroup of stage IIIA patients that does not do well with standard upper mantle and inverted-Y radiotherapy. Several workers (28,29), including ourselves (30), have reported that patients who have generalized abdominal nodal involvement have a poorer disease-free and overall survival than patients whose disease is confined to upper abdominal nodes or spleen when radiotherapy alone is the treatment. In our study (30), patients with stage IIIA whose disease was confined in the abdomen to the spleen or splenic hilar nodes had a significantly better disease-free and overall survival after radiotherapy alone compared with patients with positive lymphangiograms. These differences were not observed in patients treated with radiotherapy followed by MOPP. Others have recently made similar observations (15).

As pointed out by Dr. Portlock in her chapter in this volume, the Stanford data do not support the implications of the data above on the prognostic import of anatomic site of abdominal disease in patients with stage IIIA. In an effort to shed more light on this controversial area we participated in a retrospective study that involved, in addition to our group, Vanderbilt University, University of Chicago, and Harvard (31). The pooled group of 130 stage IIIA patients was divided into stage III_1A (spleen, or splenic hilar, or celiac, or hepatic portal nodes, or any combination of these sites) and stage III_2A (para-aortic, iliac, or mesenteric nodes with or without upper abdominal involvement. The median follow-up of all patients was almost five years. Disease-free and total survival were significantly better for stage III_1A patients. Disease-free survival was significantly better when radiotherapy-chemotherapy was the treatment for stage III_1A patients than when radiotherapy alone was the treatment. However, total survival was similar for both treatment groups. When stage III_2A patients treated with radiotherapy alone were compared with stage III_2A patients treated with a combined modality approach, significant differences in disease-free and overall survival in favor of the combined modality groups were noted.

Dr. Portlock attributes the differences between the Stanford data and all other available data to radiotherapy technique. She states in her chapter in this volume that the Stanford patients with stage IIIA received prophylactic irradiation to the ipsilateral lung if hilar disease was present and to the liver when the spleen was involved. She also points out that radiation doses 400 to 800 rad greater than those used in the collaborative study (28) described above were used at Stanford. It seems clear to me from Table 3 in Dr. Portlock's chapter that neither the additional ports nor additional doses of radiation are necessary for stage III_1A patients, since the Stanford and collaborative study data (31) are identical for stage III_1A patients. It may very well be that such additional radiotherapy accounts for the better results with radiotherapy for stage III_2A patients at

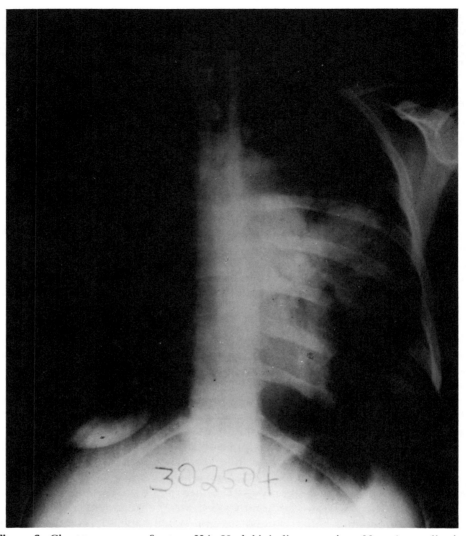

Figure 6. Chest tomogram of a stage IIA_E Hodgkin's disease patient. Note the mediastinal mass and E stage disease of lung. The patient was treated with radiotherapy alone and received 4,000 R in four weeks to an upper mantle and high periaortic nodes. The entire mass and E lung disease received the full dose. The patient sustained a marginal pulmonary parenchynal relapse 14 months after completely responding to initial therapy. She then had a complete response to MOPP but relapsed in the contralateral lung 18 months later. After several responses to additional chemotherapy, she died with active Hodgkin's disease almost four years after her first relapse.

Table 1. Proposed Classification of and Treatment Recommendations for Hodgkin's Disease

Proposed New Stage	Ann Arbor Stage	Recommended Treatment
I	IA, IIA, III$_1$A (spleen or upper abdominal nodes represent only intra-abdominal involvement). Patients must have no mediastinal mass, or a mediastinal mass < 1/3 the diameter of the chest. No E stage of lung (may be E stage elsewhere, such as thyroid, bone, etc.).	Extended field radiotherapy alone. Pelvic nodes need not be treated (48).
II	Any I, II, or IIIA patient with E stage of lung or mediastinal mass > 1/3 chest diameter. All IB and IIB. All III$_2$A (lower abdominal node involvement).	Extended field radiotherapy followed by six courses of MOPP. Pelvic nodes irradiated only for III$_2$A.
III	IIIB, IVA, IVB.	MOPP alone.

Stanford compared with the collaborative study data (see Table 3, Dr. Portlock's chapter). There may be two ways of improving results with stage III$_2$A disease: radiation therapy according to the Stanford method, or combined modality treatment using smaller radiation ports and less radiation dose. Only time will tell which method is associated with the least acute and long-term morbidity and the best long-term result.

On the basis of the considerations above, a new Hodgkin's disease staging system outlined in Table 1 is proposed. Patients are grouped according to what is likely to be optimal therapy in this system.

POST-THERAPY SECOND NEOPLASMS

There is legitimate concern over the development of acute leukemia after treatment for Hodgkin's disease, since both modalities of treatment are known to be leukemogenic in man. However, close scrutiny of relevant data reveals that, although combined modality treatment may be associated with a higher secondary acute leukemia incidence than either modality alone, the incidence of leukemia is highest in patients who are treated with one modality, relapse after initial response, and receive the second modality of treatment in the form of "salvage" therapy for active Hodgkin's disease (32–37). The majority of the rest of patients with Hodgkin's disease who have developed acute leukemia are patients who have received initial treatment with one or more modalities that has been excessive in either intensity or duration (38) or patients who have been placed on long-term maintenance chemotherapy after achieving complete remission (39). The number of patients initially treated with extended field radiotherapy to a total dose of 4,000 rad or less, followed by a maximum of six courses of MOPP that have developed acute leukemia is small. In our own study of 74 patients discussed above there have been two cases of posttreatment acute leukemia. One of 41 patients treated with radiotherapy alone and 1 of 33 patients treated with radiotherapy followed by MOPP developed acute leukemia in that study after a minimum observation period of six years. The patient initially treated with radiotherapy alone had relapsed and received multiple secondary treatments before developing acute leukemia, and the patient who initially received combined modality treatment (stage IIIA, mixed cellularity histology) developed acute leukemia while in first remission 46 months after completion of initial treatment. In the past 14 years we have treated 463 patients with Hodgkin's disease on a variety of studies. Acute leukemia has developed in 7 patients. Two of 101 patients initially treated with a combined modality approach developed acute leukemia while in remission, 2 of 142 patients treated only with chemotherapy developed acute leukemia after treatment for relapse (chemotherapy only), and 3 of 220 patients treated initially with radiotherapy alone developed acute leukemia after receiving chemotherapy for relapse.

It should be pointed out that, even when one includes deaths from acute leukemia or other second malignancies, there has never been a study published in which the disease-free or overall survival curves for Hodgkin's disease patients treated initially with radiotherapy and chemotherapy are poorer than those for patients treated initially with radiotherapy alone.

A report from the Southwest Oncology Group (40) supports the comments above. In that report, the incidence of acute leukemia in 643 Hodgkin's disease patients treated on several different protocols was assessed. None of 210 stage I, IIA, or IIB previously untreated patients who were treated with extended-field irradiation alone or involved field irradiation followed by six courses of MOPP, as in our study, has developed acute leukemia. In another study examined in the same report, 4 of 179 (2.2%) stage IIIA and IIIB patients treated with three courses of MOPP followed by total nodal irradiation developed acute leukemia. It is not stated whether any of these patients were in relapse at the time acute leukemia developed, but it is implied in the article that the majority of the 179 patients had B symptoms before treatment of Hodgkin's disease. In a third study included in that report, 254 patients with stage IIIB, IVA, or IVB were examined. Patients with or without prior treatment were placed on study and randomizd to receive MOPP or MOPP plus bleomycin. Those patients who achieved complete remission were randomly assigned to MOPP every other month for 18 months, involved field radiotherapy to major initial nodal sites of involvement followed by MOPP every other month for 18 months, or MOPP monthly for 18 months. Acute leukemia developed in 7 of the 254 patients (2.8%). Some of those patients who developed acute leukemia had been treated before entry into the SWOG protocol. Thus, the SWOG data are similar to our own and similar to the majority of data in the literature on the subject. The highest incidence of acute leukemia in Hodgkin's disease patients is in patients who have received "salvage" chemotherapy or who have been placed on long-term maintenance chemotherapy schemes that we now know to be inappropriate for a variety of reasons. In the SWOG experience as in our own, patients with early stage disease who are asymptomatic have an entirely acceptable incidence of acute leukemia following extended field radiotherapy and six or fewer courses of MOPP.

OTHER SECOND NEOPLASMS

Since the incidence of secondary solid tumors is not related to the intensity of Hodgkin's disease treatment (40), it is difficult to ascribe these tumors to treatment rather than to an increased likelihood of cancer occurring in a patient with Hodgkin's disease. In the SWOG experience (40) 7 of the 643 patients reviewed (1.1%) developed a second neoplasm other than acute leukemia. We reported similar data (4). Thus, it would appear that the probability of the development of second tumors other than acute leukemia in patients with Hodgkin's disease is low irrespective of treatment.

CONSIDERATIONS FOR THE FUTURE

MOPP combination chemotherapy has been eminently successful in advanced Hodgkin's disease in terms of complete remission induction rate (41) and long-term survival (42). The augmentation of results achieved in early stage disease by combined modality therapy provides evidence of the efficacy of MOPP combination chemotherapy in early Hodgkin's disease. It is necessary, therefore, to ask whether the superior results achieved with radiotherapy followed by MOPP compared with radiotherapy alone might be accomplished with MOPP alone. Some pilot data that bear on that point are available. Ziegler et al. treated a small group of Ugandan children with MOPP alone for early stage Hodgkin's disease and achieved results comparable with those reported for radiotherapy (43). In addition, 20 of 22 patients with stage IIIA or IVA treated at the National Cancer Institute have remained disease-free with up to 12 years of observation (44). Recently, similar British data have been reported (45). Those results are comparable with results with combined modality treatment reported by others.

We have demonstrated in a prospective, randomized pilot study that patients with stages IIA, IIB, and IIIA Hodgkin's disease have the same complete response rate with combined modality therapy or MOPP alone (46). It is too early to evaluate remission duration differences fully, if any, in that study. However, the latest data reveal a 100% overall survival for both groups with a maximum observation period of three years (Figs. 7 and 8). During that time none of the 18 patients who has received combined modality treatment has relapsed, whereas 3 of the 14 patients treated with MOPP alone have relapsed, all in the first year after treatment. These relapsed patients all had nodular sclerosing histology, and, as pointed out by DeVita (44), patients with that histology may be more likely to relapse after MOPP alone treatment. Therefore, it may be that combined modality treatment is more appropriate for that histologic group. In addition, patients with symptoms (B disease) may not be optimally treated with MOPP

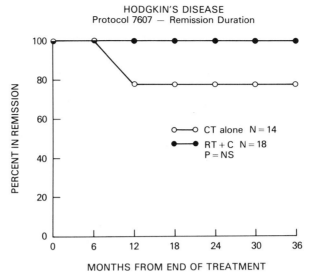

Figure 7. Early complete remission duration results of a Baltimore Cancer Research Center pilot study in which patients with stage II or IIIA were randomized to treatment with extended field radiotherapy followed by six courses of MOPP chemotherapy or MOPP chemotherapy alone.

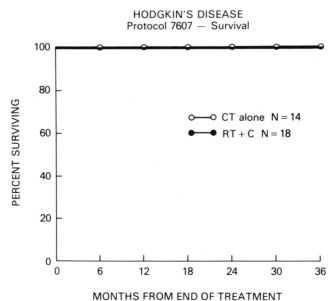

Figure 8. Early survival curves for patients in Figure 7.

alone (44), and early stage patients who are symptomatic may fare better with combined modality treatment as patients with stage IIIB (47) may.

The resolution of these issues is of paramount importance to patients with Hodgkin's disease confined primarily to lymph nodes. Therefore, the clinical branches of the Division of Cancer Treatment, NCI, in Baltimore and Bethesda are collaborating in a major study in which such patients are randomly allocated to treatment with extended field radiotherapy alone, MOPP chemotherapy alone, or combined modality therapy. Patients are stratified for randomization according to stage, histology, and the presence or absence of a large mediastinal mass. It may be a decade before the therapeutic and toxicity results of this study are known, but when available they may provide significant guidance in the management of early Hodgkin's disease.

In summary, my interpretation of available data is that patients with large mediastinal masses or lower abdominal nodal disease or both have a better disease-free and overall survival with combined modality treatment than with radiotherapy alone. Second malignancies cause fewer deaths in combined modality treatment patients than the number of deaths from Hodgkin's disease that have been avoided by such treatment. Research into the feasibility of MOPP alone treatment for Hodgkin's disease is warranted, but research should also continue to determine minimum fields and doses of radiotherapy that, when combined with MOPP, yield maximal long-term results.

REFERENCES

1. Portlock CS, Rosenberg SA, Glatstein E, Kaplan HS: Impact of salvage treatment on initial relapses in patients with Hodgkin's disease, Stages I-II. *Blood* 51:825–833, 1978.

2. Jenkin D, Freedman M, McClure P, Peters V, et al: Hodgkin's disease in children: treatment with low dose radiation and MOPP without staging laparotomy. *Cancer* 44:80–86, 1979.

3. Rosenberg SA, Kaplan HS, Brown BW Jr: The role of adjuvant MOPP in the therapy of Hodgkin's disease: an analysis after ten years, in Jones SA, Salmon SE (eds): *Adjuvant Therapy of Cancer II*. New York, Grune & Stratton, 1979, pp 109–117.

4. Wiernik PH, Gustafson J, Schimpff SC, Diggs C: Combined modality treatment of Hodgkin's disease confined to lymph nodes. *Am J Med* 67:183–193, 1979.

5. O'Connell MJ, Wiernik PH, Brace KC, Byhardt RW, et al: A combined modality approach to the treatment of Hodgkin's disease. *Cancer* 35:1055–1065, 1975.

6. Levi JA, Wiernik PH: Limited extranodal Hodgkin's disease. *Am J Med* 63:365–372, 1977.

7. Levi JA, Wiernik PH, O'Connell MJ: Patterns of relapse in stages I, II and IIIA Hodgkin's disease: influence of initial therapy and implications for the future. *Int J Rad Oncol Biol Phys* 2:853–862, 1977.

8. Mauch P, Goodman R, Hellman S: The significance of mediastinal involvement in early stage Hodgkin's disease. *Cancer* 42:1039–1045, 1978.

9. Thar TL, Million RR, Hausner RJ, McKetty MHB: Hodgkin's disease, Stages I and II. Relationship of recurrence to size of disease, radiation dose, and number of sites involved. *Cancer* 43:1101–1105, 1979.

10. Prosnitz LR, Curtis AM, Knowlton AH, Peters LM, et al: Supradiaphragmatic Hodgkin's disease: significance of large mediastinal masses. *Int J Rad Oncol Biol Phys* 6:809–813, 1980.

11. Mauch P, Hellman S: Supradiaphragmatic Hodgkin's disease: is there a role for MOPP chemotherapy in patients with bulky mediastinal disease? *Int J Rad Oncol Biol Phys* 6:947–949, 1980.

12. Fuller LM, Madoc-Jones H, Hagemeister FB, Rodgers RW, et al: Further follow-up of results

of treatment in 90 laparotomy-negative stage I and II Hodgkin's disease patients: significance of mediastinal and non-mediastinal presentation. *Int J Rad Oncol Biol Phys* 6:799–808, 1980.

13. Lange B, Littman P, Schnaufer L, Evans A: Treatment of advanced Hodgkin's disease in pediatric patients. *Cancer* 42:1141–1145, 1978.

14. Timothy AR, Sutcliffe SBJ, Stansfeld AG, Wrigley PG, et al: Radiotherapy in the treatment of Hodgkin's disease. *Br Med J* 1(6122):1246–1249, May 13, 1978.

15. Aisenberg AC, Linggood RM, Lew RA: The changing face of Hodgkin's disease. *Am J Med* 67:921–928, 1979.

16. Fletcher GH: Local results of irradiation in the primary management of localized breast cancer. *Cancer* 19:545–551, 1972.

17. Fletcher GH: Clinical dose-response curves of human malignant epithelial tumors. *Br J Radiol* 46:1–12, 1973.

18. Fletcher GH, Shukovsky LJ: The interplay of radiocurability and tolerance in the irradiation of human cancers. *J Radiol Electrol* 56:383–400, 1975.

19. Shukovsky LJ: Dose, time, volume relationships in squamous cell carcinoma of the supraglottic larynx. *Am J Roentgenol* 108:2–29, 1970.

20. Shukovsky LJ, Fletcher GH: Time-dose and tumor volume relationships in squamous cell carcinoma of the tonsillar fossa. *Radiol* 107:621–626, 1973.

21. Martin RG, Ruckdeschel JC, Chang P, Byhardt R, et al: Radiation-related pericarditis. *Am J Cardiol* 35:216–220, 1975.

22. McReynolds RA, Gold GL, Roberts WC: Coronary heart disease after mediastinal irradiation for Hodgkin's disease. *Am J Med* 60:39–45, 1976.

23. Brosius III FC, Waller BF, Roberts WC: Heavy mediastinal irradiation causing severe coronary narrowing in patients 15 to 33 years of age: A poorly appreciated cause of coronary heart disease in young people. *Am J Cardiol* 45:476, 1980.

24. Gottdiener JS, Katin MJ, Borer JS, Bacharach SL, et al: Identification of subclinical cardiac abnormality 5–15 years after therapeutic mediastinal irradiation. *Am J Cardiol* 45:475, 1980.

25. Do Pico GA, Wiley AL Jr, Rao P, Dickie HA: Pulmonary reaction to upper mantle radiation therapy for Hodgkin's disease. *Chest* 75:688–692, 1979.

26. Hoppe RT, Coleman CN, Kaplan HS, Rosenberg SA: Hodgkin's disease (HD), pathologic stage (PS) I-II: The prognostic importance of initial sites of disease and extent of mediastinal (Med) involvement. *Proc Am Soc Clin Oncol* 21:471, 1980.

27. Hoppe RT: Radiation therapy in the treatment of Hodgkin's disease. *Semin Oncol,* 7:144–154, 1980.

28. Desser RK, Golomb HM, Ultmann JE, Ferguson DJ, et al: Prognostic classification of Hodgkin's disease in pathologic stage III, based on anatomic considerations. *Blood* 49:883–893, 1977.

29. Stein RS, Hilborn RM, Flexner JM, Bolin M, et al: Anatomical substages of stage III Hodgkin's disease. *Cancer* 42:429–436, 1978.

30. Levi JA, Wiernik PH: The therapeutic implications of splenic involvement in stage IIIA Hodgkin's disease. *Cancer* 39:2158–2165, 1977.

31. Stein RS, Golomb HM, Diggs CH, Mauch P, et al: Anatomic substages of Stage IIIA Hodgkin's disease. *Ann Intern Med* 92:159–165, 1980.

32. Cadman EC, Capizzi RL, Bertino JR: Acute nonlymphocytic leukemia. A delayed complication of Hodgkin's disease therapy: Analysis of 109 cases. *Cancer* 40:1280–1296, 1977.

33. Cavallin-Ståhl E, Landberg T, Ottow Z, Mitelman F: Hodgkin's disease and acute leukemia. *Scand J Haematol* 19:273–280, 1977.

34. Coleman CN, Williams CJ, Flint A, Glatstein EJ, et al: Hematologic neoplasia in patients treated for Hodgkin's disease. *N Eng J Med* 297:1249–1252, 1977.

35. Boucheix C, Zittoun R, Reynes M, Diebold J, et al: Atypical T-cell leukemia terminating Hodgkin's disease. *Cancer* 44:1403–1407, 1979.

36. Auclerc G, Jaquillat C, Auclerc MF, Weil M, et al: Post-therapeutic acute leukemia. *Cancer* 44:2017–2025, 1979.

37. Valagussa P, Santoro A, Kenda R, Fossati-Bellani F, et al: Second malignancies in Hodgkin's disease: A complication of certain forms of treatment. *Br Med J* 1:216–219, 1980.

38. Kapadia SB, Krause JR, Ellis LD, Pan SF, et al: Induced acute non-lymphocytic leukemia following long-term chemotherapy. *Cancer* 45:1315–1321, 1980.

39. Pajak TF, Nissen NI, Stutzman L, Hoogstraten B, et al: Acute myeloid leukemia occurring during complete remission in Hodgkin's disease. *Proc Am Soc Clin Oncol* 20:394, 1979.

40. Toland DM, Coltman CA Jr, Moon TE: Second malignancies complicating Hodgkin's disease: The Southwest Oncology Group experience. *Cancer Clin Trials* 1:27–33, 1978.

41. DeVita VT Jr, Serick AA, Carbone PP: Combination chemotherapy in the treatment of advanced Hodgkin's disease. *Ann Intern Med* 73:881–895, 1970.

42. DeVita VT Jr, Simon RM, Hubbard SM, Young RC, et al: Curability of advanced Hodgkin's disease with chemotherapy. *Ann Intern Med* 92:587–595, 1980.

43. Olweny CML, Katongole-Mbidde E, Kiire C, Lwanga SK, et al: Childhood Hodgkin's disease in Uganda: A ten year experience. *Cancer* 42:787–792, 1978.

44. DeVita VT Jr: The role of combined modality therapy in the treatment of stage IIIA Hodgkin's disease. *Int J Rad Oncol Biol Phys* 5:913–914, 1979.

45. Timothy AR, Sutcliffe SBJ, Lister TA, Wrigley PFM, et al: The management of stage IIIA Hodgkin's disease. *Int J Radiol Biol Phys* 6:135–142, 1980.

46. Wiernik PH, Slawson RG, Burks LC, Diggs CH: A randomized trial of radiotherapy (RT) and MOPP (C) vs MOPP alone for stages IB-IIIA Hodgkin's disease. *Proc Am Soc Clin Oncol* 20:315, 1979.

47. Hoppe RT, Portlock CS, Glatstein E, Rosenberg SA, et al: Alternating chemotherapy and irradiation in the treatment of advanced Hodgkin's disease. *Cancer* 43:472–481, 1979.

48. Goodman RL, Piro AJ, Hellman S: Can pelvic irradiation be omitted in patients with pathologic stages IA and IIA Hodgkin's disease? *Cancer* 37:2834–2839, 1976.

2

Is Combined Modality Treatment of Early Stage Hodgkin's Disease Necessary?

Carol S. Portlock

The prognosis for patients with Hodgkin's disease has improved dramatically over the last 20 years. It is now possible to cure the majority of patients with radiation therapy alone in early stage disease and combination chemotherapy alone in advanced disease. Whether the excellent results already obtainable with irradiation in nodal Hodgkin's disease can be further improved by the addition of combination chemotherapy remains the subject of controversy.

RADIATION THERAPY

Advances in the treatment of nodal Hodgkin's disease have resulted from the elucidation of its patterns of spread and histopathology, the use of thorough clinical and pathological staging, and the development of sophisticated irradiation techniques. Some of the features that are pivotal in the delivery of curative radiation therapy (1) include the use of megavoltage beam energies (4–8 meV) as achieved with linear accelerator or ^{60}Co teletherapy; the ability to encompass large shaped fields; the use of tumoricidal doses with opposed field techniques; accurate treatment delivery with the routine use of simulation and frequent verification during treatment; and close follow-up care of all patients. Failure to observe these and other aspects of irradiation technique may lead to poorer treatment results or increased radiation complications.

The typical radiotherapy fields used in the treatment of Hodgkin's disease include the mantle (encompassing the cervical, supraclavicular, infraclavicular, axillary, mediastinal, and hilar lymph nodes); the inverted Y (encompassing the spleen or splenic pedicle, para-aortic, iliac, and inguinal-femoral lymph nodes); the spade (an inverted-Y field without irradiation to the pelvis or groin); and Waldeyer's ring (encompassing preauricular lymph nodes). Treatment may be delivered to the involved field (IF) only, irradiating only those areas involved clinically or pathologically; to the extended field (EF), irradiating the involved regions as well as all uninvolved contiguous sites; or to all major lymphoid regions both above and below the diaphragm. Total nodal irradiation (TNI) refers to the mantle and inverted-Y fields, and subtotal nodal irradiation (sTNI) refers to the mantle and spade fields.

The tumoricidal dose for Hodgkin's disease is 3,500 to 4,400 rad delivered at a dose rate of 1,000 to 1,100 rad per week (2). It may be that lower radiation doses are adequate to control occult disease in the prophylactic treatment of uninvolved regions at risk or when irradiation is combined with chemotherapy for the treatment of known disease; however, this has yet to be established.

Modifications in treatment techniques may be required for specific disease presentations, and such changes may subsequently influence treatment outcome. For example, with massive mediastinal disease dose fractionation is often modified and treatment interrupted in order to allow tumor shrinkage and subsequent shielding of normal lung. With prolonged courses of irradiation and interruption of standard technique it may be necessary to deliver local "boost" therapy to involved regions (up to total doses of 5,000 rad). With pulmonary hilar involvement there is an increased risk of occult ipsilateral lung disease. In such cases, prophylactic whole lung irradiation may be delivered during mantle therapy with a thin lung block technique, achieving a dose of 1,500 to 1,650 rad in four to five weeks to the lung at risk. This therapy has been reported to reduce the incidence of later pulmonary extensions in such patients (3). Another treatment modification that may be used is prophylactic liver irradiation when there is documented splenic involvement. In this case, the whole liver is treated to a dose of 2,000 to 2,200 rad by means of a 50% transmission block during inverted-Y therapy (4).

The toxicities of radiation therapy for Hodgkin's disease depend on such factors as the treatment portals, beam energy, dose and fractionation, and treatment technique. With the mantle field, acute toxicities may include nausea, dysphagia, esophagitis, tracheitis, and transient skin erythema. Fibrosis of paramediastinal and apical pulmonary parenchyma may be noted on radiographs following the conclusion of therapy and usually follows the contour of the radiation portal. Radiation pneumonitis and pericarditis are rare complications with proper shielding of normal structures. Other toxicities may include occipital alopecia, L'Hermittes sign, and hypothyroidism. The inverted-Y field is associated with nausea and transient hematologic depression. Radiation to the gonads may lead to temporary or permanent sterility. In the male, special shielding may be of value; in the female, oophoropexy (surgically placing the ovaries in the low midline pelvis) may permit adequate ovarian shielding. The spade field omits irradiation to the pelvis; consequently, hematologic toxicity is reduced, and there is less likelihood of radiation-induced sterility. Xerostomia is the major treatment complication associated with Waldeyer's ring irradiation.

The results of radiation therapy alone in pathologic stages IA and IIA Hodgkin's disease are presented in Table 1. As reported by Glatstein (5), involved

Table 1. Results of Radiation Therapy: Stages IA and IIA

Pathologic Stage	Number of Patients	Extent of Radiation	Dose (rad)	Five-Year Relapse-free Survival	Five-Year Actuarial Survival	Reference
IA, IIA	28	IF	4,000	38% P < .05	90%	5
IA, IIA	34	TNI	4,000	80%	90%	5
IA, IIA	56	IF, sTNI	4,000	75%	91%	6
IA	38	sTNI	3,500–4,000	97%	100%	7
IIA	81	sTNI	3,500–4,000	80%	93%	7
IA, IIA	199	sTNI, TNI	4,400	78%	95%	1

field irradiation was associated with significantly poorer relapse-free survival (38% at five years) as compared with total nodal irradiation (80% at five years) (P < .05) when studied prospectively in 62 pathologically staged patients. In spite of poorer relapse-free survival, patients receiving IF had a similar actuarial survival (90% at five years) to those receiving TNI. This disparity between relapse-free survival and survival results is attributable to the excellent ability to "salvage" patients after radiation therapy relapse and is discussed in greater detail subsequently. Several groups have retrospectively analyzed their experience with subtotal nodal irradiation and reported relapse-free and survival results that are similar to those achieved with TNI (1,6,7). Goodman et al. (8) reported a relapse-free survival of 88% and an actuarial survival of 96% at five years for 81 patients with supradiaphragmatic PS IA and IIA treated with sTNI. None of the six patients who relapsed had extension of disease to unirradiated pelvic or inguinal lymph nodes. Since subtotal nodal irradiation is associated with as good treatment results as TNI while sparing the pelvis and has little additional morbidity as compared with IF while achieving a marked improvement in relapse-free survival, sTNI has become the standard approach to patients with supradiaphragmatic PS IA and IIA disease.

Fewer data are available on the necessary radiation portals for the treatment of patients with PS IB and IIB disease. In a prospective trial comparing involved field with extended field irradiation in 21 clinically staged patients with stages IB and IIB disease, Kaplan and Rosenberg (9) reported significantly poorer relapse-free survival (25% versus 80% at one year) and survival (40% versus 90% at four years) with IF as compared with EF. A subsequent analysis of sTNI in pathologically staged IB and IIB patients by Hellman et al. (7) revealed a relapse-free survival of 82% and an actuarial survival of 86% at five years. These results compare favorably with those for total nodal irradiation (75% relapse-free survival and 86% actuarial survival at five years) recently reported by Hoppe (1).

Factors that have been reported to affect the prognosis of patients with stages I and II Hodgkin's disease adversely include bulky mediastinal disease and the presence of extranodal extension. Mauch et al. (10) have reported that of 18 patients with PS IA and IIA who had mediastinal enlargement greater than one-third of the chest diameter 9 relapsed after radiation alone compared with 5 of 93 with no mediastinal involvement ($P < .01$). Relapses were intrathoracic in 8 of these 9 patients, and 2 patients have died of progressive disease. Recently Hoppe et al. (11) have confirmed these observations. The freedom from relapse of 19 PS I and II patients with large mediastinal masses (a mediastinal mass to thoracic ratio of ≥ 0.3) was significantly poorer than 28 patients with lesser mediastinal disease (39% versus 86% at five years, $P = .007$) treated with radiation therapy alone. In addition, actuarial survival was also poorer (80% versus 100%, $P = .10$) in the group with large mediastinal disease.

Levi and Wiernik (12) have reported that extranodal extension (II_EA, II_EB, and III_EA) is also associated with a significantly higher relapse rate and poorer survival. They retrospectively analyzed 18 patients with extranodal lesions treated with either extended field irradiation or involved field irradiation plus MOPP. Ten of 18 patients relapsed, all of whom had extranodal lesions of lung and 7 of whom had large mediastinal masses in addition. Radiation technique did not permit tumoricidal doses to all areas of known or suspected pulmonary disease. Consequently it is difficult to assess the role of radiation therapy alone in this study. Hoppe (1) has recently reported the experience with radiation therapy alone in 24 patients with PS II_EA and II_EB disease. All sites of extranodal extension were treated with tumoricidal doses of irradiation, and all patients received either sTNI or TNI. The five-year freedom from relapse (65%) and actuarial survival (83%) were not significantly different from that achieved for patients with IIA and IIB disease. Therefore, it would appear that the presence of extranodal extension does not, by itself, confer a higher relapse rate or poorer survival when treated with adequate irradiation, whereas large mediastinal disease, with or without pulmonary extension, is associated with a significantly higher relapse rate and poorer survival in spite of adequate irradiation.

Although the extent (TNI) and dose (3,500 to 4,500 rad) of radiation therapy are similar for all studies of PS IIIA and III_SA Hodgkin's disease, the relapse-free survival results are markedly varied, ranging from 25 to 66% at five years (see Table 2) (1,10,13). On the other hand, the actuarial survival for all patients is 80 to 92% at five years, once again reflecting the excellent ability to "salvage" patients after radiation therapy relapse. In an attempt to identify prognostic factors that might explain this variability in the relapse-free survival of patients with PS IIIA disease, Desser et al. (14) analyzed their treatment results according to the extent of abdominal involvement. They reported that patients with disease limited to the spleen or splenic, celiac, or portal lymph nodes ("anatomic sub-

Table 2. Results of Radiation Therapy: Stages IIIA and III_SA

Pathologic Stage	Number of Patients	Extent of Radiation	Dose (rad)	Five-Year Relapse-free Survival	Five-Year Actuarial Survival	Reference
III, III_SA	86	TNI	4,400	66%	86%	1
IIIA, III_SA	48	TNI	3,500–4,500	35%	80%	13
IIIA, III_SA	37	TNI	3,600–4,000	51%	92%	10

Table 3. Results of Radiation Therapy: Stages III_1A and III_2A

Anatomic Substage	Number of Patients	Extent of Irradiation	Dose (rad)	Five-Year Relapse-free Survival	Five-Year Survival	Reference
III_1	48	sTNI, TNI	3,600–4,000	63%	91%	15
III_1	46	TNI	4,400	64%	90%	16
III_2	37	TNI	3,600–4,000	32%	56%	15
III_2	40	TNI	4,400	69%	88%	16

stage" III_1) had fewer relapses and deaths than those with disease involving the para-aortic, iliac, or mesenteric lymph nodes ("anatomic substage" III_2). A subsequent collaborative study reported by Stein et al. (15) has confirmed these data (see Table 3). With total nodal irradiation in 85 patients treated at four institutions, the relapse-free survival at five years was 63% for those patients with substage III_1 disease and only 32% for those with III_2 presentations ($P < .001$). Futhermore, five-year actuarial survival was also significantly poorer ror those with III_2 (56%) as compared with III_1 disease (91%) ($P < .001$). Hoppe et al. (16) have recently reported their results of TNI in 86 patients treated at a single institution, and their data do not support the prognostic variable of anatomic substage. The five-year relapse-free survival was 64% for patients with III_1 and 69% for III_2; similarly five-year actuarial survival was 90% for III_1 and 88% for III_2. Differences in radiation technique may account, at least in part, for the better treatment results reported by Hoppe et al. Although all patients received TNI in both series, those reported by Hoppe et al. received prophylactic irradiation to the ipsilateral lung when hilar disease was identified and to the liver when splenic disease was documented. In addition, the radiation dose to all regions was 4,400 rad in the series by Hoppe et al. and 3,600 to 4,000 rad in that reported by Stein et al.

As a single modality, radiation therapy offers essentially no curative potential for patients with stages IIIB and IV Hodgkin's disease. As reported by Rosenberg et al. (17) the relapse-free survival was 7%, and the actuarial survival 44% at eight years in 44 patients with PS IIIB disease treated with TNI. In contrast to these dismal results with radiation alone, combination chemotherapy alone in patients with stages IIIB and IV yields complete remission rates of 45 to 81% with approximately two-thirds of patients remaining disease-free at five years (18). Although there has been little experience with MOPP* alone in early stage Hodgkin's disease, the initial results are highly favorable. The complete response rates range from 70 to 100% with fewer than 25% of patients relapsing (19,20). Toxicities of combination chemotherapy may include transient bone marrow depression, nausea, vomiting, alopecia, neuropathy, effects of corticosteroids (diabetes, hypertension, osteoporosis, peptic ulcer), and infertility.

To date, only one prospective trial has been conducted comparing radiation therapy alone with combination chemotherapy alone in early stage disease (21).

*MOPP—nitrogen mustard, vincristine, procarbazine, and prednisone.

The British National Lymphoma Investigation group treated 81 pathologically staged IIIA patients with either TNI or MOPP. The complete response rate was 95% after TNI and 74% after MOPP; relapse-free survival at four years for all patients was 65% for TNI and 40% for MOPP. Survival at four years was 85% for both groups. As pointed out by De Vita (19), the chemotherapy results of this trial are poorer than what has been observed preliminarily by others. Several prospective trials are currently under way to test the relative roles of each single modality in early stage disease.

COMBINED MODALITY THERAPY

Combined modality approaches of radiation therapy plus combination chemo-therapy have been applied to all stages of Hodgkin's disease. Prospective studies in early stage disease compare "standard" radiation therapy with "standard" or modified radiation therapy followed by combination chemotherapy. The results of these studies are outlined in Table 4 (22–25). For stages IA, IIA, and IIIA disease, all studies with five or more years follow-up have demonstrated significant improvement in relapse-free survival using the combined modality approach as compared with radiation therapy alone. For stages IA and IIA, approximately 90% of patients are relapse-free at 5 and 10 years with combined modality therapy versus 65% with radiation alone. For stage IIA, 55 to 70% of patients are relapse-free at 5 and 10 years after TNI as compared with more than 90% after combined modality. In one study of patients with IB and IIB disease treated with TNI, no improvement in relapse-free survival (80% at 10 years) was observed with the addition of chemotherapy (22). Although almost all the prospective trials listed in Table 4 show significant improvement in relapse-free survival with the combined modality approach, only one study (in patients with stage IIIA disease) has shown significant improvement in actuarial survival during the 5 to 10 years of follow-up (24).

This disparity between relapse-free survival and survival has been attributed to the ability to "salvage" patients after radiation therapy relapse. Results of combination chemotherapy do not appear to be adversely influenced by prior radiation therapy as they are by prior chemotherapy (18). Consequently, one would expect that approximately 80% of patients relapsing after irradiation could achieve a second complete remission with chemotherapy alone and that more than half would have long-term disease-free survival. In a retrospective study of 64 relapsing patients reported by Portlock et al. (26), 45% of those relapsing after irradiation were free of progressive disease at four years after salvage therapy. Somewhat surprising was the observation that 30% of those relapsing after combined modality therapy were also free of progressive disease and that the probability of progression-free survival was not significantly different for the two groups ($P = .24$). Another approach to assessing the impact of salvage therapy on survival is to analyze the actuarial probability of second relapse (the time from initial therapy to failure of salvage treatment). Rosenberg et al. (17) demonstrated that freedom from second relapse closely paralleled actuarial survival in a group of 244 patients with nodal Hodgkin's disease prospectively randomized to radiation therapy alone or combined modality therapy.

following combined modality therapy was 15.2% (4.4 to 52.0, 95% confidence limits) at 10 years. None of 221 patients treated with radiation alone and none of 13 treated with chemotherapy alone have had this complication. The risk of nonhematologic second tumors also appears to be increased in those receiving combined modality therapy (30,31).

For patients with stages IA and IIA disease, subtotal nodal irradiation alone offers an initial relapse-free survival ("cure" rate) of more than 65%. Likewise, total nodal irradiation offers similar results for patients with stages IB, IIB, and III_1A disease. Therefore, if these patients had received combined modality therapy, the majority would have been subjected to adjuvant combination chemotherapy unnecessarily, since radiation therapy alone can achieve cure in more than 65% as a single modality. Not only would they incur unnecessarily the acute and chronic toxicities of chemotherapy, including infertility, but they would also incur the increased potential for the delayed occurrence of second malignancies. Therefore, it would seem more prudent to identify those patients who would not benefit from radiation therapy alone as initial treatment rather than to treat all patients initially with combined modality therapy. As discussed earlier, patients with large mediastinal masses (greater than one-third the thoracic diameter) appear to be at increased risk of relapse after radiation alone. Hoppe et al. (11) have reported a five-year freedom from relapse of 80% for 28 patients treated with combined modality therapy as compared with 39% for 19 patients treated with radiation alone ($P = .15$). Nevertheless the survival for both groups was similar (88% versus 80% at five years). Another group of patients who have been reported to have poor relapse-free survival after radiation therapy alone are those with III_2A disease. Using TNI, Stein et al. (15) and Prosnitz et al. (13) have reported five-year relapse-free survivals of only 32% and 25%, respectively. In the Stein series, with combined modality therapy, the five-year relapse-free survival was 76% in 19 patients and the five-year actuarial survival 84% as compared with 56% with TNI alone ($P < .03$). However, one must remember the results recently reported by Hoppe et al. (16) in which 40 patients with III_2 disease received TNI, including prophylactic irradiation of lungs or liver at risk. This group has reported a five-year relapse-free survival of 69% and survival of 88% with radiation therapy alone. Therefore, a modification of radiation therapy technique, associated with little if any additional morbidity, has yielded results comparable with those of combined modality therapy in III_2A disease.

For those patients who relapse following initial radiation therapy, salvage regimens must be maximally effective. This requires close follow-up and early detection of disease relapse as well as optimal therapeutic management. Both combination chemotherapy alone (18) and combined chemotherapy plus low dose irradiation programs (32) have been reported to yield second long-term disease-free survivals in the majority of such patients. Unfortunately, like patients treated with combined modality therapy at presentation, those who relapse after radiation therapy and subsequently receive chemotherapy also have an increased risk of developing second malignancies.

Another single modality approach to the treatment of early stage Hodgkin's disease is combination chemotherapy alone. Whether this modality can be used in place of radiation therapy is yet to be tested prospectively. As with studies of combined modality therapy, one will need to consider not only the end results of treatment but the relative acute and chronic toxicities of treatment and the ability to salvage relapsing patients as well.

Radiation therapy alone remains the standard of treatment in early stage Hodgkin's disease. With optimal management more than two-thirds of all patients with stages I, II, and IIIA disease can be cured with irradiation alone. Such treatment offers the majority of patients long-term disease-free survival and probable cure, while exposing them to the least risk of acute and chronic morbidity.

REFERENCES

1. Hoppe RT: Radiation therapy in the treatment of Hodgkin's disease. *Semin Oncol* 7:56, 1980.

2. Kaplan HS: Evidence for a tumoricidal dose level in the radiotherapy of Hodgkin's disease. *Cancer Res* 26:1221, 1966.

3. Palos B, Kaplan HS, Karzmark CJ: The use of thin lung shields to deliver limited whole-lung irradiation during mantle-field treatment of Hodgkin's disease. *Radiology* 101:441, 1971.

4. Schultz HP, Glatstein E, Kaplan HS: Management of presumptive or proven Hodgkin's disease of the liver: A new radiotherapy technique. *Int J Radiat Oncol Biol Phys* 1:1, 1975.

5. Glatstein E: Radiotherapy in Hodgkin's disease: Past achievements and future progress. *Cancer* 39:837, 1977.

6. Mintz U, Miller JB, Golomb HM, et al: Pathologic stage I and II Hodgkin's disease, 1968–1975: Relapses and results of retreatment. *Cancer* 44:72, 1979.

7. Hellman S, Mauch P, Goodman RL, et al: The place of radiation therapy in the treatment of Hodgkin's disease. *Cancer* 42:971, 1978.

8. Goodman RL, Piro AJ, Hellman S: Can pelvic irradiation be omitted in patients with pathologic stages IA and IIA Hodgkin's disease? *Cancer* 37:2834, 1976.

9. Kaplan HS, Rosenberg SA: Current status of clinical trials: The Stanford experience, 1962–1972. *International Symposium on Hodgkin's disease.* NCI Monograph 36, Bethesda, 1973.

10. Mauch P, Goodman R, Hellman S: The significance of mediastinal involvement in early stage Hodgkin's disease. *Cancer* 42:1039, 1978.

11. Hoppe RT, Coleman CN, Kaplan HS, et al: Hodgkin's disease (HD), pathologic stage (PS) I-II: The prognostic importance of initial sites of disease and extent of mediastinal (med.) involvement. *Proc Amer Soc Clin Oncol* 21:471, 1980.

12. Levi JA, Wiernik PH: Limited extranodal Hodgkin's disease: Unfavorable prognosis and therapeutic implications. *Am J Med* 63:365, 1977.

13. Prosnitz LR, Montalvo RL, Fischer DB: Treatment of stage IIIA Hodgkin's disease: Is radiotherapy alone adequate? *Int J Radiat Oncol Biol Phys* 4:781, 1978.

14. Desser RK, Golomb HM, Ultmann JE, et al: Prognostic classification of Hodgkin disease in pathologic stage III, based on anatomic considerations. *Blood* 49:883, 1977.

15. Stein RS, Golomb HM, Diggs CH, et al: Anatomical substages of stage III-A Hodgkin's disease: A collaborative study. *Ann Intern Med* 92:159, 1980.

16. Hoppe RT, Rosenberg SA, Kaplan HS, et al: Prognostic factors in pathological stage IIIA Hodgkin's disease. *Cancer* 46:1240, 1980.

17. Rosenberg SA, Kaplan HS, Glatstein EJ, et al: Combined modality therapy of Hodgkin's disease: A report on the Stanford trials. *Cancer* 42:991, 1978.

18. De Vita VT Jr, Lewis BJ, Rozencweig M, et al: The chemotherapy of Hodgkin's disease: Past experiences and future directions. *Cancer* 42:979, 1978.

19. De Vita VT Jr: The role of combined modality therapy in the treatment of stage IIIA Hodgkin's disease. *Int J Radiat Oncol Biol Phys* 5:913, 1979.

20. Olweny CLM, Katongole-Mbidde E, Kiire C, et al: Childhood Hodgkin's disease in Uganda: A ten year experience. *Cancer* 42:787, 1978.

21. British National Lymphoma Investigation: Initial Treatment of Stage IIIA Hodgkin's disease: Comparison of radiotherapy with combined chemotherapy. *Lancet* II:991, 1976.

22. Rosenberg SA, Kaplan HS, Brown BW Jr: The role of adjuvant MOPP in the therapy of Hodgkin's disease: An analysis after ten years, in Jones SA, Salmon SE (eds): *Adjuvant Therapy of Cancer II*. New York, Grune & Stratton, 1979.

23. Hoppe RT, Rosenberg SA, Kaplan HS, et al: The treatment of Hodgkin's disease stage I-IIA: Subtotal lymphoid irradiation vs involved field irradiation plus adjuvant MOP(P), in Jones SE, Salmon SE (eds): *Adjuvant Therapy of Cancer II*. New York, Grune & Stratton, 1979.

24. Wiernik PH, Gustafson J, Schimpff SC, et al: Combined modality treatment of Hodgkin's disease confined to lymph nodes: Results eight years later. *Am J Med* 67:183, 1979.

25. Coltman CA Jr, Fuller LA, Fisher R, et al: Extended field radiotherapy versus involved field radiotherapy plus MOPP in stage I and II Hodgkin's disease, in Jones SE, Salmon SE (eds): *Adjuvant Therapy of Cancer II*. New York, Grune & Stratton, 1979.

26. Portlock CS, Rosenberg SA, Glatstein E, et al: Impact of salvage treatment on initial relapses in patients with Hodgkin's disease, stages I-III. *Blood* 51:825, 1978.

27. Cadman EC, Capizzi RL, Bertino JR: Acute nonlymphocytic leukemia. A delayed complication of Hodgkin's disease therapy: Analysis of 109 cases. *Cancer* 40:1280, 1977.

28. Coleman CN, Williams CJ, Fline A, et al: Hematologic neoplasia in patients treated for Hodgkin's disease. *N Engl J Med* 297:1249, 1977.

29. Kirkorian JG, Burke JS, Rosenberg SA, et al: Occurrence of non-Hodgkin's lymphoma after therapy for Hodgkin's disease. *N Engl J Med* 300:452, 1979.

30. Arseneau JC, Sponzo RW, Levin DL, et al: Nonlymphomatous malignant tumors complicating Hodgkin's disease: Possible association with intensive therapy. *N Engl J Med* 287:1119, 1975.

31. Canellos GP, De Vita VT, Arseneau JC, et al: Second malignancies complicating Hodgkin's disease in remission. *Lancet* I:947, 1975.

32. Prosnitz LR, Farber LR, Fischer JJ, et al: Long term remissions with combined modality therapy for advanced Hodgkin's disease. *Cancer* 37:2826, 1976.

3

Intensive Treatment of Nodular Non-Hodgkin's Lymphoma

Fernando Cabanillas

Emil J. Freireich

INTRODUCTION

The major contribution of the Rappaport classification of malignant lymphomas was the recognition of two basic morphologic patterns: nodular and diffuse (1). The malignant lymphomas of nodular pattern, in general, grow more slowly and respond more favorably to chemotherapy than their diffuse counterparts (2). This group includes the nodular poorly differentiated lymphocytic, nodular mixed, and nodular histiocytic lymphomas. Of these, by far the most frequently observed subtype is the nodular poorly differentiated lymphocytic. Asymptomatic or minimally symptomatic presentations are common in the nodular varieties, especially in the nodular poorly differentiated lymphocytic and nodular mixed subtypes. These clinical characteristics have led to the grouping of these two histologic subtypes under a special category of so-called favorable types of lymphoma (3). Long survival times are common in these types, sometimes even after relapse from a chemotherapy-induced remission. For this reason, some investigators have advocated mild treatment or even no treatment at all in asymptomatic patients with these types of lymphoma (4). Eventually, however, the majority of patients managed this way develop symptoms of progression and succumb to their disease. We have also learned that the natural history of patients with these nodular tumor types who enter complete remission, in contrast to most of those with the diffuse varieties, is characterized by late relapses (5). Consequently, even though the overall survival can be relatively long, the cure rate of patients with nodular lymphomas is low. This has motivated us to seek other alternatives to improve the current situation. In view of the superiority of combination chemotherapy over single agent treatment in the vast majority of tumor types studied so far, we have used that approach for the malignant lymphomas. The purpose of this chapter is to review our experience with two different combination regimens of varying intensity and to draw conclusions as to which we consider is currently the best strategy for the treatment of malignant nodular lymphomas.

Historical Aspects

The validity of the Rappaport classification was not well recognized until the series of papers from Stanford published by Jones et al. in 1972 demonstrated conclusively that this classification offers an excellent correlation with the clinical course not provided by previous methods (2). It became evident from these papers that patients with nodular poorly differentiated lymphocytic, nodular mixed, and nodular histiocytic lymphoma treated with single agents had a more favorable outcome than their counterparts with the diffuse histological patterns. The complete response rate of patients with the above types of nodular lymphomas treated with single agents was 38% in contrast to only 12% for the corresponding diffuse histologic subtypes (2). Not only was the complete remission rate superior, but also the duration of response was significantly longer. Furthermore, the overall survival of patients with nodular tumors who achieved a complete remission was superior to those who achieved only a partial remission.

This study was followed by a prospective therapeutic trial at Stanford in which the patients with the so-called *favorable histologic types* (NPDL, NMX, DWDLL) were randomized to receive one of three regimens: (*1*) chemotherapy alone with single agents, (*2*) combination chemotherapy alone with CVP (cyclophosphamide, vincristine, prednisone), or (*3*) CVP in addition to total lymphoid radiation (3). Several interesting conclusions can be drawn from this Stanford J6 study: (*1*) Treatment with combination chemotherapy alone (CVP) yielded a higher complete remission rate (83%) compared with 65% for single agents. (*2*) With single agent treatment, a complete remission rate of 65% was obtained, but in the report by Jones the single agent complete remission rate was only 38%. This marked difference in the complete remission rate cannot be explained by an imbalance in the distribution of histologic subtypes, since the vast majority of patients in both studies had a diagnosis of either NPDL or NMX. (*3*) Even though the complete remission rate was higher for the CVP arm, this did not result in any advantage in the overall survival when compared with the single agent arm. This implies that overall survival is not affected by the quality of the response; that is, achievement of a complete remission does not offer any advantage over a partial remission. Again, this finding is in contrast with the first study in which patients who achieved a complete remission survived longer than those with a partial remission.

This lack of advantage in achieving a complete remission implied in the Stanford J6 study has been widely disputed. The data presented by Anderson et al. (6) from the National Cancer Institute and by Diggs et al. (7) from the Baltimore Cancer Research Center clearly show a superior survival for patients who achieve a complete remission over those with only a partial remission. Our own data also clearly show such a difference, as described below.

The Problem of Comparability of Populations

The marked difference in complete response rate between the single agent arm of the Stanford J6 study and their first study, in addition to the other discrepancies mentioned above, clearly points out the problem of comparing different studies even in the same institution. Without an adequate knowledge of the prognostic factors that predict response and survival, it is impossible to attribute a positive result to a particular chemotherapy regimen when other important factors might also influence the outcome. The technique of prospective randomization has been offered as a solution to the problems of comparing historical data. However, randomization does not guarantee equal distribution of prognostic factors among the different arms of a study. The problems become more pronounced when data from different institutions are compared because of additional factors such as differences in supportive care facilities, treatment philosophy, and patient selection, which may vary greatly.

Consequently, we have chosen to evaluate our data using the technique of multivariate analysis in order to account for the influence of other variables, aside from treatment, on the final results.

Treatment Programs

From 1967 to 1977, 109 consecutive patients with nodular lymphomas were entered into various protocols that used combination chemotherapy. During the first five years of this period, the COP regimen or one of its variations was used. In essence, the COP 1, 2, and 3 regimens were used in this period. Details of these regimens have been described before (8,9). The major difference between the COP 1 and 2 studies was that the latter used oral cyclophosphamide instead of intravenous. The COP 3 study involved a three-arm randomization among COP 1, MOPP, and COAP (COP + Ara − C). The doses used in these COP trials were in general relatively low, and myelosuppression was usually mild.

From 1972 to 1977, we investigated a more intense regimen consisting of different combinations of adriamycin (hydroxyldaunomycin), which we have called the CHOP protocols. The first one of these was the CHOP-HOP regimen, which involved a randomization between CHOP and HOP (10). When bleomycin became available, this drug was added to the CHOP regimen in the CHOP-Bleo protocol (11). Recently, we investigated the CHOP-Bleo-Levamisole regimen, which included the latter immunopotentiating agent (12). From 1974 to 1977, whenever a laminar air flow room was available, patients were randomized to be treated inside or outside of such rooms with higher doses of CHOP-Bleo (13). Maintenance chemotherapy with CHOP was given to all patients for at least one year after achievement of complete remission. Patients who were treated with the CHOP-HOP protocols or with standard dosage CHOP-Bleo received immunotherapy with 6×10^8 BCG Pasteur strain organisms given by scarification weekly for three months and then every other week subsequently after chemotherapy was discontinued. Patients who were treated with high dose CHOP-Bleo either inside or outside of a laminar air flow room did not receive immunotherapy after the chemotherapy was discontinued. Patients treated with CHOP-Bleo-Levamisole were maintained on levamisole immunotherapy after chemotherapy was discontinued.

Patient Population

One hundred nine patients ranging in age from 20 to 81 years old were entered on these studies. The median age was 55 years. No age limit was established for entering patients on these studies. The male to female ratio was 57:52 or 1.1.

The distribution of histological subtypes showed a predominance of patients with nodular poorly differentiated lymphocytic lymphoma (78) with the other types occurring less frequently (nodular histiocytic 16, nodular mixed 14).

Prognostic Factors Associated with Complete Remission

When dealing with a population of patients with variable factors such as age, sex, and treatment that are potentially important variables that could influence the complete remission rate and survival, the technique of multivariate analysis is a very useful tool. Such a model can discern the interrelations among the different variables and has the capacity of ranking them in order of importance (14).

Twelve factors were considered for analysis of their impact on the complete remission rate. These variables, together with the complete remission rate associated with each one, are shown in Table 1. Of these 12 factors, the only ones found to be significantly associated with a difference in complete remission rates were history of prior chemotherapy, hemoglobin level, bulky disease, and type of chemotherapy given (either COP or CHOP). Some of these variables, however, were closely linked or interrelated. For example, patients who received treatment with the COP regimens had a higher frequency of exposure to prior treatment than those who received treatment with the CHOP regimens. In order to adjust for the influence of these variables on the complete remission rate and for their possible interactions, a logistic regression model was used. By using this method, only three of the factors above were found to be significant at a level of less than 0.05. In order of decreasing importance, these are (1) type of chemotherapy, (2) tumor bulkiness, (3) exposure to prior treatment. The type of chemotherapy regimen found to be associated with a higher complete remission rate was the CHOP regimen. This factor carried the most weight in predicting achievement of complete remission. The absence of a bulky tumor and no prior exposure to treatment were also factors associated with a higher complete response rate.

With the knowledge of these prognostic factors, a predicted probability of complete response can be calculated for each patient in the study, and a regression equation can be derived from this analysis. Thus, the patients were grouped into three distinct categories according to their predicted probability of complete remission for each of these three groups (Table 2). A good correlation between the predicted and the observed complete response rate is evident from this table.

Prognostic Factors Associated with Length of Survival

The factors that predict length of survival are different from those that predict complete remission. A method proposed by Cox (15) was used to determine the characteristics related to length of survival. Of the 12 factors tested, this model identified the following as important in predicting prolonged survival: normal pretreatment hemoglobin, CHOP chemotherapy, female sex, and no exposure to prior treatment of any type. In the case of survival, hemoglobin turned out to be the most important variable, but in the logistic regression analysis for response, this variable was not judged important at all. Treatment with the CHOP regimen was found to be the second most important variable that predicted prolonged survival.

Table 1. Complete Response Rate by Prognostic Variables

Characteristic	Number	CR (%)	P Value
Diagnosis			
NPDL	78	54 (69%)	
NH	16	12 (75%)	> 0.5
NMX	14	11 (79%)	
Other	1	1 (—)	
Sex			
Male	57	41 (72%)	> 0.5
Female	52	37 (71%)	
Age			
< 50	42	31 (74%)	
50–60	37	26 (70%)	> 0.5
> 60	30	21 (70%)	
Absolute lymphocyte count			
0–1,000	43	30 (70%)	
1,000–1,500	21	14 (67%)	> 0.5
> 1,500	42	32 (76%)	
Blood involvement			
Yes	9	6 (67%)	> 0.5
No	100	71 (71%)	
Bone marrow positive (biopsy)			
Yes	32	23 (72%)	0.16
No	43	36 (84%)	
Symptoms			
Yes	29	18 (63%)	0.47
No	80	58 (73%)	
Prior chemotherapy			
Yes	13	4 (31%)	< 0.01
No	96	74 (77%)	
Hemoglobin			
< 10	14	5 (36%)	
10–12	24	16 (67%)	< 0.01
> 12	71	57 (80%)	
Bulky disease			
Yes	36	19 (53%)	< 0.01
No	73	59 (81%)	
Type of chemotherapy			
COP	40	21 (53%)	< 0.01
CHOP	69	57 (83%)	

Adapted from Cabanillas F, Smith T, Bodey G: Nodular malignant lymphomas: Factors affecting complete response rate and survival. *Cancer* 44:1983, 1979.

Table 2. Comparison of Predicted Versus Observed Complete Response Rates

Number of Patients	Predicted Complete Remission Rate	Observed Complete Remission Rate
20	<60%	30%
44	60–79%	73%
45	80–100%	89%

Adapted from Cabanillas F, Smith T, Bodey G: Nodular malignant lymphomas: Factors affecting complete response rate and survival. *Cancer* 44:1983, 1979.

In order to test the ability of this model to categorize patients into various prognostic groups with different predicted survival times, the model was applied to the same group of patients from which it was derived. Figure 1 shows the results of applying such a model. The patients were divided into four categories based on their predicted median survival time, and the actual survival times were then plotted. At least three prognostic categories of patients could be discerned: the group of 27 patients predicted to have a median survival of 40 or more months in which only three deaths have occurred, the group predicted to survive less than 15 months in which the actual or observed median was only nine months, and an intermediate group consisting of those in the 15 to 26 and 27 to 39 months categories.

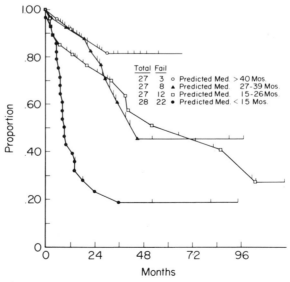

Figure 1. Nodular lymphoma; predicted vs. observed survival. Adapted from Cabanillas F, Smith T, Bodey G: Nodular malignant lymphomas: Factors affecting complete response rate and survival. *Cancer* 44:1983, 1979.

Effect of Second-Line Therapy on Survival after Relapse

When results of chemotherapy trials are reported, one important point seldom mentioned is the effect of subsequent treatments on survival following relapse from complete remission. The usefulness of a certain regimen could be over-estimated if the reader fails to realize that length of survival might not always reflect the effectiveness of the first treatment regimen alone. When second-line regimens of considerable efficacy are used for the treatment of recurrent disease, this can result in prolongation of survival that might be incorrectly attributed to the primary treatment regimen. Of the patients in our COP studies who relapsed from complete remission, six were retreated with adriamycin as a single agent or in combination with other drugs. Five of these six achieved a second complete remission that has lasted a median of 71 + months. The effectiveness of adriamycin even in the face of relapse is clear from these data. The superiority of the CHOP regimen over COP could be even more evident if the six patients relapsing after induction with COP had not received adriamycin subsequently.

Effect of Complete Response on Survival

The favorable effect of achieving a complete remission on the length of survival has been shown before for rapidly growing tumor types such as diffuse histiocytic lymphoma. However, for favorable types, the importance of attaining a complete remission has been questioned. Figure 2 shows the survival of our patients with nodular lymphoma as related to the quality of response, that is, complete re-

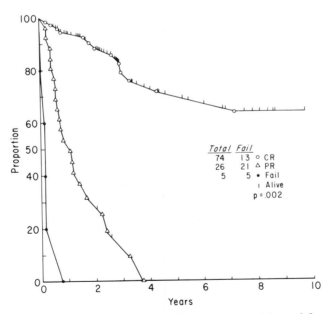

Figure 2. Nodular lymphomas survival related to response. Adapted from Cabanillas F, Smith T, Bodey G: Nodular malignant lymphomas: Factors affecting complete response rate and survival. *Cancer* 44:1983, 1979.

mission, partial remission, or failure. The survival of those patients who attained a complete remission is clearly superior to those who achieved only a partial remission or who failed to respond to treatment. Only the patients who achieved complete remission are still alive, some of them for periods as long as 8 to 10 years. These results attest to the desirability of achieving a complete remission if prolongation of survival is to be a major goal of treatment.

Effect of Immunotherapy and Other Prognostic Factors on Duration of Complete Remission

Two different types of immunotherapy agents were used in our studies. First, we investigated BCG in a group of 16 patients who were in complete remission after chemotherapy with the CHOP regimen. Levamisole was used more recently in a second group of 17 patients who were induced into complete remission after chemotherapy with the CHOP regimen but who did not receive any type of immunotherapy. Figure 3 shows the duration of complete remission of these four treatment groups. A statistically significant advantage in disease-free survival is evident for the group that received CHOP + BCG when compared with

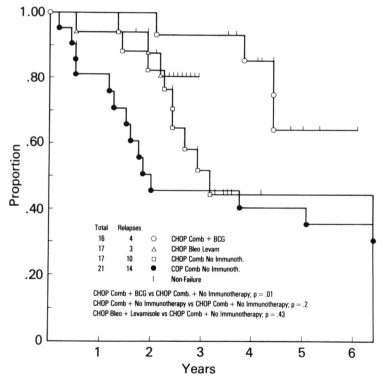

Figure 3. Disease-free survival of patients treated with immunotherapy vs. no immunotherapy. Adapted from Cabanillas F, Smith T, Bodey G: Nodular malignant lymphomas: Factors affecting complete response rate and survival. *Cancer* 44:1983, 1979.

those who received CHOP without immunotherapy. In the levamisole group, no significant differences are yet evident, although longer follow-up might reveal some differences, since a plateau is beginning to form at 26 months. Two groups of patients did not receive immunotherapy, one whose initial induction therapy consisted of COP and a second one who received CHOP. An initial advantage in the length of disease-free survival is evident for the CHOP group. This advantage, however, is lost at three years, at which time the curves approximate each other.

The issue of comparability can also be applied to these three treatment groups. A comparison like the one above is not acceptable without knowledge of which factors can influence the duration of complete remission. Such an analysis has been carried out, and the results show that only two factors are important in predicting the length of complete remission: the presence of B symptoms and history of prior therapy. The presence of either one of these significantly shortens the length of complete remission. The frequency with which these adverse factors occurred was then analyzed for these three treatment groups. The results are summarized in Table 3. There were some differences among the three groups in terms of the frequency in which these two factors were observed. In comparison with the other two groups, the BCG treated patients had a higher incidence of adverse factors present. In spite of this, however, their duration of complete remission was strikingly superior to the control group.

Effect of Histology on Duration of Complete Response

The only histological subtype in this study for which a difference in the relapse pattern is present is for the nodular mixed type in which only one relapse has occurred in 11 patients (Table 4). The pattern observed in the NPDL and NH types is similar with a constant trend for late relapses. The differences are not statistically significant as calculated by the Wilcoxon test. It is of interest to note that only one relapse has occurred after two years in the NH group. The induction therapy of this particular patient consisted of COP.

Table 3. Distribution of Adverse Prognostic Factors Associated with Duration of Complete Remission in Patients Treated with Immunotherapy or No Immunotherapy

		Number of Patients With	
Type of Therapy	*Total Number of Patients*	*B Symptoms*	*Prior Therapy*
CHOP + BCG	16	3	5
CHOP-Bleo + Levamisole	17	1	4
CHOP–no immunotherapy	17	4	1

Table 4. Relapses from Complete Remission According to Histological Types[a]

Histology	Total Number	Relapses	Time of Relapse
NPDL	54	20	2–61 mo
NHL	12	6	5, 6, 7, 7, 24, 77 mo
NMxL	11	1	6 mo

[a]P value (Wilcoxon) NPDL versus NMx = 0.28; NHL versus NMx = 0.12.

DISCUSSION

Most investigators today accept the important role of intensive treatment for the aggressive subtypes of malignant lymphoma. Particularly, adriamycin has made a significant contribution that has resulted in a higher complete remission rate and longer survival for patients with these aggressive subtypes. In the more indolent lymphomas of the nodular varieties, the issue of intensive treatment has remained controversial. In order to clarify some of these controversial points, we have used the technique of multivariate analysis to determine the relative influence of several factors on the following parameters: complete remission rate, survival, and duration of complete remission. This technique has the advantage that it can actually weigh the contribution and influence of each factor on the parameters above. Consequently, it reduces the possibility of incorrectly attributing a positive outcome to treatment differences when it could actually be due to random differences in the distribution of prognostic variables.

In our hands, the use of the adriamycin combination regimen of CHOP was selected by this technique of multivariate analysis as the single most influential factor in achieving a complete remission. It is clear from our results that the only possible explanation for the higher complete remission rate observed with the CHOP regimen in the nodular lymphomas is the treatment itself and not any other factor. Whether achieving a complete remission per se confers any advantage in survival to a patient with nodular lymphoma has also been questioned before. That issue has been settled for the group of patients with aggressive histologic subtypes but has remained controversial in the nodular lymphomas. Our data again show that achievement of a complete remission has a strikingly favorable effect on the duration of survival, as can be observed in Figure 2. In this regard, our results agree with those of Anderson et al. (6) and Diggs et al. (7), who have shown a significant improvement in the length of survival of patients with nodular lymphoma who achieved a complete remission over those who reached only a partial remission.

In view of the higher complete response rate obtained with the CHOP regimen in our patient population, it is not surprising that it was also selected by the logistic regression model as the second most important factor associated with longer survival. However, an interesting finding was that the hemoglobin level was identified as the most important variable associated with length of survival.

Regarding duration of complete remission, the data in Figure 3 show that patients who were induced into complete remission with the CHOP regimen and subsequently received BCG immunotherapy have benefited from a longer period of disease-free survival. This superiority in the duration of complete remission cannot be attributed to differences in the prognostic variables among the treatment groups. If anything, the patients in the BCG group showed a higher frequency of adverse prognostic variables present, and in spite of this their disease-free survival was longer than for the rest of the groups. Jones et al. have recently reported an improvement in the overall survival of patients with nodular lymphoma who received treatment with BCG after chemotherapy over those who received only chemotherapy. What is missing in this trial is an attempt at comparing both treatment groups as to the distribution of prognostic variables. Another conclusion that can be drawn from our study is that as long as a complete remission is achieved, it does not matter much in the long run whether it is obtained with an adriamycin-containing regimen or not. The disease-free survival of the complete remitters after COP with BCG has been comparable with that obtained with the adriamycin-containing regimen of CHOP without BCG. There is, however, an initial advantage in duration of complete remission for those treated with CHOP, but the difference between those two groups is not statistically significant (Fig. 3).

One important question recently raised is whether patients with the relatively rare subtype of nodular mixed lymphoma behave similarly to those with nodular poorly differentiated lymphocytic lymphoma, particularly with regard to the relapse pattern. Our data in 11 patients with nodular mixed lymphoma show that only one relapse was seen in this group of patients, and it occurred within one year (Table 4). These data are analogous to those reported by Anderson et al. in the group of patients with nodular mixed lymphoma treated with combination chemotherapy at the National Cancer Institute (6). In regard to the nodular histiocytic lymphomas, only one relapse after two years of complete remission was seen in this group, and it occurred in a patient who did not receive adriamycin as part of his induction chemotherapy (Table 4). None of the patients who received induction with CHOP manifested late relapses in the nodular histiocytic subgroup. Thus, the major problem in the area of nodular lymphomas is mostly limited to the nodular poorly differentiated lymphocytic group, in which a continuous pattern of relapse is observed. However, even in this subgroup of NPDL, those patients who received BCG immunotherapy experienced a longer disease-free survival than those who did not.

From our data, we must conclude that the treatment of choice for nodular lymphomas is combination chemotherapy with a regimen that includes an alkylating agent such as cyclophosphamide in addition to adriamycin, vincristine, and prednisone. Maintenance chemotherapy with COP is recommended after a cumulative dose of 450 mg/M^2 of adriamycin is reached. This should be continued for a total of one year after complete remission is achieved. Following discontinuation of chemotherapy, BCG scarification with Pasteur strain organisms has been helpful in maintaining patients in complete remission. This approach, in addition to offering the advantage of a higher complete remission rate and longer duration of survival, has also been associated with a relatively rapid response. Occasionally, a rapid response is desirable even in patients with nodular lymphomas, particularly when they have compromise of vital structures such as the ureters, intestinal tract, and bladder.

Even though we advocate the use of adriamycin-containing regimens for the management of nodular lymphomas, we nevertheless recognize that some patients are not candidates for this type of treatment. Adequate supportive care facilities as well as experience in treating infectious complications are mandatory prerequisites to undertake this treatment. Even though serious complications such as severe infections are not extremely frequent with the CHOP regimen, occasionally they occur, mostly when there is compromise of the bone marrow by tumor or by prior radiation therapy.

Patients with congestive heart failure or borderline cardiac status should also be excluded from receiving adriamycin as initial treatment. This decision, of course, has to be individualized, and factors such as the histologic subtype have to be considered, since it might be necessary to pursue initial treatment with adriamycin in a patient with nodular lymphoma of the histiocytic type, which can behave more aggressively. However, patients with more indolent tumors who have cardiovascular problems are better managed without adriamycin. This drug should be held and used only if necessary as second-line treatment in this particular situation.

In patients with asymptomatic stage I or II disease not compromising vital structures, other avenues of treatment such as non-adriamycin-containing chemotherapy regimens, radiation treatment, or maybe even watchful waiting could be considered as reasonable alternatives. These decisions have to be individualized and factors such as age and treatment facilities have to be weighed. It is not reasonable to commit an 80-year-old patient with asymptomatic and slow-growing nodular poorly differentiated lymphocytic lymphoma to intensive treatment with an adriamycin-containing regimen. There is little likelihood that such a patient will ever require treatment for his lymphoma, and, in such a case, no treatment might be the best treatment.

At this point, it appears that the major problem in the management of nodular lymphomas is the maintenance of the complete remission state rather than its achievement. With adequate treatment, most patients with these histologic subtypes should be able to achieve disease-free status. Immunotherapy with BCG has made a contribution in maintaining or prolonging the duration of complete remission in these patients, but the problem is, however, far from solved. New approaches as well as new treatment agents need to be investigated. At present, we are studying two different possibilities: (1) the use of late intensification treatment using a non-cross-resistant combination chemotherapy regimen after complete remission is achieved; (2) the role of interferon in the management of these nodular lymphomas. The latter compound has shown promising results in preliminary studies and could find a very important role in the future (16). We are hopeful that either one or both of these modalities, if rationally combined with already existing modalities of treatment, will result in the cure of a larger proportion of patients by totally eradicating all residual viable tumor cells.

REFERENCES

1. Rappaport H: Tumors of the hematopoietic system, in *Atlas of Tumor Pathology,* section 3, fascicle 8. Washington, DC, US Armed Forces Institute of Pathology, 1966, p 270.
2. Jones SE, Rosenberg SA, Kaplan HS, et al: Non-Hodgkin's lymphomas, II: Single agent chemotherapy. *Cancer* 30:31, 1972.

3. Portlock CS, Rosenberg SA: Chemotherapy of the non-Hodgkin's lymphomas: The Stanford experience. *Cancer Treat Rep* 61:1049, 1977.

4. Portlock CS, Rosenberg SA: No initial therapy for stage III and IV non-Hodgkin's lymphomas of favorable histologic types. *Ann Intern Med* 90:10, 1979.

5. McKelvey EM, Moon TE: Curability of non-Hodgkin's lymphomas. *Cancer Treat Rep* 61:1185, 1977.

6. Anderson T, Bender RA, Fisher RI, et al: Combination chemotherapy in non-Hodgkin's lymphoma: Results of long term follow-up. *Cancer Treat Rep* 61:1057, 1977.

7. Diggs CH, Wiernik PH, Sutherland JC: Nodular lymphomas: Prolongation of survival by complete remission (abstract 843). *Proc Am Assoc Cancer Res* 20:208, 1979.

8. Luce JK, Gehan EA, Gamble JF, et al: High rate and long duration of complete remission in malignant lymphoma treated with combined oral cyclophosphamide (CTX) and prednisone (PRED) and IV vincristine (VCR) (abstract 514). *Proc Am Assoc Cancer Res* 16:129, 1975.

9. Luce JK, Gamble JF, Wilson HE, et al: Combined cyclophosphamide, vincristine, and prednisone therapy of malignant lymphoma. *Cancer* 28:306, 1971.

10. McKelvey EM, Gottlieb JA, Wilson HE, et al: Hydroxyldaunomycin (adriamycin) combination chemotherapy in malignant lymphoma. *Cancer* 38:1484, 1976.

11. Rodriguez V, Cabanillas F, Burgess MA, et al: Combination chemotherapy "CHOP-BLEO" in advanced (non-Hodgkin's) malignant lymphoma. *Blood* 49:325, 1977.

12. Cabanillas F, Rodriguez V, Hersh EM, et al: Chemoimmunotherapy of advanced non-Hodgkin's lymphoma (NHL) with CHOP-Bleo + Levamisole (abstract C-248). *Proc Am Soc Clin Oncology* 18:328, 1977.

13. Bodey GP, Rodriguez V, Cabanillas F, et al: Protected environment prophylactic antibiotic program for malignant lymphoma: Randomized trial during chemotherapy to induce remission. *Am J Med* 66:74, 1979.

14. Cox DR: *The Analysis of Binary Data*. London, Methuen and Co., Ltd., 1970, p 87.

15. Cox DR: Regression models and life tables. *J R Statist Soc* 34:187, 1972.

16. Gutterman J, Yap Y, Buzdar A, et al: Leukocyte interferon (IF) induced tumor regression in patients (PTS) with breast cancer and B cell neoplasms (abstract 674). *Proc Am Assoc Cancer Res* 20:167, 1979.

4

Is Intensive Treatment of Favorable Non-Hodgkin's Lymphoma Necessary?

Saul A. Rosenberg

INTRODUCTION

The management of patients with malignant lymphomas other than Hodgkin's disease is controversial only for those with histologic types associated with a favorable natural history. Patients who have the histologic types associated with an unfavorable or poor natural history should have appropriate diagnostic studies and prompt therapy. There may be debate and differences of opinion regarding the diagnostic studies and procedures indicated and the choice of radiation therapy and chemotherapy programs for the various stages and settings for patients with unfavorable disease; but since cure is a potential for all stages of these patients (1,2) and the natural history of the unfavorable types is predictably poor, the standard of therapy is to treat them early and with maximally tolerated treatment programs.

The problem is very different for patients with the favorable histologic types. For these patients, paradoxically, there are no established curative programs. Moreover, early and aggressive treatment programs have failed to result in survival benefits in any study that has been properly controlled (3–5).

The controversies in this field are complicated by the following factors:

1. Experienced and precise histopathologic skills are necessary to separate patients with non-Hodgkin's lymphomas into the various Rappaport subtypes (2,6,–8). Clinical series reported before 1970 are very difficult to evaluate because of inadequate pathologic criteria and terminology. Even among major medical centers involved in clinical trials in the United States and Europe

Studies were supported in part from Grants CA-05838, CA-08122, CA-21555, and CA-09287 from the National Institutes of Health, Bethesda, Maryland, and a gift from the Bristol-Myers Company.

45

since 1970, the criteria and reproducibility of the pathologic subgroups are variable. Only when members of the Lymphoma Pathology Panel (8) have reviewed the diagnostic material can a measure of comparability between and among series be expected.

2. The diagnostic methods and skills used to determine the initial extent and stage of the disease and to establish the remission status of the patients have been extremely varied in the reported studies. Patients with these lymphomas usually have widespread disease, often clinically occult in many sites (9,10). Since occult or minimal disease is well tolerated and slowly growing in the majority of these patients, the accuracy and significance of a so-called complete remission (CR) is seriously questioned. For these reasons, survival benefits and the toxicity of various treatment programs are the only acceptable measures of the relative value and indications for these programs.

3. The majority of patients with these lymphomas respond very well to a variety of treatment programs. Even without treatment, a significant number of these patients may have perfectly stable or only very slowly growing disease (11). A minority but significant number of these patients may experience spontaneous regression of their disease for various periods of time (12).

4. Controlled clinical trials are only rarely used and reported, comparing conservative or standard therapies with new proposed aggressive treatments. Because of patient selection factors, probable important geographical differences in the incidence of these diseases, variable histopathologic and staging methods, and patient tolerance of occult disease for prolonged periods, concurrent randomized, controlled trials establishing survival benefits are sorely needed.

Physicians who treat patients with malignant diseases are not usually prepared to allow tumors to persist or slowly progress when a variety of more or less well-tolerated treatment programs can cause regression, even apparent disappearance, of the malignant disease for significant periods of time. There may be no parallel position in the field of oncology that argues that patients with obvious disease, responsive to therapy, should be individualized and often managed without prompt intervention. But that is exactly my current recommendation. Until clear survival benefits are demonstrated for routine and aggressive treatment programs when compared with individualized and conservative treatment programs, they cannot be accepted beyond the study setting.

Histopathologic Considerations

Patients with malignant lymphomas have a continuous spectrum of natural history and prognosis, depending on the histologic subtype. The most favorable group of patients, in terms of natural history, are those with the diffuse, well-differentiated lymphocytic type of Rappaport (DLWD) (13). All histopathologic classifications recognize this group of patients who, by relatively arbitrary criteria, are separated from patients with chronic lymphocytic leukemia and Waldenstrom's macroglobulinemia. The major group of patients with favorable natural histories are those with a nodular lymphoma composed of poorly differentiated lymphocytes in the Rappaport system (NLPD). This group corresponds to the follicular type composed of small cleaved follicular center cells of Lukes and Collins (14) and the centrocytic-centroblastic type of the Kiel classification (15). Most studies indicate that patients with nodular lymphomas composed of significant numbers of both poorly differentiated lymphocytes and histiocytes, the nodular mixed type of Rappaport (NM), also have good prognoses. More rarely, the nodules are composed primarily of large or histiocytic cells, the nodular histiocytic type of Rappaport (NH). These patients have a poorer natural history and behave more like patients with the diffuse histiocytic type (DH) and are generally not included in studies or recommendations for patients with favorable histologies. There are some patients with diffuse lymphomas of relatively poorly differentiated lymphocytes of Rappaport (DLPD) that correspond to the diffuse, small cleaved follicular center cell type of Lukes and Collins and the centrocytic type of the Kiel classification who have a relatively poor prognosis. However, these patients are not usually included in the favorable histologic grouping.

It is generally accepted that any degree of nodular or follicular structure in the NLPD and NM subtypes is associated with a favorable natural history (16).

The problem is further complicated by the not infrequent occurrence of two or more histopathologic subtypes in the same patient, even of the same site, at the time of initial diagnostic studies. This occurs in at least 10% of patients who have had two biopsies at the time of diagnosis (17). If a histologic subtype associated with a poor natural history, such as DH, is combined with a favorable type, such as NLPD, patients should be treated for the unfavorable type.

During the course of the disease, patients with favorable histologic subtypes, such as NLPD, often transform to a more aggressive and unfavorable type after various periods of time (18,19). The majority of patients who die of their disease, which was histologically favorable at onset, have transformed to an unfavorable histologic type at autopsy (20). This is true whether or not initial aggressive treatment programs are used early in the course of the disease.

For the purpose of this discussion, the Rappaport system and nomenclature are used, and the favorable histologic types are DLWD, NLPD, and NM.

Stanford Series

Controlled clinical trials directed at improving the therapy of patients with lymphomas have been underway at Stanford University since 1962 (21). Since 1971, trials involving patients with the non-Hodgkin's lymphomas have used the Rappaport system of classification, routine lower extremity lymphography, bone marrow biopsy for staging and restaging, and exploratory laparotomy for patients with less than stage IV disease. Various treatment programs have been used, usually comparing new, aggressive treatment plans of combination chemotherapy or total lymphoid irradiation with standard treatment programs. Whole body irradiation (WBI) was introduced in 1974, replacing the program of combined total lymphoid irradiation and chemotherapy. The philosophy of the new treatment arms of the randomized protocol studies has been to attempt to cure the patients with the best known diagnostic and therapeutic programs. The details of these studies have been described in prior publications (21).

In addition to these "protocol" patients, a group of patients has been followed who were ineligible because of advanced age (over 65 years) or unwillingness

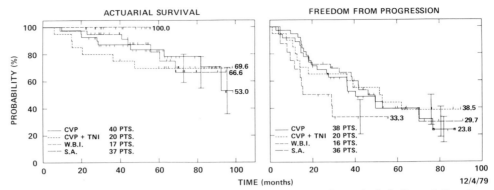

Figure 1. Favorable non-Hodgkin's lymphomas. Actuarial survival (left) and freedom from progression (right), of four randomized treatment groups; CVP (cyclophosphamide, vincristine, prednisone), CVP and TNI (total nodal irradiation), WBI (whole body irradiation), and SA (single agent, cyclophosphamide or chlorambucil). (indicates an event occurring with fewer than three patients at risk.)

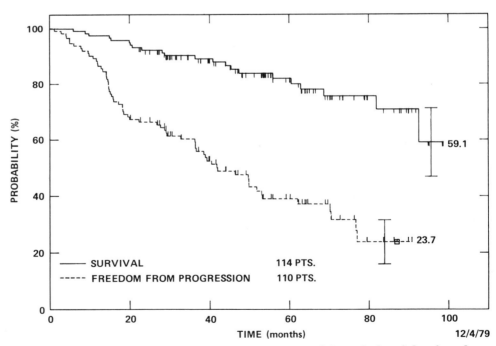

Figure 2. Favorable non-Hodgkin's lymphomas. Actuarial survival and freedom from progression of 114 protocol patients, 16 stage III and 98 stage IV. (—— indicates an event occurring with fewer than three patients at risk.)

48

to participate in randomized studies. A group of 44 of these patients followed since 1963 was managed with an individualized program of no initial active therapy, treating them as necessary for progressive or symptomatic diseases (11).

Figure 1, left, shows the actuarial survival of the four randomly selected treatment programs for patients with stages III and IV favorable non-Hodgkin's lymphoma. The results in all four arms are excellent, and no program is clearly superior to another, including a group treated with conservative single agent chemotherapy (oral chlorambucil or cyclophosphamide).

Figure 1, right, shows the actuarial freedom from progression of these four treatment groups, demonstrating no differences among the groups and no group with a low risk of recurrence, indicating a probable cured population.

Figure 2 combines these previously untreated patients between the ages of 16 and 65 years of age. The 5-year survival is 80%, with a 5-year disease-free survival of 40%. With the longest follow-up at 8½ years, the 10-year figures can be projected to be about 50% survival and 20% still free from relapse in all treatment groups. Most studies in the literature do not provide 5-year figures for proposed treatment programs, but some have 3-year data. The Stanford protocol figures at 3 years indicate a 90% survival and 60% disease-free survival, for comparison purposes.

Figure 3 indicates the lack of differences in survival or disease-free survival among the three histologic subtypes, DLWD, NLPD, and NM.

The 44 patients reported in detail by Portlock and Rosenberg (11), managed with no initial therapy, have been updated an additional 21 months, as of December, 1979. Though there are valid objections in comparing these selected patients with the protocol patients, Figure 4 shows the survival of the protocol patients and the group managed with no initial therapy. Their survival is virtually the same, with 3-, 5-, and 10-year survivals of 92, 75, and 60%, respectively.

Among the 44 patients with no initial therapy, there is no influence of histologic type on survival (Fig. 5).

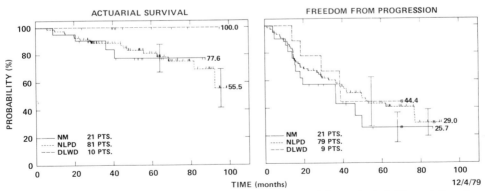

Figure 3. Favorable non-Hodgkin's lymphomas. Actuarial survival (left) and freedom from progression (right) of 112 protocol patients. Effect of histologic subtype. (——— indicates an event occurring with fewer than three patients at risk.)

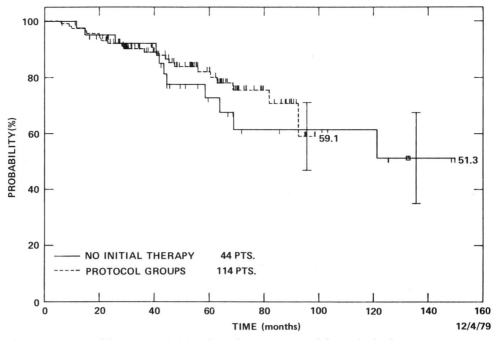

Figure 4. Favorable non-Hodgkin's lymphomas. Actuarial survival of 114 patients on protocol studies compared with 44 patients managed with no initial therapy. (——— indicates an event occurring with fewer than three patients at risk.)

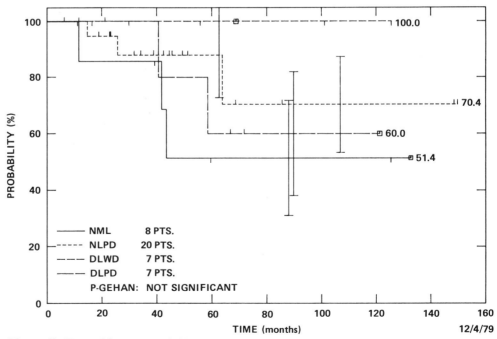

Figure 5. Favorable non-Hodgkin's lymphomas. Actuarial survival of patients managed with no initial therapy. Effect of histologic subtype. (——— indicates an event with fewer than three patients at risk.)

These studies have demonstrated the relatively good survival experience of these patients treated at a major medical center, independent of the initial therapeutic philosophy. At least 75% of the patients should survive for 5 years, and the median survival has yet to be reached in 8 to 12 years, in two different patient groups. These survival figures can serve as a standard for any group proposing a new management program.

The studies have also demonstrated the failure to cure these patients. Though there remains a group of patients who have yet to demonstrate a recurrence, even as long as 8 to 10 years after therapy, inspection of the disease-free survival cures shows a continuous relapse experience with time for as long as 10 years after initial apparent complete remission. This is quite different from the experience with Hodgkin's disease (HD), diffuse histiocytic lymphoma (DH), and almost all other human neoplasms. There is usually a period of 2 to 5 years after treatment completion when the probability of recurrence becomes very small and clinical cure can be projected (22,23). This is not the case with these favorable non-Hodgkin's lymphomas for any treatment program studied at Stanford or for those reported in the literature from elsewhere. One possible as yet unconfirmed exception is a subgroup of patients with NM lymphoma treated at the National Cancer Institute (NCI), to be discussed below (24).

Results of Others

It is extremely difficult to review and analyze the literature describing treatment programs for the non-Hodgkin's lymphomas of favorable histologic types. In some series, histopathologic criteria and expertise are not evident. Necessary diagnostic methods using lymphography and bone marrow biopsy for initial staging and restaging have not often been used (25). Quite often, results of treatment programs are given in terms of complete and partial remissions and their duration, rather than survival data. Often survival of complete responders is compared with those who did not achieve a response with the assumption that the complete response was responsible for the improved survival observed. Rarely are survival data given for more than three years, with some studies reporting data at two years or less.

In only several recent studies have controlled randomized trials been reported with a group receiving conservative treatment programs (26).

Table 1 lists a number of the major reports of the treatment of stages III and IV favorable non-Hodgkin's lymphomas. This is not a comprehensive listing but is representative of the modern literature since 1970. The range of three-year actuarial survival is 50 to 90%, with the exception of a 100% survival of a stage III group reported by Cox (27). The disease-free survival at three years ranges from 15 to 60%. No results are superior to the Stanford protocol series and the Stanford no initial therapy group.

Table 2 lists the several reports that give five-year actuarial survival figures. The range is 40 to 80%. Disease-free survival ranges from 20 to 60%, with only the NCI group of NM patients achieving the 60% figure (24). The survival of this group of NM patients is not superior to the NCI group of NLPD patients or to the Stanford experience.

Table 1. Three-Year Treatment Results

Group	Number Points	Histologic Types	Stage	Therapy Programs	Survival (%)	Disease-Free Survival (%)	Reference Number
Stanford, "Protocol" Randomized studies	114	NLPD, NM, DLWD	III (16), IV (98)	SA, CCT, CMT, WBI	90	60	Present series
Stanford, "No initial Rx" Selected patients	44	NLPD, NM, DLWD, DLPD	III (4), IV (40)	Delayed	92	—	11 Present series
NCI	50	NLPD, DLWD	III, IV	CVP	80	30	24
	31	NM	III, IV	C-MOPP	70	56	
NCI Randomized study CT vs. RT	29	NLPD	III, IV	CVP	} 85	25	30
	13	NM	III, IV	C-MOPP	}		
	25	NLPD	III, IV	RT	} 70	25	
ECOG	8	NM	III, IV	RT	60	N.A.	35
	35	DLWD	III (6), IV (28)	} CCT	} 70		
	104	NLPD	III, IV	}			
Joint Center, Boston	32	} "Lymphocytic and mixed"	III, IV	WBI	85	45	36
Nonrandomized study	25		III, IV	CVP	60	N.A.	
St. Bartholomew, London	66	NLPD, NM, DLWD	III (10), IV (56)	SA, CVP	85 (responders)	} 58 35 (est.)	26

Randomized study	No.	Histology	Stage	Treatment			Reference
Tufts	57	Nodular	III (19) } IV (38) }	TNI (3) SA (6) Remainder—CCT	35 (nonresponders) III 85 IV 45	N.A. 58 N.A.	29
Villejuif (Misset)	19	Nodular	III, IV	Chemo-immuno. Rx	80 (2 yr est)	65 (2 yr est)	37
Univ. Chicago	86	Nodular	?III, IV	Variable	80–87 2 yr, palliative 76–93 2 yr, comb. chemo.	70 (CRs only)	38
Univ. Florida	26	Nodular	II, III, IV	WBI	65	45	32
Paris (Gorin)	32	Nodular	II (4), III (8), IV (20)	CCT	90 (2 yr)	75 (2 yr)	39
SWOG	206	Nodular	III, IV	CHOP-BCG	95 } }	} 40	
				CHOP-Bleo	85 }(2 yr est.) }	} 30 (est.)	
				CPO-Bleo	85 }	}	
Stanford 1961–73 Radiotherapy series	48	Nodular	III only	TNI, TLI	88	60	34
Wisconsin	21	Nodular	III only	TLI	100	75	27

NLPD Nodular, Lymphocytic, Poorly Differentiated
NM Nodular, Mixed, Lymphocytic and Histiocytic
DLWD Diffuse, Lymphocytic, Well Differentiated
DLPD Diffuse, Lymphocytic, Poorly Differentiated
SA Single Agent Chemotherapy
CCT Combination Chemotherapy
CMT Combined Modality Therapy
RT Radiotherapy

TNI Total Nodal Irradiation
TLI Total Lymphoid Irradiation
WBI Whole Body Irradiation
N.A. Not Available
CR Complete Remission
CVP, COP Cyclophosphamide, Vincristine, Prednisone
C-MOPP Cyclophosphamide, Vincristine, Procarbazine, Prednisone
CMT Cyclophosphamide, Vincristine, Prednisone
CHOP-BCG Cyclophosphamide, Doxorubicin, Vincristine, Prednisone, BCG

Table 2. Five-Year Treatment Results

Group	Number Points	Histologic Types	Stage	Therapy Programs	Survival (%)	Disease-Free Survival (%)	Reference Number
Stanford, "Protocol" Randomized studies	114	NLPD, NM, DLWD	III (16), IV (98)	SA, CCT, CMT, WBI	80	40	Present series
Stanford, "No Initial Rx"	44	NLPD, NM, DLWD, DLPD	III (4), IV (40)	Delayed	75	—	11 Present series
NCI	50	NLPD, DLWD	III, IV	CVP	70	20	24
	31	NM	III, IV	C-MOPP	70	60	
NCI Randomized study CT vs. RT	29	NLPD	III, IV	CVP	} 85	} 25	30
	13	NM	III, IV	C-MOPP	}	}	
	25	NLPD	III, IV	RT	} 70	} 25	
	8	NM	III, IV	RT	}	}	
Tufts	57	Nodular	III (19)	}TNI (3)	III 85 } 45	N.A.	29
			IV (38)	}SA (6)	IV 25 }	N.A.	

Stanford 1961–73 radiotherapy series		} Remainder— CCT		
		III only	TNI, TLI	
48 Nodular		75	45	34

NLPD Nodular, Lymphocytic, Poorly Differentiated
NM Nodular, Mixed, Lymphocytic and Histiocytic
DLWD Diffuse, Lymphocytic, Well Differentiated
DLPD Diffuse, Lymphocytic, Poorly Differentiated
SA Single Agent Chemotherapy
CCT Combination Chemotherapy
CMT Combined Modality Therapy
RT Radiotherapy

TNI Total Nodal Irradiation
TLI Total Lymphoid Irradiation
WBI Whole Body Irradiation
N.A. Not Available
CR Complete Remission
CVP, COP Cyclophosphamide, Vincristine, Prednisone
C-MOPP Cyclophosphamide, Vincristine, Procarbazine, Prednisone
CHOP-BCG Cyclophosphamide, Doxorubicin, Vincristine, Prednisone, BCG

DISCUSSION

It is surprising that a group of patients who are so responsive to various treatment programs with very high apparent complete remission rates are not cured by their treatment. Management programs, including three- or four-drug combination chemotherapy, one- or two-drug conservative programs, combined irradiation with chemotherapy, and whole body irradiation, have all resulted in comparable survival figures, with no aggressive program superior to conservative programs.

The only data arguing for aggressive treatment programs are those series which show that patients achieving a complete remission survive longer than those who do not. Several groups have made this observation and conclude that the achievement of the complete remission is responsible for the improved survival observed (26,28). This fallacious reasoning does not consider the probability that prognostic factors that may be responsible for the lack of complete response are probably also responsible for the observed poorer survival. Recently appreciated prognostic factors, such as systemic symptoms, bulk of disease, site of stage IV disease, occult histologic conversion, or as yet unknown prognostic factors, may be responsible for the observation (22,29). Only if the combined survival experience of the entire treatment group is superior to a proper control group receiving another treatment can the proposed treatment be concluded to be superior. This basic tenet of clinical medicine should not be overlooked.

No data have been presented or discussed concerning patients with stage I or II non-Hodgkin's lymphoma of favorable histologies. These lymphomas are usually widespread when discovered, only about 10% being localized after proper diagnostic studies have been performed (9,10). Radiation therapy is usually used for these patients, but no randomized studies are available that indicate the required radiation fields, whether or not chemotherapy should be used, or if any therapy is really of benefit. These patients will enjoy a relatively long survival on the order of 10 to 20 years, and, in the Stanford series, 80% remain disease-free for 8 plus years after irradiation alone (21) (Fig. 6). It is impossible, however, to conclude that these patients are, in fact, cured of their disease.

The one group of patients that differs from the general experience is that reported by the NCI using C-MOPP (cyclophosphamide, vincristine, procarbazine, and prednisone) for patients with NM histology (24). This series of 31 patients experienced a 77% complete response rate, with 60% still in complete remission for up to 101 months, as of the report in 1977. In a subsequent study of NM patients, also treated at the NCI with C-MOPP, only 7 of 13, or 54%, had a complete response (30). Their duration of response is not reported separately, but only 25% of their combined group of NLPD and NM were disease-free at four years. It appears that the NCI group has not been able to repeat its initial good, unique result in the NM patients, but the confirmation of others should be sought.

CONCLUSIONS

Can it be concluded that early aggressive treatment programs are harmful for these patients with favorable histologic subtypes? The survival data of most of the studies in the literature are poorer than for the Stanford series. However,

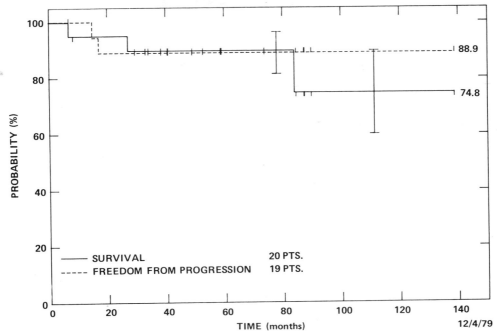

Figure 6. Favorable non-Hodgkin's lymphomas. Actuarial survival and freedom from progression of 20 protocol patients with pathologic stages I and II managed with irradiation only.

factors other than aggressive therapy, such as patient selection, histologic criteria, and previous treatment, may be responsible. Generally, when randomized studies are reported, the results of the aggressive program are the same or only slightly worse than the results of the conservative program, in terms of survival. What are clearly worse, however, are the greater mobidity, toxicity, and costs of the aggressive program, which argue against its use.

The case for conservative management is especially strong for the older patient with these diseases who is asymptomatic and who has no immediate threat because of the location and size of the lymph node masses. This situation occurs in more than half of the patients seen at Stanford (11). If the patient is over the age of 50 and meets these criteria, a period of observation, without therapy, can be of great value. Many patients are relieved by the observation that the lymph nodes do not enlarge rapidly, sometimes regress spontaneously, and they can function quite normally without therapy. Baseline lymphography is of great value in evaluating these patients, providing objective evidence of tumor growth or stability by comparing routine abdominal roentgenograms for several years.

If the patient is, or becomes, symptomatic or if there is a relatively rapid growth of lymph node masses, treatment should be initiated. The choice of treatment depends on the clinical situation and, to some extent, on the facilities and experience available. For localized problems, such as growing symptomatic adenopathy in the groin, axilla, or neck, local irradiation may be the best palliative treatment. For slowly growing, widespread lymphadenopathy associated with mild symptoms of night sweats or fatigue, oral alkylating agent therapy or whole body irradiation can be very satisfactory. Some patients have rapid growth of tumor masses with the onset of more severe systemic symptoms, pain, neuropathies, and other serious problems. These patients should receive prompt combination chemotherapy programs, usually with an alkylating agent, vincristine, and prednisone. There is no evidence that adding doxorubicin or bleomycin improves the treatment result. Whole body irradiation is an acceptable, well-tolerated alternative to single-agent chemotherapy for widespread, slowly progressing disease if the blood counts are adequate, if there has been no prior therapy, and if radiotherapists experienced with the technique are available (31–33). Total lymphoid irradiation, including treatment of Waldeyer's ring and whole abdominal fields, is acceptable therapy for carefully staged patients with pathologic stage III disease in the younger age group (below 50 years) (27,34).

It is more readily accepted to use a palliative treatment program for these diseases for patients over the age of 50 than for younger patients, because the median survival will be at least 10 years. The younger the patient, the more likely he or she will die of these relatively favorable lymphomas. Unfortunately, no known therapy can result in the cure of the disease. Physicians and patients should acknowledge this fact before embarking on a treatment program.

Despite the frustrations in developing therapies to cure or prolong the life of patients with favorable non-Hodgkin's lymphomas, the efforts should be continued. These are relatively common tumors and they are highly responsive to a wide variety of treatment modalities. In the clinical trial setting, new and even more aggressive treatment programs should be developed and attempted. Possibilities of combined irradiation and chemotherapy, multiple combination chemotherapy programs, and immunotherapy approaches should be considered and initiated when appropriate. However, such clinical trials must acknowledge the long, favorable natural history of the majority of these patients, use proper controls to establish the superiority of new treatment programs in terms of survival benefits, and use patients in such studies only with their informed consent.

ACKNOWLEDGMENTS

Studies reported herein were performed in collaboration with Henry S. Kaplan, M.D., Eli Glatstein, M.D., Richard Hoppe, M.D., Ronald Dorfman, M.D., Carol S. Portlock, M.D., Paula Kushlan, M.D., and other colleagues in the Divisions of Medical Oncology, Radiotherapy, Surgical Pathology, and Diagnostic Radiology at Stanford University.

REFERENCES

1. DeVita VT Jr, Glatstein EJ, Young RC, et al: Changing concepts: The lymphomas, in Jones SE, Salmon SE (eds): *Adjuvant Therapy of Cancer II*. New York, Grune & Stratton, 1979, pp 173–190.

2. Lewis BJ, Devita VT Jr.: Combination therapy of the lymphomas. *Semin Hemat* 15:431–457, 1978.

3. Portlock CS, Rosenberg SA, Glatstein E, et al: Treatment of advanced non-Hodgkin's lymphomas with favorable histologies: Preliminary results of a prospective trial. *Blood* 47:747–756, 1976.

4. Glatstein E, Donaldson SS, Rosenberg SA, et al: Combined modality therapy in malignant lymphomas. *Cancer Treat Rep* 61:1199–1208, 1977.

5. Bonadonna G, Narduzzi E, Monfardini S: Chemotherapy of non-Hodgkin's lymphomas with favorable histologies. *Antibiotics Chemother* 24:112–124, 1978.

6. Rappaport H, Winter WJ, Hicks EB: Follicular lymphoma: A re-evaluation of its position in the scheme of malignant lymphoma, based on a survey of 253 cases. *Cancer* 9:792–821, 1956.

7. Rappaport H: Tumors of the hematopoietic system, in *Atlas of Tumor Pathology*, section III, fascicle 8. Washington, DC, US Armed Forces Institute of Pathology, 1966.

8. Jones SE, Butler JJ, Byrne GE Jr, et al: Histopathologic review of lymphoma cases from the Southwest Oncology Group. *Cancer* 39:1071–1076, 1977.

9. Goffinet DR, Warnke R, Dunnick NR, et al: Clinical and surgical (laparotomy) evaluation of patients with non-Hodgkin's lymphomas. *Cancer Treat Rep* 61:981–992, 1977.

10. Chabner BA, Johnson RE, Chretien PB, et al: Percutaneous liver biopsy, peritoneoscopy and laparotomy: An assessment of relative merits in the lymphomata. *Br. J Cancer* 31(suppl II):242–247, 1975.

11. Portlock CS, Rosenberg SA: No initial therapy for stage III and IV non-Hodgkin's lymphomas of favorable histologic types. *Ann Intern Med* 90:10–13, 1979.

12. Krikorian JG, Portlock CS, Cooney DP, et al: Spontaneous regression of non-Hodgkin's lymphoma: A report of nine cases. *Cancer* 46:2093–2099, 1980.

13. Pangalis GA, Nathwani BN, Rappaport H: Malignant lymphoma, well differentiated lymphocytic: Its relationship with chronic lymphocytic leukemia and macroglobulinemia of Waldenstrom. *Cancer* 39:999–1010, 1977.

14. Lukes RJ, Collins RD: New approaches to the classification of the lymphomata. *Br J Cancer* 31(suppl II):1–28, 1975.

15. Lennert K, Mohri N, Stein H, et al: The histopathology of malignant lymphoma. *Br J Haematol* 31(suppl):193–203, 1975.

16. Warnke RA, Kim H, Fuks Z, et al: The coexistence of nodular and diffuse patterns innodular non-Hodgkin's lymphomas: Significance and clinicopathologic correlation. *Cancer*40:1229–1233, 1977.

17. Kim H, Hendrickson MR, Dorfman RF: Composite lymphomas. *Cancer* 40:959–976, 1977.

18. Cullen MH, Lister TA, Brearley RL, et al: Histological transformation of non-Hodgkin's lymphoma: A prospective study. *Cancer* 44:645–651, 1979.

19. Jones R, Young RC, Berard CW, et al: Histologic progression in non-Hodgkin's lymphoma (NHL): Implications for survival and clinical trials. *Proc Am Assoc Cancer Res–Am Soc Clin Oncol* 17:353, 1979 (C-257).

20. Risdall R, Hoppe RT, Warnke R: Non-Hodgkin's lymphoma: A study of evolution of the disease based upon 92 autopsied cases. *Cancer* 44:529–542, 1979.

21. Glatstein E, Donaldson SS, Rosenberg SA, et al: Combined modality therapy in malignant lymphomas. *Cancer Treat Rep* 61:1199–1208, 1977.

22. DeVita VT Jr, Canellos GP, Chabner B, et al: Advanced diffuse histiocytic lymphoma: A potentially curable disease. *Lancet* 1:248–250, 1975.

23. Kaplan HS: *Hodgkin's Disease*, ed. 2. Cambridge, Mass., Harvard University Press, 1980.

24. Anderson T, Bender RA, Fisher RI, et al: Combination chemotherapy in non-Hodgkin's lymphoma: Results of long-term follow-up. *Cancer Treat Rep* 61:1057–1066, 1977.

25. Herman TS, Jones SE: Systematic re-staging in the management of non-Hodgkin's lymphomas. *Cancer Treat Rep* 66:1009–1015, 1977.

26. Lister TA, Cullen MH, Beard MEJ, et al: Comparison of combined and single agent chemotherapy in non-Hodgkin's lymphoma of favorable histological type. *Br Med J* 1:533–537, 1978.

27. Cox JD: Total central lymphatic irradiation for stage III nodular malignant lymphoreticular tumors. *Int J Radia Oncol Biol Phys* 1:491–496, 1976.

28. Cabanillas F, Burke JS, Smith TL, et al: Factors predicting for response and survival in adults with advanced non-Hodgkin's lymphoma. *Arch Intern Med* 138:413–418, 1978.

29. Rudders RA, Kaddis M, DeLellis RA, et al: Nodular non-Hodgkin's lymphoma (NHL): Factors influencing prognosis and indications for aggressive treatment. *Cancer* 43:1643–1651, 1979.

30. Young RC, Johnson RE, Canellos GP, et al: Advanced lymphocytic lymphoma: Randomized comparisons of chemotherapy and radiotherapy, alone or in combination. *Cancer Treat Rep* 61:1153–1159, 1977.

31. Johnson RE: Management of generalized malignant lymphomata with "systemic" radiotherapy. *Br J Cancer* 31(suppl II):450–455, 1975.

32. Chaffey JT, Hellman S, Rosenthal DS, et al: Total-body irradiation in the treatment of lymphocytic lymphoma. *Cancer Treat Rep* 61:1149–1152, 1977.

33. Thar TL, Million RR: Total body radiation in non-Hodgkin's lymphoma. *Cancer* 42:926–931, 1978.

34. Glatstein E, Fuks Z, Goffinet DR, et al: Non-Hodgkin's lymphomas of stage III extent. Is total lymphoid irradiation appropriate treatment? *Cancer* 37:2806–2812, 1976.

35. Icle F, Ezdinli EZ, Costello W, et al: Diffuse well-differentiated lymphocytic lymphoma (DLWD): Response and survival. *Cancer* 42:1936–1942, 1978.

36. Hellman S, Rosenthal DS, Moloney WC, et al: The treatment of non-Hodgkin's lymphoma. *Cancer* 36:804–808, 1975.

37. Misset JL, Mathe G, Tubiana M, et al: Preliminary results of chemoradiotherapy followed or not by active immunotherapy of stage III and IV lymphosarcoma and reticulosarcoma: Correlation of the results of WHO categorisation. *Cancer Chemother Pharmacol* 1:197–202, 1978.

38. Britan JD, Golomb HM, Ultmann JE, et al: Non-Hodgkin's lymphoma, poorly differentiated lymphocytic and mixed cell types: Results of sequential staging procedures, response to therapy, and survival of 100 patients. *Cancer* 42:88–95, 1978.

39. Gorin NC, David R, Stachowiak J, et al: Combination of cyclophosphamide, vincristine, and prednisone, with and without radiotherapy, in the management of patients with non-Hodgkin's lymphomas. *Med Pediatr Oncol* 3:41–51, 1977.

40. Jones SE, Salmon SE, Fisher R: Adjuvant immunotherapy with BCG in non-Hodgkin's lymphoma: A Southwest Oncology Group controlled trial, in Jones SE, Salmon SE (eds): *Adjuvant Therapy of Cancer II*. New York, Grune & Stratton, 1979, pp 163–171.

5

Intensive Treatment of Multiple Myeloma

Burton J. Lee

Diana Lake-Lewin

Jane E. Myers

Multiple myeloma (MM) is a neoplasm of plasma cell origin. It is an old term (1,2), seeking to describe the multiple areas of diseased bone noted by the pathologist and clinician. It was only later (3) that it was fully appreciated that the disease was one of plasma cell origin. Physicians have been intrigued by the triad of anemia, renal disease with proteinuria, and lytic bone disease. Studies of the excessive immunoglobulins produced by the malignant clone of plasma cells have clarified many of the details of normal immunoglobulin structure and function. But it is important to understand the basic fact that MM defines a plasma cell malignancy and that the abnormal protein production in serum and urine, renal disease, anemia, bone pain, lytic bone disease noted on x-ray films, and all the other peripheral manifestations of the disease may individually or collectively be absent. The diagnosis is made histologically, usually by marrow aspiration or biopsy.

Dr. Osserman has coined the term *plasma cell dyscrasias* (4), which encompasses the spectrum of the plasma cell malignancies, extending from solitary plasmacytomas on one end to plasma cell leukemia on the other. This is a more useful term than MM, because it focuses the attention of the physician on the primary aberration that he must face, that is, the malignant transformation of one or more clones of plasma cells in a given patient.

The peripheral manifestations of disease, especially the monoclonal immunoglobulin (Ig) production, are useful criteria of evaluation. The Igs are an unusually valuable tumor marker. But the therapist should not be misled that the disappearance of the protein means the disappearance of disease or that relatively minor decreases in protein production signal an absence of therapeutic response.

Improvement in cancer therapies revolves around increase in malignant cell kill. Our problem is how to kill the maximum number of malignant plasma cells most rapidly and maintain the advantage we have gained. Most major advances in cancer chemotherapy have been a product of research into combinations of biologically active drugs, drugs to which the tumor cells do not develop cross resistance and which have different mechanisms of action. Advances in treatment (5) demonstrate this consistent principle again and again.

Response rates in any cancer relate to total cell kill, to the efficacy of the drugs used. It is also very nearly axiomatic that drug responders always live longer than nonresponders. The task, then, is first to get as high a response rate as possible.

Let us look at some of the rationale for combination drug therapy of any cancer, myeloma included.

RATIONALE FOR COMBINATION CHEMOTHERAPY

The growth pattern of human tumors is now generally accepted to be Gompertzian-like (6,7), which means that initial growth is exponential, followed by a progressively slower growth rate as the tumor enlarges and a plateau phase is reached. In other words, as the tumor mass increases, the time it takes to double its volume increases. If one assumed exponential growth and compared the number of cells in the tumor mass with the number of doublings, one might obtain a theoretical growth curve that would show that for a tumor mass of 1 mm, 20 doublings would have occurred; for a tumor first visualized on x-ray film (0.5 cm mass), 27 doublings would have occurred, and so on (8,9). The most important fact here is to know that, with our current means of detection, we recognize tumors only after they have already undergone a large number of doublings. Estimates of doubling times (DT) for various human histologic cell types have been quite different. For example, the average DT is 27 days for embryonal tumors (lung metastases) and 166 days for primary adenocarcinomas. Lymphomas, depending on histological type, have been found to have various DTs (10–12), for example, the mean DT for Burkitt's lymphoma is approximately 2.8 days and nodular lymphomas 400 days (10,11). Human IgG myeloma in its clinical phase has been estimated to have an average tumor DT of four to six months (13–15).

To understand and characterize the growth kinetics of tumors further, one must look at the individual cells making up the tumor mass. All proliferating cells go through a cell cycle that is divided into four phases. The events taking place during these phases of the cell cycle have been previously described in detail (8,16–20). Briefly, the stage of actual division is known as the mitotic (M) phase. Following this, there is the G1 postmitotic phase, which is of various length. Cells in this period may either differentiate, remain in a resting state, or continue on to the S phase of the cell cycle, in which DNA synthesis occurs. Following the DNA synthesis period, the cell enters the G2, or premitotic, phase in which the DNA content of the cells remains constant for a short period and then again enters mitosis (M). The variability of the G1 phase is the main determinant of the duration of the cell cycle. If this phase is short, the cells cycle rapidly. If they have a very long G1 phase, and do not reenter S, the term G0 has been used to describe a long postmitotic resting state. This implies that the resting cell during the course of observation is not in active cycle, but it does retain proliferative capacity (8,20). By definition, the growth fraction of a tumor mass is the number of cells in the mass that is actively participating in the cell cycle. It is most commonly defined as all cells in G1, S, G2, and M and excludes cells in a prolonged resting phase or G0. The value of the growth fraction is dynamic, and, depending on the stage in the Gompertzian curve that one is measuring, the value varies.

The pulse ^{3}H-thymidine labeling index (LI) represents the fraction of cells in S phase, since only cells engaged in DNA synthesis incorporate this labeled precursor. Labeling indices in myeloma are generally low and were reported by Drewinko (20) in a study of 13 previously untreated patients to range from 0.1 to 18% (median of 2.4). These values included patients with both high and low tumor cell burdens. It was shown that patients with low tumor mass had a median LI of 8.4% (range 4 to 18), and the median LI in the high tumor mass group was 1.2% (range of 0.1 to 4). Myeloma is a low growth fraction tumor comparable with chronic lymphocytic leukemia (CLL) and nodular lymphomas and distinct from other more rapidly proliferating hematopoietic tumors such as Burkitt's lymphoma and some cases of acute leukemia and Histiocytic Lymphoma. Our experience at Memorial Hospital in 12 previously untreated patients has shown the LI to vary from 0.2 to 12% with a median value of 1.0%. In 34 previously treated patients, the LIs ranged from 0 to 16% with a median of 1.3%. The two highest LIs in both these groups, 12 and 16%, respectively, were from patients with plasma cell leukemia.

It has previously been suggested that the LI varies with changes in the tumor mass. Drewinko (20) studied the effect of chemotherapy and reduced tumor cell mass on LIs. Tumor mass reduction induced by chemotherapy was assessed from changes in the myeloma protein production rate. When the reduction in tumor mass was greater than 50%, the median LI was 15 (range of 1 to 28) for nine patients in the high tumor mass category and 26 (range of 11 to 50) in patients in the low tumor mass group.

Salmon (13) has also observed progressive and significant rises in the percentage of myeloma cells in DNA synthesis, from 3% initially to 30% after treatment, after repetitive courses of chemotherapy. Pileri (21) reports that the increased thymidine LIs, a few days after the initiation of cytostatic treatment, may be indicative of the early recruitment of nonproliferating cells into the proliferating compartment. He stresses it is the increase in proliferative activity that makes the use of a cell cycle specific agent desirable.

Hokanson has found that the growth of myeloma can be expressed in terms of two cell populations, the drug-sensitive and drug-resistant cells (22). The tumor growth curve and response to chemotherapy would then represent various sizes of these two populations. Longer tumor doubling times are associated with a higher pretreatment fraction of resistant cells (the median tumor doubling time for responders was 2.9 months, and for unresponsive patients the median tumor doubling time was 6.9 months).

The growth kinetics of various tumors have been well studied in order to achieve optimum benefit from chemotherapy. There are many features about myeloma that make it an ideal model for a marker-kinetic approach to chemotherapy that has been well described by Salmon and Durie (15):

1. Myeloma is a monoclonal neoplasm that usually arises from a single tumor stem cell (23).
2. The plasma cells are easily accessible by bone marrow aspirations.
3. The majority of myeloma cells secrete an available characteristic protein marker.
4. The metabolism of these immunoglobulins has been well described (24).
5. Myeloma can be readily induced in the mouse. Tumor-colony-forming assays can be carried out both in vivo and in vitro in mice and humans (25,26).

Salmon et al. have pioneered most of the work capitalizing on some of the features of myeloma in order to provide insight into the pathophysiology and kinetics of the disease. They have been instrumental in developing a quantitative system to aid the clinical oncologist in evaluating the extent of disease and magnitude of response to chemotherapy (27–30).

With findings of the constancy of the in vitro rates of cellular M component, Salmon et al. then assumed that synthetic rates measured in vitro approximated the in vivo immunosynthetic behavior of tumor cells. A relationship could then be developed that would express the total body myeloma cell number (TBMC no.).

$$\text{TBMC no.} = \frac{\text{Total body M component synthetic rate}}{\text{Cellular M component synthetic rate}}$$

Initially the numerator in this equation was measured in vivo, using radioiodinated immunoglobulins and metabolic turnover study techniques. Total body myeloma cell numbers were found to be in the range of 0.2×10^{12} to 3×10^{12} cells (13,29).

Patients with clinical evidence of hyperviscosity were in the high immunosynthetic rate range (13). It was found that there was no correlation between plasma cell morphology and the immunoglobulin synthetic rate (6). Ghanta and Hiramoto (31), using a subcutaneous plasmacytoma model in mice, confirmed the general validity of the approach by showing that tumor burden and drug-induced changes in tumor mass, as calculated from serum M component levels, can be closely correlated with the measured weights of the subcutaneous plasmacytoma. Through studying patients with IgG myeloma (13,29), it was noted that the clinical diagnosis is never early. At least 0.2×10^{12} (200 g) of myeloma cells are present in the body in early cases. In most instances, more that 1×10^{12} myeloma cells are present at the time of diagnosis, and patients with multiple lytic lytic bone lesions have in excess of 2×10^{12} tumor cells in the body. Salmon has estimated that the lethal burden of myeloma cells is in the range of 5 to 7% of body weight, assuming 10^{12} myeloma cells equals 1 kg.

From several measurements of serum M components and other parameters of M component metabolism, it was possible to construct a graph of calculated myeloma cell mass against time. With careful analysis of growth curves in untreated patients, and regression curves after chemotherapy, it was confirmed that the myeloma growth pattern is indeed Gompertzian-like (13,22,29,31,32). It is now thought that myeloma growth occurs over one to two years and at the time of clinical presentation it has almost plateaued (13). The reverse occurs in response to chemotherapy. There is an initial exponential regression followed by a plateaued response to chemotherapy. In a good response to chemotherapy, the plateau tumor load is just one to two logs smaller than the pretreatment tumor cell number (13). If one considered the Hokanson model (22), this plateau phase would consist primarily of surviving drug-resistent cells. Clinically, responses of this magnitude are associated with relief of symptoms and prolongation of survival; however, a considerable tumor burden still resides. This clinical observation supports the laboratory findings of Pileri and Conte (33) and Mellested et al. (34) that the tumor mass of untreated patients and patients in remission is maintained by a very small fraction of proliferating cells.

Our experience at Memorial Hospital with the M2 protocol (35) further supports these findings. The average maximum tumor cell regression in 40 responders was 76% or 0.8 log kill. After the plateau phase had been reached, the tumor cell number remained stable without any appreciable change until relapse. These patients clinically had relief of symptoms and prolonged survival.

Young (8) has pointed out that in animal tumor systems, the survival of the animal is inversely proportional to the number of tumor cells implanted or to the size of the tumor at the time the study is initiated. Chemotherapeutic agents are effective by virtue of first-order kinetics; that is, they kill a constant fraction of the cells exposed to the agent rather than a constant number of cells (36). For example, for a tumor weighing 1 kg that contains approximately 10^{12} cells, a treatment killing 90% of the cells (i.e., 1 $\log_{10}$) would reduce the tumor population to 10^{11} cells. If the tumor weighed only 1 g (10^9 cells), the same treatment would produce the same 90% cell kill and would reduce the population to 10^8 cells. Thereafter, the tumor regrows at a relatively constant rate after exposure to the drug. It is only when a very large cell kill (e.g., 99.999%) is produced that one finds a significant delay in the regrowth of the tumor mass and prolongation of survival. One of the major reasons for the development of combination chemotherapy protocols and intermittent courses of chemotherapy is to accomplish maximum tumor cell kill while causing the least amount of damage to sensitive normal tissues.

As Zubrod (5) has pointed out, of key importance for the development of combination chemotherapy were the observations of Frei and colleagues (37) that a combination of 6-MP and methotrexate produced a greater percentage of complete remission in ALL than either drug alone and the observations of Selawry and Frei (38) that vincristine and prednisone were an extremely active comination for remission induction in that disease. The concept slowly developed that combinations of drugs with different toxicities and mechanisms of action could be used to give added tumor kill without synergistic bone marrow damage. This is the underlying rationale for the construction of the M2 protocol.

It is an accepted fact in the management of oncology patients that improved response rates almost invariably correlate with improved survival (39,40). Drug responders, in any cancer, live longer than patients who fail treatment. With almost all neoplastic disorders, both a higher remission rate and a better quality of remission are obtained with combination chemotherapy than with single agents (SA).

Treatment with melphalan and prednisone (MP) has been reported to produce marked tumor regression and symptomatic improvement in 30 to 70% of patients with multiple myeloma (41–46). At Memorial Hospital, we have consistently obtained a response rate of 30 to 35% with MP (47). With the knowledge that even with significant improvement a significant tumor cell burden remains, the quest for other combinations of active chemotherapeutic agents continued. Based on the initial favorable results reported by Harley (48), in 1972 we instituted a five-drug regimen (M2 protocol), consisting of melphalan, cyclophosphamide, vincristine, prednisone, and 1,3-bis(2-chlorethyl) 1-nitrosourea (BCNU). As Bergsagel and others have shown, the clinical rationale for this drug regimen includes the fact that BCNU, melphalan, and cyclophosphamide have all been shown to be effective and non-cross-resistant agents in the treatment of myeloma (45). Even though melphalan, cyclophosphamide, and BCNU act primarily as alkylating agents, they appear to have somewhat different modes of action. Prednisone has been noted to cause a fall in serum protein concentration and to cause a rise in hemoglobin in patients with myeloma (49). Vincristine is effective following an initial cell kill by alkylating agents when the LI rises; that is, it appears to be killing the cells in active DNA synthesis (13).

Alberts et al. (50) individually used four-cycle specific drugs, azathioprine, cytosine arabinoside, hydroxyurea, and vincristine to treat 12 patients with myeloma who were already in partial remission (plateau phase) after treatment with cell cycle nonspecific agents. In this study, cytosine arabinoside and hydroxyurea were unsuccessful in further reducing tumor cell burdens. Azathioprine had limited activity. Vincristine induced statistically significant reductions in total body myeloma cell number (24 to 60% reductions) in six of eight patients. From this, the authors concluded that vincristine is a useful agent for multiple myeloma and should be added to cell cycle nonspecific agents for the treatment of this disease. Whether vincristine is acting as a cycle specific agent or as a "helper" agent, by increasing the permiability of the myeloma cell to the other drugs, is not clear. The latter phenomenon has been described for the combination of vincristine and methotrexate (51).

The value of the nitrosoureas in the treatment of multiple myeloma has been well documented (52,53). They are now incorporated into multiple-treatment regimens, with various response rates: 50 to 55% for BCNU, cyclophosphamide, and prednisone (54), 87% in previously untreated patients (M2 protocol) (35), and 46% for oral methylCCNU and prednisone in previously treated alkylating-agent-resistant multiple-myeloma patients (53). Azam and Delamore (55) obtained a greater than 62% response rate using BCNU, cyclophosphamide, melphalan, and prednisone. In addition, they found this regimen most useful in patients with elevated BUNs or who were very ill when first seen.

One of the most promising trials reporting improved survival in myeloma is from the Southwest Oncology Group (56). Between March, 1977, and June 1979, a randomized trial was conducted. Two hundred seventy-five patients were evaluable. Three treatment arms were used: (1) melphalan and prednisone (MP); (2) vincristine, melphalan, cyclophosphamide, and prednisone (VMCP) alternating with vincristine, cyclophosphamide, Adriamycin, and prednisone (VCAP); and (3) (VMCP) for three cycles followed by vincristine, BCNU, Adriamycin, and prednisone (VBAP) for three cycles. Similar response rates were found in the three arms; however, the two-year survival was much better for the combination chemotherapy arms, with the VMCP-VBAP being the superior regimen, especially in stage III patients.

Alexanian and SWOG have shown that drug combinations including vincristine, given at three-week intervals, were associated with a higher response rate and longer survival times (57). Six different regimens were evaluated. The two regimens containing vincristine (VMCP, VCAP) produced response rates of 62 and 57% and produced survival times of 34 months, which appeared to be significantly longer than those produced by MP or their other combination chemotherapy control groups. Alexanian has repeatedly stressed that maximum degrees of myeloma protein reduction were associated with longer remissions and survival (40), and we have consistently shown, with the help of Drs. Durie and Salmon, that combination chemotherapy produces faster and higher cell kills and a greater reduction in paraprotein levels than does MP or any SA therapy (35).

Kyle also has shown that his objective drug responders lived a median of 31 months and patients who did not respond lived a median of 9.4 months (58).

Cohen (54) has shown that melphalan-resistant patients have had good responses to a combination of BCNU, cyclophosphamide, and prednisone and suggests that perhaps the addition of this regimen to melphalan might produce improved response rates. He also points out that patients who fail to achieve an initial response have less of a chance of responding to subsequent therapy, thus jeopardizing their chance for maximal survival. Presant suggests much the same thing (59).

Salmon has shown that nitrosoureas, in combination with other alkylating agents or adriamycin, are effective treatment for melphalan-resistant cases (52). Belpomme concludes that a better survival is apparent when one uses two alkylating agents instead of one as initial therapy for the disease (60). Ösby demonstrates a definite advantage with improved survival for combination chemotherapy patients with stage III myeloma (61). Harley and Cancer and Acute Leukemia Group B have recently shown much improved response rates and survival times in poor risk stage III patients treated with BMCP (BCNU, melphalan, cytoxan, and prednisone) over those patients treated with MP, (24 versus 12 months) (62). There are thus an increasing number of reports, both from single institutions and from cooperative groups, that are beginning to confirm the Memorial experience, that is, that combination chemotherapy of myeloma produces better response rates and better survival.

DETAILS OF M2 STUDY AT MEMORIAL HOSPITAL

Since 1972, the standard treatment of multiple myeloma on the Lymphoma Service at Memorial Sloan-Kettering Cancer Center has been the M2 protocol. The results of our initial pilot study were so good (63) that our plans for a subsequent randomized trial, against MP, were abandoned on ethical grounds. This treatment regimen has now been used with 204 patients. No patients have been excluded from treatment and subsequent study because of poor risk factors such as age or accompanying life-threatening illnesses. A total of 167 patients are suitable for analysis. Included in the group are 101 males and 66 females. Median age is 57 years. Eighty-six patients (51%) were treated before. Eighty-one patients (49%) had had no previous chemotherapy. Thirty-seven (18%) of the patients are excluded from the analysis for the following reasons: protocol violations (3), absence of objective disease parameters to follow (3), lack of follow-up of the extent of disease (1), misdiagnosis (1), patients lost to follow (17), and patients presenting with plasma cell leukemia (4) or primary amyloidosis (8). We have not had a response of amyloidosis to chemotherapy, though this has been reported in the literature (64,65).

Diagnosis was confirmed in all patients by bone marrow aspiration. Initial work-up included chest x-ray films, skeletal survey, CBC and differential, SMA-12, and serum and urine electrophoresis, immunoelectrophoresis, and creatinine levels. Treatment was easily administered as an outpatient and well tolerated by almost all patients, with only rare occurrences of increased nausea and vomiting, necessitating attenuation of the drug schedule. Hematologic toxicity for all patients, including those previously treated, was also acceptable. The median nadir counts for leukocytes is 2,500/mm^3, for hemoglobin 9.2 g%, and for platelets 98,000/mm^3.

Terminal acute leukemia developed in three patients (2 myelomonocytic and 1 erythroblastic), or 1.7 of the 167 studied. Two of these patients were previously treated over a two-year period before coming to Memorial Hospital for treatment with the M2 protocol. They subsequently went on to receive 9 and 29 cycles of therapy at this institution. The other patient with no previous therapy received 34 cycles of the M2 before relapse and further therapy with other agents.

Of greatest interest is the previously untreated group, and our analysis is concentrated on this group of 81 patients. All patients were clinically staged according to Salmon and Durie (66). Among the 81 patients with no previous therapy, 58 (71%) had stage III disease, 16 (20%) had stage II, and 7 (9%) had stage I. These percentages are similar to those for the previously treated segment of the patient population in which there were 64 stage III patients (74%), 19 stage II patients (22%), and 3 stage I patients (4%). Further breakdown of the previously untreated group showed that 83% (67) exhibited an abnormal monoclonal paraprotein and 11 (13%) manifested light chains only in serum and urine. Three, or 4% of the patients, were nonsecretors in whom no paraprotein or light chain component could be identified. Sixteen percent of the group (13:81) had a hemoglobin $\leq$ 8.5, and 17% (14) a BUN $\geq$ 30. Elevated calcium levels to $\geq$ 12 were present in only 9% of the patients (7) on presentation.

Patient response was evaluated in accordance with criteria set up by the Myeloma Task Force (67). A reduction in calculated cell mass, as well as improvement in, or maintenance of, a hemoglobin above 9.0 g/100 ml, a serum albumin above 3.0 g/100 ml, and a calcium level below 12 mg/100 ml were requirements for status as responders. Results showed the median time to response from the start of therapy was 3.1 months. Among the previously untreated patients, 78% were responders (63:81), 18% were nonresponders (15:81), and 4% (3:81) were too early in their treatment course to be adequately evaluated. This is a significant improvement over our earlier experience in the 1960s, when our response rate with melphalan alone, or melphalan plus prednisone, in 46 previously untreated patients was 33% (47). This melphalan treated group was composed of 85% (39:46) stage III patients. Six (13%) were stage II, and one (2%) was stage I.

A response rate of 51% (44:86) was achieved in those M2 patients who had had previous chemotherapy.

Analysis of survival in the previously untreated group included all 81 evaluable patients, including all early deaths, for whatever reason. A comparison was then made between the 81 previously untreated myeloma patients recently treated with the M2 protocol and the 46 previously untreated patients treated with melphalan alone in the decade of the 1960s.

The survival experience of the previously untreated patients for the two groups, M2 and melphalan, was compared both from time of diagnosis and from the entry on protocol until death. Median survival times, from diagnosis, respectively, are 48 months and 18 months. From the start of treatment, they are, respectively, 38 months and 15 months. In both cases, there was a statistically significant difference between the two treatment groups ($p < .0001$) (Figs. 1 and 2).

A comparison of the total survival experience from the time of diagnosis of the kappa light chain only, lambda light chain only, and all other patients was carried out separately for the previously untreated patients and then for the previously treated patients for both M2 and melphalan patients combined. In both cases, no statistically significant differences were observed (Figs. 3 and 4). Neither M2 therapy nor melphalan produced different response rates or survival times in patients with different types of immunoglobulin production.

Grouping stage I and II previously untreated patients, there was a statistically significant difference between the survival distributions for the two therapies both from the time of diagnosis and from the onset of therapy ($P < .01$). These results should be noted with caution in view of the fact that the sample sizes were small: for the M2 ($n = 23$) and for the melphalan group ($n = 7$). The median survival times from diagnosis has not been reached for the M2 and was 21 months for the melphalan group (Fig. 5). From the onset of therapy, they were 60 and 20 months, respectively (Fig. 6). Considering only previously untreated stage III patients, a difference was observed both from the time of diagnosis ($P = > .0003$) and from the time of the onset of therapy ($P = >$

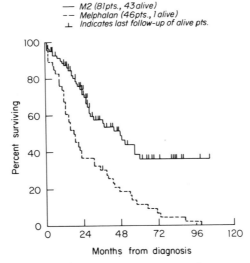

— M2 (81pts., 43 alive)
-- Melphalan (46pts., 1 alive)
⊥ Indicates last follow-up of alive pts.

Figure 1. Survival from diagnosis of previously untreated patients.

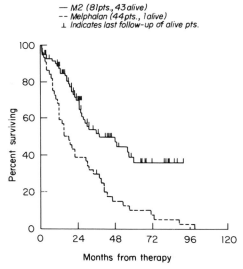

Figure 2. Survival from start of therapy of previously untreated patients.

.0005). The median survival times from the time of diagnosis were 31 months for the M2 group and 18 months for the melphalan group (Fig. 7). From the onset of therapy, they were 29 months and 15 months, respectively (Fig. 8).

Comparisons of survival times with other groups are somewhat difficult. Kyle (68) reports on 869 patients from the Mayo Clinic, none of whom was presumably treated with combination chemotherapy. These patients were seen from 1960

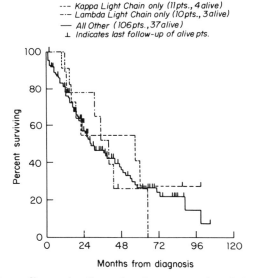

Figure 3. Survival from diagnosis of previously untreated melphalan and M2 patients combined.

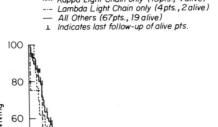

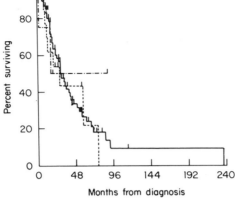

Figure 4. Survival from diagnosis of previously treated melphalan and M2 patients combined.

to 1971, the same time period as our Memorial melphalan-treated group. Our results are similar to Kyle's, that is, 18 versus 20 months from diagnosis. Bergsagel, in 1972 (46), published similar statistics, citing 20 months from the start of single-agent therapy, which in his hands apparently very nearly coincides with the time of diagnosis. In 1979, using various sequences and combinations of melphalan, cytoxan, BCNU, and prednisone, his three treatment groups lived a median of 30 months from therapy (69).

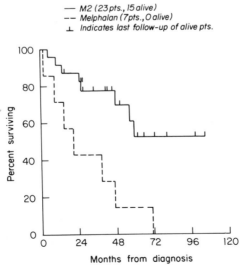

Figure 5. Survival from diagnosis of previously untreated stage I and II patients.

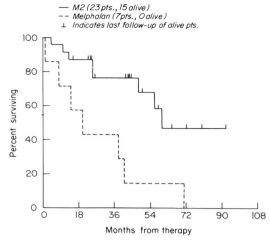

Figure 6. Survival from start of therapy of previously untreated stage I and II patients.

DISCUSSION

Bergsagel, among others, has given us an excellent rationale for multiple-drug combination chemotherapy of myeloma (46). Some of his rationale for this therapy has been explained above. At Memorial Hospital, our experience has borne out these theories. Since the decade when we treated our patients with melphalan and prednisone, we have more than doubled our response rates and doubled our survival times with the M2. Our experience in showing the superiority of combination chemotherapy is now being confirmed by others, both single institutions and cooperative groups. Some of these reports have been cited. Progress

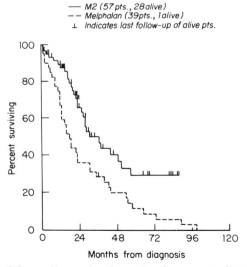

Figure 7. Survival from diagnosis of previously untreated stage III patients.

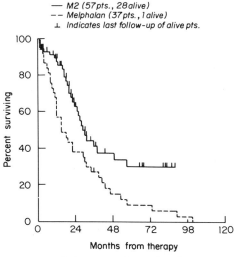

— M2 (57 pts., 28 alive)
-- Melphalan (37 pts., 1 alive)
⊥ Indicates last follow-up of alive pts.

Figure 8. Survival from start of therapy of previously untreated stage III patients.

has been made (70); yet we wonder why recognition that combination chemotherapy of myeloma is better treatment has come along so slowly. Let us explore some of the possible reasons.

Myeloma is one of the most difficult lymphomas to treat. The patients have multiple critical problems that require instant expert management, much of which is available only in an academic medical center. Most of the difficult problems arise during the first three months of therapy. Myeloma patients go into remission slowly. It may take three to six months for the patient's condition to stabilize and for the disease to show a significant response. But when remission is achieved, it may last several years. Much of the difficulty then lies in getting the patients through the first few months. At Memorial Hospital, we lose very few patients during the first induction months. Dr. Elliot Osserman, at the College of Physicians and Surgeons of Columbia University, has had the same experience (71). In the days of single-agent (SA) chemotherapy this was a more discouraging matter, because only a third of our patients responded, and then for a shorter period. However, if the patient can be brought through the first few months, approximately 80% of myeloma patients respond to the M2, and the yield in high-quality longer survival is significant.

During the first few months of therapy, first of all the patient needs an excellent house staff. Sepsis, shock, hemorrhage, hyperviscosity, renal shutdown, myocardial infarcts, pulmonary emboli, critical electrolyte disturbances, and so on, usually do not occur between 8 A.M. and 6 P.M. These complications occur in the setting of pancytopenia, severe renal disease, broken bones, and pain that may be difficult to control except with the use of high-dose narcotics and in older age patients who are bedridden. The patients require excellent sophisticated blood banking, the services of a special care unit, and multiple specialized consulting services. Infectious disease, physiology, and clotting experts must be available around the clock. A 24-hour capability for plasmaphoresis and renal dialysis will save many critically ill patients and allow them to continue therapy that will produce a remission a month or two later.

It is particularly important that all this specialized care be available at the start of therapy. This is the dangerous time. This is when unexpected drops in blood counts occur. This is when the patient's disease is not yet under control and when he is most vulnerable to a fatal complication. It may well be that, like acute leukemia, these patients should all be referred to centers particularly devoted to the care of their disease. It has been repeatedly said that patients with untreated Hodgkin's disease should all be referred to cancer centers. If this is true, certainly it is true of patients with myeloma. Myeloma is far more difficult to treat initially than Hodgkin's disease, and, yet, if the patients can be handled properly at the beginning, nearly the same percentage of patients will respond with current combination chemotherapy.

It is axiomatic that drug responders do better (higher quality and longer survival) than nonresponders. This is demonstrable in almost every malignant disease studied, even the nodular lymphocytic lymphomas (72,73), in which the favorable consequence of combination chemotherapy has been particularly difficult to demonstrate.

There is another reason why there has been difficulty demonstrating the benefit of combination chemotherapy over SA treatment of myeloma. It is probable that the spectrum of plasma cell dyscrasias is similar to the lymphoproliferative spectrum in that combination chemotherapy is particularly effective in the more aggressive forms of the disease. It may not be easy to show the benefit of combination chemotherapy in the less aggressive, stage I or II form of the disease. Our M2 series has a particularly high percentage of stage III patients. The Canadian Cooperative Study (69), which was unable to demonstrate multiple-drug superiority, has a considerably higher proportion of stage I and II patients. As noted before, other investigators also have had difficulty showing the superiority of combination chemotherapy in stage I and II disease, although this is not true in our experience. All myeloma patients at Memorial Hospital have had higher response rates and survival times with the M2.

Another problem in myeloma is how to define accurately the easy to treat or indolent cases that may go into remission on SA therapy and stay in remission. In myeloma, there is a big penalty for administering inadequate initial therapy. If the patient fails SA therapy, he is much more likely to fail combination therapy subsequently, and the chance for maximum survival may be jeopardized. The oncologist knows that by far the best chance for obtaining maximal control and optimal response rates in any given cancer is the first chance. If myeloma rebounds through therapy, or after successful therapy has been discontinued, there is at least a 50% chance that the rebound of the disease will be uncontrollable (74). We stopped successful M2 therapy in eight patients in our M2 series, and instituted melphalan-prednisone maintenance therapy. Four of the patients died within six months. Three limped slowly back into a less successful remission. One did very well on melphalan alone. There are no obvious predictive factors, including stage, for selecting those patients who can be put into a satisfactory second remission after successful chemotherapy has been stopped (74). We are strongly opposed to the cessation of therapy in myeloma patients who are responding to chemotherapy. Drewinko (20) has demonstrated the rapid rises in labeling indices and in the active growth fraction of the tumor cells after initial alkylating agent cell kills are obtained. If successful chemotherapy is stopped at this point, the disease may accelerate and be refractory to all attempts at containment. To experiment will result in a few patient deaths. Therefore, it is particularly vital in this disease to start off with the best therapy possible and to continue therapy in drug responders. We can see then that it is not in the patient's best interest to start therapy before it is necessary, because once successful therapy starts, it has to be continued. This is especially important when one is treating aggressive stage III disease and when studies of cell mass reveal rapid turnover of the malignant cell population.

At Memorial Hospital, we have long taken the position, since 1960, that since complete remission or cure is impossible in myeloma with current available chemotherapy (1 or 2 log cell kill is the best we can do), we do not start chemotherapy until the patient demonstrates generalized progressing disease, usually symptomatic as well. We therefore do not often start stable, asymptomatic stage I or II patients on drugs, especially a vigorous five-drug combination regimen. The alkylating agents are oncogenic. Bergsagel reports the alarming statistic that in his Canadian series 14 out of 364 patients have so far developed acute leukemia (69). He calculates the actuarial risk of developing acute leukemia is 17.4% at 50 months.

If a patient with "indolent" myeloma has no symptoms, shows no progression of his disease, and is stage I or II, it has been shown that he will probably live five to seven years (66) on minimal therapy. This is the type of case in which it is most difficult to show the benefit of combination chemotherapy and indeed in which early aggressive therapy may be of almost no use (similar to the nodular lymphocytic lymphoma model). It has never been shown that aggressive "prophylactic" therapy of the asymptomatic myeloma patient prolongs life, and if one notes the incidence of acute leukemia in the Canadian experience, one should be loathe to put a patient on aggressive alkylating-agent therapy before therapy becomes necessary. We start patients on chemotherapy if they are symptomatic or their disease gives evidence of progression.

In our M2 series, we have not had this high acute leukemia or second primary cancer experience. This may be partially due to our limited use of radiation therapy. When more and better drugs become available and when better control of the disease or cure becomes a possible reality, we shall start giving treatment routinely at the time of diagnosis.

The age of combination chemotherapy of myeloma is here. The clock will not be turned back to SA therapy in this disease until we are able to identify that minority of patients who will not be penalized by it. The SWOG group is now studying the next generation of combinations, that is, alternating one non-cross-resistant combination of drugs with another (VMCP-VMAP). This alternating non-cross-resistant combination type of approach has already been of great value in Hodgkin's disease (75) and represents in our hands a real advance in the therapy of patients with stage III and IV Hodgkin's disease over our previous results with MOPP alone. We have enough drugs now, effective in the therapy of myeloma, so that this alternating combination chemotherapy concept will compose the myeloma drug trials of the 1980s. In our hands, Pyrazofurin (76), cis-platinum (currently under study), and Adriamycin (77) are all effective drugs and have different mechanisms of action than the drugs used in the M2. MethylCCNU is noted to be effective in the setting of BCNU resistance (53). Changing the route of administration of some of the drugs may enhance results further (62,78–80). We now have nine drugs, all with somewhat different mechanisms of action. Two new four- or five-drug alternating combination regimens would appear to be most promising for out next trial, particularly for the poor prognosis stage III myeloma patients who represent the bulk of our referrals at Memorial Hospital.

In 1973, an editorial in the *British Medical Journal* was entitled "Progress in Myeloma at Last" (70). It was an excellent brief summary of some of the early recent advances in the therapy of the disease through the use of combination chemotherapy. These advances have been further documented and consolidated over the past seven years. It now seems unlikely that medical centers devoted to improvement in the treatment of myeloma will revert back to single-agent therapy of this very difficult and challenging disease.

REFERENCES

1. Rustizky J: Multiple myeloma. *Dtsch Z Chir* 3:162, 1873.
2. Kahler O: Zur Symptomatologie des multiplen Myeloms; Beobachtung von Albumosurie. *Prag Med Wochenschr* 14:33, 1889.
3. Wright JH: A case of multiple myeloma. *Trans Assoc Am Physicians* 15:137, 1900.
4. Osserman E: The plasmocytic dyscrasias, editorial. *Am J Med* 31:671, 1961.
5. Zubrod C: Historic milestones in curative chemotherapy. *Semin Oncol* 6:490, 1979.
6. Laird AK: Dynamics of tumor growth. *Br J Cancer* 18:490, 1964.
7. Simpson-Herren L, Lloyd HH: Kinetic parameters and growth curves for experimental tumor systems. *Cancer Chemother Rep* 54:143, 1970.
8. Silver R, Young RC, Holland J: Some new aspects of modern cancer chemotherapy. *Am J Med* 63:772, 1977.
9. Collins VP, Loeffler RK, Tivey H: Observations on growth rates of human tumors. *Am J Roentgenology* 76:988, 1956.
10. Iversen O, Iversen V, Ziegler J, Bluming A: Cell kinetics in Burkitt lymphoma. *Eur J Cancer* 10:155, 1974.
11. Nishikori M, Shirakawa S: Cell proliferation kinetics of human malignant lymphoma. *Recent Adv RES Res* 17:133, 1977.
12. Charbit A, Malaise EP, Tubiana M: Relation between the pathological nature and the growth rate of human tumors. *Eur J Cancer* 7:307, 1971.
13. Salmon S: Immunoglobulin synthesis and tumor kinetics of multiple myeloma. *Semin Hematol* 10:135, 1973.
14. Salmon S: Expansion of the growth fraction in multiple myeloma with alkylating agents. *Blood* 45:119, 1975.
15. Salmon S, Durie B: Cellular kinetics in multiple myeloma. *Arch Internal Med* 135:131, 1975.
16. Howard A, Pelc S: Nuclear incorporation of P-32 as demonstrated by autoradiographs. *Exp Cell Res* 2:178, 1951.
17. Karnofsky DA, Clarkson B: Annual review: Cellular aspects of anticancer drugs. *Pharmacology* 3:357, 1963.
18. Hill BT, Baserga R: The cell cycle and its significance for cancer treatment. *Cancer Treat Rev* 2:159, 1975.
19. Baserga R: *Multiplication and Division in Mammalian Cells.* Dekker, New York, 1976.

20. Drewinko B, Brown B, Humphrey R, Alexanian R: Effect of chemotherapy on the labeling index of myeloma cells. *Cancer* 34:526, 1974.

21. Pileri A, Bernengo M, Buccadoro M, Pierfranco C, et al: Early recruitment in the human myeloma cell population after cytostatic treatment. *Haematologica* 61:184, 1976.

22. Hokanson J, Brown B, Thompson J, Drewinko B, et al: Tumor growth patterns in multiple myeloma. *Cancer* 39:1077, 1977.

23. Waldenstrom J: Hypergammaglobulinemia as a clinical hematological problem: A study in the gammopathies. *Prog Hematol* 3:266, 1962.

24. Waldman TA, Strober W: Metabolism of immunoglobulins. *Progr Allergy* 13:1, 1969.

25. Bergsagel D, Ogawa M, Librach S: Mouse myeloma: A model for studies of cell kinetics. *Arch Int Med* 135:109, 1975.

26. Salmon S, Hamberger A, Soehnlen B, Durie B, et al: Quantitation of differential sensitivity of human-tumor stem cells to anti-cancer drugs. *N Engl J Med* 298:1321, 1978.

27. Salmon S, Mackey G, Fudenberg H: "Sandwich" solid phase radioimmunoassay for the quantitative determination of human immunoglobulins. *J Immunol* 103:129, 1969.

28. Salmon S, Smith B: Sandwich solid phase radioimmunoassay for the characterization of human immunoglobulins synthesized in vitro. *J Immunol* 101:665, 1970.

29. Salmon SE, Smith BA: Immunoglobulin synthesis and total body tumor cell number in IgG multiple myeloma. *J Clin Invest* 49:1114, 1970.

30. Hammerton K, Cooper D, Duckett M, Penny R: Biosynthesis of immunoglobulin in human immunoproliferative diseases: I. Kinetics of synthesis and secretion of immunoglobulin and protein by bone marrow cells in myeloma. *J Immunol* 121:409, 1978.

31. Ghanta V, Hiramoto R: Quantitation of total-body tumor cells (MOPC 104E): I. Subcutaneous tumor model. *J Natl Canc Inst* 52:1199, 1974.

32. Sullivan P, Salmon S: Kinetics of tumor growth and regression in IgG multiple myeloma. *J Clin Invest* 51:1697, 1972.

33. Pileri A, Conte P: The biological and clinical features of human myeloma. *Haematologica* 62:202, 1977.

34. Mellested H, Killander D, Pallerson D: Bone marrow kinetic studies of three patients with myelomatosis. *Acta Med Scand* 202:413, 1977.

35. Case DC, Lee BJ III, Clarkson BD: Improved survival times in multiple myeloma treated with Melphalan, Prednisone, Cyclophosphamide, Vincristine, and BCNU: M-2 protocol. *Am J Med* 63:897, 1977.

36. Skipper HE: Pharmacological basis of cancer chemotherapy: Closing remarks, in *Pharmacological Basis of Cancer Chemotherapy in A Collection of Papers Presented at the 27th Annual Symposium on Fundamental Cancer Research*, 1974, University of Texas, M.D. Anderson Hospital and Tumor Institute at Houston. Baltimore, Md., Williams & Wilkins Co. 1975, p 756.

37. Frei E III, Freireich ET, Gehan E, the Acute Leukemia Group B: Studies of sequential and combination antimetabolite therapy in acute leukemia: 6-Mercaptopurine and methotrexate. *Blood* 18:431, 1961.

38. Selawry OS, Frei E III: Prolongation of remission in acute lymphocytic leukemia by alteration in dose schedule and route of administration of methotrexate. *Clin Res* 12:231, 1964.

39. Cuttner J, Wasserman L, Martz G, Sunnhal R, et al: The use of low-dose Prednisone and Melphalan in the treatment of poor-risk patients with multiple myeloma. *Med Pediatr Oncol* 1:207, 1975.

40. Alexanian R, Bonnet J, Gettani E, Haut A, et al: Combination chemotherapy for multiple myeloma. *Cancer* 30:382, 1972.

41. Alexanian R, Haut A, Khan A: Treatment for multiple myeloma. *J Am Med Assoc* 208:1680, 1969.

42. Alexanian R, Bergsagel DE, Philip DE, Migliore PJ, et al: Melphalan therapy for plasma cell myeloma. *Blood* 37:1, 1968.

43. McArthur JR, Athens JW, Wintrobe MM, Cartwright GE: Melphalan and myeloma: Experience with a low dose continuous regimen. *Ann Int Med* 72:665, 1970.

44. Hoogstraten B, Costa J, Cuttner J, Forcier RJ, et al: Intermittent melphalan therapy in multiple myeloma. *J Am Med Assoc* 209:251, 1969.

45. Costa G, Engle RL Jr, Schillim A, Cavbone R, et al: Melphalan and Prednisone: An effective combination for the treatment of multiple myeloma. *Am J Med* 54:589, 1973.

46. Bergsagel DE: Plasma cell myeloma: An interpretive review. *Cancer* 30:1588, 1972.

47. Pinsky CM, Lee BJ III: Melphalan treatment of multiple myeloma. *Memorial Sloan-Kettering Cancer Center Bulletin* 6:142, 1976.

48. Harley JB, Ramanan SV, Kim I, et al: The cyclic use of multiple alkylating agents in multiple myeloma. *W Va Med J* 68:1, 1971.

49. Salmon SE, Shadduck RD, Schilling A: Intermittent high dose Prednisone (nsc-10023) therapy for multiple myeloma. *Cancer Chemother Rep* 51:179, 1967.

50. Alberts P, Durie B, Salmon S: Treatment of multiple myeloma in remission with anticancer drugs having cell cycle specific characteristics. *Cancer Treat Rep* 61:381, 1977.

51. Goldman I, Gupta V, White J, Loftfield S: Exchangeable intracellular methotrexate levels in the presence and absence of vincristine at extracellular drug concentrations relevant to those achieved in high-dose methotrexate-folinic acid "rescue" protocols. *Cancer Res* 36:276, 1976.

52. Salmon S: Nitrosoureas in multiple myeloma. *Cancer Treat Rep* 60:789, 1976.

53. Tornyos K, Silberman H, Solomon A: Phase II study of oral methyl-CCNU and Prednisone in previously treated alkylating agent-resistant multiple myeloma. *Cancer Treat Rep* 61:785, 1977.

54. Cohen H, Silberman H, Larsen W, Johnson L, et al: Combination chemotherapy with intermittent 1-3-bis (2-chloroethyl) 1-nitrosourea (BCNU), Cyclophosphamide, and Prednisone for multiple myeloma. *Blood* 54:824, 1979.

55. Azam L, Delamore IW: Combination therapy for myelomatosis. *Br Med J* 4:560, 1974.

56. Salmon SE, Alexanian R, Dixon D: Non-cross resistant combination chemotherapy improves survival in multiple myeloma. *Blood* 54:207A, 1979.

57. Alexanian R, Salmon S, Bonnet J, Gehan E, et al: Combination therapy for multiple myeloma. *Cancer* 40:2765, 1977.

58. Kyle RA, Gailani S, Seligman BR, Blom J, et al: Multiple myeloma resistant to Melphalan: Treatment with Cyclophosphamide, Prednisone, and BCNU. *Cancer Treat Rep* 63:1265, 1979.

59. Presant CA, Klahr C: Adriamycin, 1,3-bis (2-chloroethyl)-1-nitrosourea (BCNU, NSC #409962), Cyclophosphamide plus Prednisone (ABC-P) in Melphalan-resistant multiple myeloma. *Cancer* 42:1222, 1978.

60. Belpomme D, Simon F, Pouillart P, Amor B, et al: Prognostic factors and treatment of multiple myeloma: Interest of a cyclic sequential chemohormonotherapy combining Cyclophosphamide, Melphalan, and Prednisone. *Cancer Res* 65:28, 1978.

61. Osby E, Carlmark B, Reizenstein P: Staging of myeloma: A preliminary study of staging factors and treatment in different stages. *Recent Results Cancer Res* 65:21, 1978.

62. Harley JB, Pajak TF, McIntyre OR, Kochwa S, et al: Improved survival of increased-risk myeloma patients on combined triple-alkylating-agent therapy: A study of the CALGB. *Blood* 54:13, 1979.

63. Lee BJ, Sahakian G, Clarkson B, Krakoff I: Combination chemotherapy of multiple myeloma with Alkeran, Cytoxan, Vincristine, Prednisone and BCNU. *Cancer* 33:2533,1974.

64. Cohen JH, Lessin LS, Hallal J, Burkholder P: Resolution of primary amyloidosis during chemotherapy: Studies in a patient with nephrotic syndrome. *Ann Int Med* 82:466, 1975.

65. Kyle RA, Greipp PR: Primary systemic amyloidosis: Comparison of Melphalan and Prednisone versus placebo. *Blood* 52:818, 1978.

66. Durie BG, Salmon SE: A clinical staging system for multiple myeloma: Correlation of measured myeloma cell mass with presenting clinical features, response to treatment, and survival. *Cancer* 36:842, 1975.

67. Committee of the Chronic Leukemia-Myeloma Task Force, National Cancer Institute: Proposed guidelines for protocol studies: II. Plasma cell myeloma. *Cancer Chemother Rep* 4:145, 1973.

68. Kyle RA: Subject review: Multiple myeloma, review of 869 cases. Mayo *Clin Proc* 50:29, 1975.

69. Bergsagel DE, Bailey AJ, Langley GR, MacDonald RN, et al: The chemotherapy of plasma-cell myeloma and the incidence of acute leukemia. *N Engl J Med* 301:743, 1979.

70. Editorial. Progress in myeloma at last. *Br Med J* June 24:1653, 1978.

71. Elliot Osserman: Personal communication.

72. Cabanillas F, Smith T, Bodey GP, Gutterman JU, et al: Nodular malignant lymphomas: Factors affecting complete response rate and survival. *Cancer* 44:1983, 1979.

73. Diggs CH, Wiernik PH, Sutherland JC: Nodular lymphoma: Prolongation of survival by complete remission. *Proc AACR,* 1979.

74. Cohen HJ, Silberman HR: Unmaintained remission after two years of combination chemotherapy in myeloma. *Proc AACR and ASCO C-476,* 1979.

75. Straus DJ, Myers J, Passe S, Young CW, et al: The eight-drug/radiation therapy program (MOPP/ABDV/RT) for advanced Hodgkin's disease: A follow-up report. *Cancer* 46:in press, 1980.

76. Lake-Lewin D, Myers J, Lee BJ, Young CW: Phase II trial of pyrazofurin in patients with multiple myeloma refractory to standard cytotoxic therapy. *Cancer Treat Rep* 63:1403, 1979.

77. Alberts DS, Salmon SE: Adriamycin (NSC-123127) in the treatment of alkylator-resistant multiple myeloma: A pilot study. *Cancer Chemother Rep* 59:345, 1975.

78. Alberts DS, Chang SY, Chen H-SG, Evans TL, et al: Systemic availability of oral melphalan. *Cancer Treat Rev* 65:51, 1979.

79. Vistica DT: Studies on the relationship between melphalan transport and cytotoxicity. *Cancer Treat Rev* 6S:51, 1979.

80. Tattersall MHN, Jarman M, Newlands ES, Holyhead L, et al: Studies with labeled melphalan in patients with malignant disease. *Cancer Treat Rev* 6S:52, 1979.

6

Is Multidrug Chemotherapy Necessary for Multiple Myeloma?

Daniel E. Bergsagel

The current status of treatment for plasma cell myeloma (PCM) is very similar to the status achieved for chronic granulocytic leukemia (CGL) after the introducation of busulfan. We have effective methods for controlling both diseases during the chronic phase, but treatment during the acute terminal phase is only sporadically effective and has little influence on the survival of groups of patients. The time of onset of the acute terminal phase is the major factor determining the survival of patients with both diseases (1). Drugs that delay, or prevent, the onset of the acute terminal phase would have a major effect on the survival of these patients. We must continue to look for drugs with this property.

The treatment of CGL with x-irradiation of the spleen, or busulfan, improved the quality of life for these patients but had only a small effect on survival (2). The treatment of PCM patients with alkylating agents has had a much greater influence on survival. Before the use of alkylating agents, the median survival of patients treated with local irradiation and urethane was only 7 months from the onset of treatment (3,4). The median survival of patients treated with melphalan and prednisone has increased to about 30 months from the start of treatment (5–8). However, these patients are not cured, and the survival curve never becomes parallel to that of an age and sex matched control group. The improvement in survival after treatment of PCM results from a 1 to 2 log decrease in the myeloma cell mass (1,9). This minor decrease in the tumor cell number is enough to relieve symptoms and improve survival by reducing the number of early deaths from complications such as hypercalcemia, renal failure, hypervolemia, and possibly infections.

If the growth of human myeloma cells followed the classical rules that have been established for the transplantable mouse leukemia L1210, one would expect to demonstrate the following:

1. A dose response effect, that is, increasing doses should destroy more tumor cells.
2. Remission duration and survival should be related directly to the myeloma cell kill achieved by a treatment.
3. Maintenance treatment should prolong the duration of a remission.
4. Surviving myeloma cells should begin to proliferate and grow exponentially as soon as treatment is stopped.

The response of human PCM to treatment does not demonstrate any of these features. Furthermore, the growth rate of PCM during relapse, as measured by the serum M-protein doubling time, increases progressively during the course of the disease until the acute terminal phase is reached (1). Thus, the regulation of growth in human PCM is much different than for L1210 and most other animal tumor models.

For these reasons it is unlikely that combination chemotherapy directed at destroying myeloma cells is more effective than less intensive treatment for PCM patients. In this chapter, I review features of the growth of PCM first and then explore selected articles that claim that combination chemotherapy is more effective than melphalan and prednisone in the treatment of PCM.

GROWTH CHARACTERISTICS OF HUMAN PCM

The growth of human PCM can be evaluated indirectly by following changes in the serum M-protein or directly by looking at the labeling of myeloma cells with H^3TdR (10–12) or the growth of myeloma stem cells in culture (13,14). The amount of M-protein in the serum (15) or ascitic fluid (16) of a mouse is directly related to tumor mass. The same statement does not apply to the amount of light chain protein excreted in the urine, because an unknown fraction is catabolized by the kidney (17) and the amount excreted is influenced by renal function (18).

We have estimated the tumor cell kill in myeloma patients by following the serum M-protein after treatment is discontinued (1). For example, the M-protein disappeared from the serum of an IgA myeloma patient after treatment with melphalan and prednisone. It took 335 days for the serum M-protein concentration to return to the pretreatment value after treatment was stopped. The serum M-protein concentration increased exponentially during the regrowth phase, with a doubling time of 98 days. If we make the reasonable assumption that the M-protein doubling time reflects the growth rate of myeloma cells, we can estimate that 335/98, or 3.4, doublings of the residual myeloma cells are required to return the tumor to its original size following four courses of melphalan and prednisone. Reducing the tumor cell number by $2^{-3.4}$ is equal to a 1 log (10^{-1}) cell kill. Salmon and Smith (19) have developed a more sophisticated method for estimating the total body myeloma cell number from measurements of the amount of M-protein produced per myeloma cell, the total amount of M-protein in the plasma volume, and the catabolic rate of the M-protein. Using this method for following changes in the myeloma cell number of patients with

IgG myeloma during chemotherapy, Sullivan and Salmon (20) found that a plateau is reached after a maximum myeloma cell reduction of 1 to 2 logs.

Can a Dose-Response Effect Be Demonstrated in the Treatment of PCM?

Unfortunately this question has not been investigated directly. Doses of chemotherapeutic agents are usually adjusted to cause acceptable hematologic toxicity. However, many have observed that objective responses occur just as frequently in patients treated with doses that produce little toxicity as with doses that cause marked toxicity. This question has been investigated indirectly by comparing the duration of maintained and unmaintained remissions (5) and is examined later. The fact that continued treatment during a remission does not influence the duration of either the remission or survival strongly suggests that the dose-response effect in PCM is weak or nonexistant.

Furthermore, the observation that continuing treatment leads to a progressive decrease in the myeloma cell mass until a plateau is reached (9) is difficult to reconcile with a simple dose-response effect of myeloma cells to treatment. Initial treatment causes a fall in the serum M-protein for three to nine months; thereafter, the serum M-protein concentration remains constant despite continued therapy. Others have observed an increase in the labeling index of myeloma cells after treatment with an alkylating agent is started (10–12); however, this persists for less than six months (21). Attempts to reduce the myeloma cell mass with cycle-active agents during the plateau phase have been largely unsuccessful, but a minor change was observed in one patient treated with vincristine (12).

Unusually long remissions observed after minimal treatment also argue against a dose-response effect in PCM. A remission that has lasted for more than nine years following 225 rad of total body irradiation has been observed (1). This dose of irradiation is estimated to be capable of reducing the tumor cell mass by about 1 log, based on the radiation sensitivity of myeloma cells. A 1 log tumor cell reduction would have resulted in a remission of about three years in this patient; the remission has far exceeded that which was predicted by the tumor cell kill that would have been expected for this dose of irradiation. Similarly, at least one long remission of more than six years has been reported after a single course of melphalan administered to a kappa light chain disease patient (22). In addition, I have observed unmaintained remissions of five years in a patient with IgG kappa myeloma, and a remission that persists for more than eight years after melphalan was discontinued in a patient producing only lambda light chains. It is difficult to explain these prolonged remissions on the basis of the tumor cell kill anticipated with melphalan.

Is There a Direct Relationship between Myeloma Cell Kill and Survival?

If the improved survival of myeloma patients who respond to treatment results from the effect of that treatment on myeloma cells, one would expect to find a correlation between the estimated cell kill and survival. We estimated the myeloma cell kill after 12 courses of treatment and found that the cell kill varied from $10^{-0.3}$ to $10^{-6.4}$, with survivals ranging from 3 months to more than 10 years. We found no correlation between cell kill and survival (1).

Does Maintenance Therapy Prolong Remission Duration or Survival?

The Southwest Oncology Group (SWOG) have examined this question and found that maintenance therapy does not prolong the duration of a remission or improve survival (5). This observation provides additional evidence that these myeloma-response parameters are not determined by the tumor cell kill achieved by treatment.

Do Surviving Myeloma Cells Begin to Grow When Treatment Is Stopped?

The status of myeloma patients during treatment-induced remissions resembles that status of patients with benign monoclonal gammopathy (BMG). The M-protein level falls progressively during remission induction to reach a plateau and then remains stable throughout the remission. The duration of this stable phase is not prolonged by maintenance therapy. As mentioned above, some of these remissions persist for unusually long periods. The M-protein persists throughout the remission, although unusually sensitive techniques such as an anti-idiotype antiserum may be required to demonstrate the M-protein. Furthermore, myeloma stem cells capable of forming colonies of plasma cells have been demonstrated in 12 of 24 remission marrows and in two of three patients with BMG (14). This evidence demonstrates that a plasma cell monoclone persists during myeloma remissions and in BMG but appears to be controlled and stable.

Thus, in both BMG and myeloma remissions there are large monoclonal populations of plasma cells ($>10^{10}$ cells) that remain stable for prolonged periods. Myeloma stem cells capable of forming colonies of plasma cells are present in both BMG and remission marrows. A recurrence of progressive, uncontrolled growth of myeloma cells ends the remission in most myeloma patients. In contrast, progression from the stable monoclone occurs in only about 20% of patients with BMG (23).

Progressive Increase in Growth Rate During Successive Relapses

The myeloma growth rate as reflected by the M-protein doubling time has been measured repeatedly on myeloma patients in unmaintained remissions. A progressive shortening in the M-protein doubling time was observed (1). Most of the patients who progressed to an M-protein doubling time of less than 30 days also developed marrow failure (24). This marrow failure apparently did not result from treatment, because the marrow remained cellular, and the pancytopenia persisted after all therapy was stopped. In a large study, 31% of myeloma patients progressed to develop marrow failure and died during the acute terminal phase of the disease (7). The M-protein doubling time during relapse correlates strongly with subsequent survival; short M-protein doubling times predict brief survival (1). The survival of myeloma patients appears to be determined largely by the time required for a progressive increase in the myeloma growth rate and the development of marrow failure to occur. For the reasons stated above, I do not think that cytotoxic therapy directed at myeloma cells during the chronic phase of the disease prolongs survival unless this treatment affects the growth control mechanisms operative in PCM and delays or prevents progression to the acute terminal phase.

COMBINATION CHEMOTHERAPY FOR PCM

In this evaluation of the effectiveness of treatment for PCM, survival from the start of treatment is used as the basis for comparison. The myeloma cell kill does not correlate with survival. For this reason response rates are of little use in judging the effectiveness of treatment.

It is important to recognize that many features of PCM influence survival. Thus, factors such as the initial hemoglobin level, serum calcium, the M-protein synthesis rate, and the extent of skeletal disease correlate with the total body myeloma cell number and have a strong influence on prognosis (25). Renal function is another important prognostic factor, which is unrelated to myeloma cell mass (25). Since death can result from complications such as infections, renal failure, and hyperviscosity, the ready availability of effective treatment such as antibiotics and leukocyte transfusions for infections, and plasmapheresis for acute renal failure and hyperviscosity, may also have an important influence on survival. When we compare the survival of groups of patients treated with different treatments, we must make sure that the treatment groups are comparable, in terms of prognostic factors, and that they have the same access to treatment for acute, life-threatening complications. The use of the log rank test (26) to control for known prognostic factors in the analysis of survival is helpful (7). The best way to ensure comparable access to emergency treatment is to specify the treatment to be used for common problems in the protocol.

The addition of prednisone to intermittent courses of melphalan doubled the response rate but had little influence on survival (27). The improved response rate could result from effects of prednisone that are not directed at myeloma cells. For example, a prednisone-stimulated increase in the catabolic rate of the M-protein (28) or a decrease in bone resorption as a result of prednisone's blocking the effects of the osteoclast-activating factor (29) could increase the response rate without changing the myeloma cell mass. Even though prednisone may not have a strong antineoplastic action against myeloma cells, its nonspecific effects are so useful that it is now included in most therapeutic drug trials for plasma cell myeloma.

Combining procarbazine with melphalan and prednisone appeared to increase the response rate but, again, had little effect on survival (27). Further experience suggests that procarbazine contributes little to the management of myeloma, and it has been dropped from subsequent SWOG myeloma trials.

The addition of adriamycin to melphalan and prednisone or cyclophosphamide and prednisone did not improve the response rate or survival (6).

The discovery that mouse (30) and human (31) plasma cell tumors that are resistant to one alkylating agent still respond to another drug of this class indicated that different alkylating agents are not necessarily cross resistant. Furthermore, combinations of alkylating agents were shown to be synergistic in the treatment of two murine tumors (32,33). These observations stimulated clinical trials of combinations of alkylating agents in the treatment of plasma cell myeloma. The SWOG found that combinations containing melphalan and cyclophosphamide or those drugs and carmustine did not significantly change the response rate or survival (6). Similarly the National Cancer Institute of Canada (NCI-C) Clinical Trials Group found no advantage for the melphalan-cyclophosphamide-carmustine-prednisone combination, administered either alternately or concurrently, over melphalan and prednisone alone (7). In contrast, the Cancer and Acute Leukemia Group (CALGB) found that the four-drug combination significantly improved the response rate in several parameters over that obtained with melphalan and prednisone but did not improve the survival of patients (34). The CALGB study of the four-drug combination differs from those of the SWOG and NCI-C in that all the alkylating agents in the combination were administered intravenously; the results were compared with the oral administration of melphalan in the two-drug group. Since the absorption of melphalan may be erratic (35,36), the improved response rate could be the result of the intravenous administration of melphalan in the four-drug group. A recent study from Argentina has shown that a combination of methyl (CCNU), cyclophosphamide, and prednisone was no more effective than melphalan and prednisone in the treatment of PCM (18).

Studies of the labeling index of myeloma marrow plasma cells before and after treatment demonstrated a marked rise in the index after treatment with alkylating agents (10–12). This observation led to a trial of cycle-specific agents in the treatment of myeloma. In a preliminary trial, vincristine caused a modest further decrease in myeloma cell number (12) and was selected for further study in drug combinations. The SWOG was encouraged by the modest improvement in the response rate and survival of patients treated with combinations containing vincristine (5,6). The M2 protocol for myeloma patients, used at Memorial Hospital in New York, combines vincristine, melphalan, cyclophosphamide, carmustine, and prednisone; this combination reportedly produces a higher response rate and longer survival than melphalan and prednisone (37). Unfortunately, no conclusions can be reached about the relative merits of the M2 protocol, because this study was uncontrolled. Additional factors make this study difficult to interpret. Asymptomatic myeloma patients are followed without treatment until there is clear evidence of progressive disease at Memorial Hospital. Patients called "asymptomatic," "stable," or "indolent" may not require treatment for intervals varying from a few months to eight years. In the M2 study, survival was measured from diagnosis, rather than from the onset of treatment. Since the size of the asymptomatic cohort of patients treated with the M2 protocol and the "control" group treated with melphalan and prednisone is not stated, it is not possible to compare these two forms of treatment.

A recent SWOG study allocates patients at random to one of three arms: (1) vincristine, melphalan, cyclophosphamide, and prednisone alternating with vincristine, adriamycin, cyclophosphamide, and prednisone; (2) vincristine, melphalan, cyclophosphamide, and prednisone for three cycles alternating with vincristine, carmustine, adriamycin, and prednisone for three cycles; and (3) melphalan and prednisone (38). The doses of these drugs were adjusted so that they could be repeated at three-week intervals. At two years the response rates on the three arms were similar. The survival at two years for all patients receiving arm 1 or arm 2 is superior to melphalan and prednisone. These combinations may be better than prednisone alone; however, longer follow-up and careful analysis, controlling for important prognostic factors, must be done before we conclude that these combinations are in fact better. It has been suggested that combination therapy may provide more uniform drug delivery than oral melphalan, which is known to have variable absorption that may reduce its toxicity and response. It should also be recognized that these drug combinations are given at three-week intervals rather than the usual four- to six-week intervals for melphalan and prednisone.

In conclusion, I am not convinced that the drug combinations mentioned in this review are more effective than melphalan and prednisone alone in the treatment of PCM. To have a major influence on the survival of PCM patients, we need to find ways for preventing or delaying the onset of the acute terminal phase.

REFERENCES

1. Bergsagel DE: Assessment of the response of mouse and human myeloma to chemotherapy and radiotherapy, in Drewinko B, and Humphrey R (eds): *Growth Kinetics and Biochemical Regulation of Normal and Malignant Cells.* Baltimore, Williams & Wilkins Co., 1977, pp 705–717.

2. Bergsagel DE: The chronic leukemias: A review of disease manifestations and the aims of therapy. *Can Med Assoc J* 96:1615, 1967.

3. Osgood EE: The survival of plasmacytic myeloma. *Cancer Chemother Rep* 9:1, 1960.

4. Holland JF, Hosely H, Scharlan C, et al: A controlled trial of urethane treatment in myeloma. *Blood* 27:328, 1966.

5. Southwest Oncology Group: Remission maintenance therapy for multiple myeloma. *Arch Intern Med* 135:147, 1975.

6. Alexanian R, Salmon S, Bonnet J, et al: Combination chemotherapy for multiple myeloma. *Cancer* 40:2765, 1977.

7. Bergsagel DE, Bailey AJ, Langley GR, et al: The chemotherapy of plasma cell myeloma and the incidence of acute leukemia. *N Engl J Med* 301:743, 1979.

8. Cavagnaro F, Lein JM, Pavlovsky S, et al: Comparison of two combination chemotherapies for multiple myeloma with MeCCNU, cyclophosphamide and prednisone versus melphalan, prednisone. *Cancer Treat Rep,* 64:73, 1980.

9. Salmon S, Durie BGM: Application of kinetics to chemotherapy for multiple myeloma, in Drewinko B, and Humphrey R (eds): *Growth Kinetics and Biochemical Regulation of Normal and Malignant Cells.* Baltimore, Williams & Wilkins Co, 1977, pp 865–878.

10. Alberts DS, Golde DW: Perturbation of DNA synthesis in multiple myeloma cells following cell-cycle-nonspecific chemotherapy. *Cancer Res* 34:2911, 1974.

11. Drewinko B, Brown BW, Humphrey R, et al: Effect of chemotherapy on the labeling index of myeloma cells. *Cancer* 34:526, 1974.

12. Salmon SE: Expansion of the growth fraction in multiple myeloma with alkylating agents. *Blood* 45:119, 1975.

13. Park CH, Bergsagel DE, McCulloch EA: Mouse myeloma tumor stem cells: A primary cell culture assay. *J Natl Cancer Inst* 46:411, 1971.

14. Hamburger A, Salmon SE: Primary bioassay of human myeloma stem cells. *J Clin Invest* 50:846, 1977.

15. Nathaus D, Fahey JL, Potter M: The formation of myeloma protein by a mouse plasma cell tumor. *J Exp Med* 108:121, 1958.

16. Hiramoto RN, Ghanta VK, Hamlin NM: Quantitation of total body tumor cells (MOPC 104E). II. Ascites tumor model. *J Natl Cancer Inst* 53:767, 1974.

17. Harrison JF, Blainey JD, Hardwicke J, et al: Proteinurea in multiple myeloma. *Clin Sci* 31:95, 1966.

18. DeFronzo RA, Cooke CR, Wright JR, et al: Renal function in patients with multiple myeloma. *Medicine* 57:151, 1978.

19. Salmon SE, Smith BA: Immunoglobulin synthesis and total body tumor cell number in IgG multiple myeloma. *J Clin Invest* 49:1114, 1970.

20. Sullivan PW, Salmon SE: Kinetics of tumor growth and regression in IgG multiple myeloma. *J Clin Invest* 51:1697, 1972.

21. Alexanian R, Hakanson JA, Drewinko B: Tumor kinetics in multiple myeloma, in Drewinko B, and Humphrey R (eds); *Growth Kinetics and Biochemical Regulation of Normal and Malignant Cells.* Baltimore, Williams & Wilkins Co, 1977, pp 629–641.

22. Von Schéele C: Light chain myeloma with features of adult Fanconi syndrome: Six years remission with one course of melphalan. *Acta Med Scand* 199:533, 1976.

23. Kyle RA: Monoclonal gammopathy of undetermined significance. *Am J Med* 64:814, 1978.

24. Bergsagel DE, Pruzanski W: Treatment of plasma cell myeloma with cytoxic agents. *Arch Intern Med* 135:172, 1975.

25. Durie BGM, Salmon SE: A clinical staging system for multiple myeloma: Correlation of measured myeloma cell mass with presenting clinical features, response to treatment and survival. *Cancer* 36:842, 1975.

26. Peto R, Pike MC, Armitage P, et al: Design and analysis of randomized clinical trials requiring prolonged observations of each patient. II. Analysis and examples. *Br J Cancer* 35:1, 1977.

27. Alexanian R, Bonnet J, Gehan E, et al: Combination chemotherapy for multiple myeloma. *Cancer* 30:382, 1972.

28. Bergsagel DE: Plasma cell myeloma: An interpretive review. *Cancer* 30:1588, 1972.

29. Raisz LG, Luben RA, Mandy GR, et al. Effect of osteoclast activating factor from human leukocytes on bone metabolism. *J Clin Invest* 56:408, 1975.

30. Bergsagel DE, Ogawa M, Librach SL: Mouse myeloma: A model for studies of cell kinetics. *Arch Intern Med* 135:109, 1975.

31. Bergsagel DE, Cowan DH, Hasselback R: Plasma cell myeloma: Response of melphalan-resistant patients to high-dose, intermittent cyclophosphamide. *Can Med Assoc J* 107:851, 1972.

32. Valeriote F, Bruce WR, Meeker BE: Synergistic action of cyclophosphamide and 1,3 bis (2-chloroethyl)-1-nitrosourea on a transplanted murine lymphoma. *J Natl Cancer Inst* 40:935, 1968.

33. Lin H, Bruce WR: Chemotherapy of the transplanted KHT fibrosarcoma in mice. *Ser Haematol* 5:89, 1972.

34. Harley JB, Pajak TF, McIntyre OR, et al: Improved survival of increased risk myeloma patients on combined triple-alkylating-agent therapy: A study of the CALGB. *Blood* 54:13, 1979.

35. Tattersall MHN, Jarman M, Newlands ES, et al: Pharmacokinetics of melphalan following oral or intravenous administration in patients with malignant disease. *Eur J Cancer* 14:507, 1978.

36. Alberts DS, Chang SV, Chen H-S, et al: Variability of melphalan absorption in man. *Proc AACR-ASCO* 19:334, 1978 (abstract).

37. Case DC Jr, Lee BG III, Clarkson BD: Improved survival times in multiple myeloma treated with melphalan, prednisone, cyclophosphamide, vincristine and BCNU: M-2 protocol. *Am J Med* 63:897, 1977.

38. Salmon SE, Alexanian R, Dixon D: Non-cross resistant combination chemotherapy improves survival in multiple myeloma. *Blood* 54 (suppl 1):207a, 1979.

7

Androgen Therapy of Hematologic Malignancies

Daniel Hollard

Monique Laurent

Jean Jacques Sotto

On the basis of clinical and experimental findings supporting the stimulating action of androgens on hemopoiesis, stanozolol was used in the treatment of AML patients in complete remission. This treatment, begun in 1973, led to the recognition of stanozolol as a possible factor in improving considerably the mean survival time of AML patients (1). This study was resumed recently (2) and has shown an unusually high number of long-surviving patients in the first group. These results, however, are disputed by some authors, especially because of the absence of a control population. Other authors, using a different treatment regimen did not find stanozolol to have a significant effect. Since the first experimental (3) and clinical (4) findings were observed, numerous studies have been conducted on the action of androgens in normal and pathological hemopoiesis. This action was first demonstrated in erythropoiesis by Nathan and Gardner (5) and initially related to an increase in the secretion of erythropoietin and later to an increase in those cells sensitive to erythropoeitin (6). The stimulating effect of androgens on granulopoiesis in vivo and in vitro was later demonstrated. It was shown experimentally by Udupa (7) that testosterone and other androstane derivatives were effective in accelerating granulopoietic recovery after different chemotherapies. On the basis of these findings androgens were used to accelerate normal hemopoiesis either during antitumoral chemotherapy (8) or in primary or secondary marrow deficiencies of various hemopathic disorders. Despite the large number of clinical and experimental obser-

This work was supported by INSERM (A.T.P. no. 79/114) and has been performed with the support of Fundamental Research Department (CEN Grenoble) (Convention Recherche CHR/CENG no. GR-759-719).

vations, the therapeutic significance of androgens remains controversial, particularly with regard to marrow aplasias (9–11). However, all experimental results obtained appear to indicate that testosterone, as well as other androstane derivatives, act on the pluripotential stem cell, investigated using the spleen colony method in mice by Byron. Given the increase in the thymidine suicide index and the sensitivity to hydroxyurea, it would seem that this action stimulates the cells to enter into the cell cycle (12). This process may be more complex, involving the stimulation of the monocytes-macrophages to secrete CSA (13,14) and also the stimulation of the GM-CFUc studied in vitro culture system (15). The mechanism involved appears somewhat different for erythropoiesis from that for granulopoiesis. In the latter case the stimulation was independent of the presence of a receptor for androgen on the stem cells (16).

Following our first clinical results, these differing clinical and experimental observations were taken into consideration. In another study being conducted in parallel, stanozolol was used in various therapeutic regimes to induce and maintain remission. These current results favor the initial theory that in the treatment of acute leukemias androgen therapy is of definite value. The stimulation of hemopoiesis by androgens, in particular by stanozolol, whatever the mode of action involved, would appear important as a therapeutic addition. However, it appears that the drugs used in obtaining induction and maintenance, particularly cytosine-arabinoside, may reverse the effects of androgens. Thus, it is probable that a group of patients can be distinguished from among the various types of acute myeloid leukemias who are potentially long- or very long-term survivors under androgen therapy.

PRESENT RESULTS OF CLINICAL STUDY

These introductory comments are developed in this chapter. Since 1975 these observations have been based on the results of three successive therapeutic tests of which the most significant results are reported here, that is, continued surveillance of those patients having received the first maintenance treatment; the failure of the multicentric test, using ARA-C together with a high dose of stanozolol to induce remission; the induction treatment test involving a high dose of stanozolol and cell-cycle-dependent drugs.

CURRENT STATE OF THE FIRST TEST

Compared with the study presented recently (2), the regular surveillance of the surviving patients contributed no further information (Fig. 1). Among the 22 patients having received the stanozolol maintenance treatment, 11 had a survival time of greater than 4 years, the mean survival time remaining the same at 45 months. Among these 11 patients, 6 remained in complete remission for 6 years, and 3 have survived 10 years and are no longer under treatment.

The most important criteria used as guidelines in these tests are as follows: The treatment used to induce complete remission involved only rubidomycine

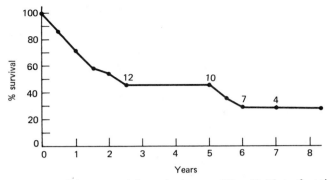

Figure 1. Present status of the actuarial survival curve (Test I). Note that time is in years.

and vincristine; the treatment used to reinduce remission involved the same drugs and was administered at four-month intervals. It has been shown previously that the AML treated in this manner shows no distinguishing characteristics. In all cases, a large number of blasts are present in the marrow and the peripheral blood. The percentage of complete remissions was 52%; however, in 80% of the cases an aplastic marrow was obtained, with the disappearance of blasts in the blood and marrow. During this period, these patients had only simple semisterile protection. However, neither leukoplatelet transfusions nor hyperalimentation was carried out (17). A significant number of patients died in the postchemotherapy stage.

The principal characteristics of this study were the small proportion of relapses during the first year of surveillance, the absence of a plateau in the survival curve, and the duration of complete remission. It was possible to propose that a maintenance chemotherapy, together with a low dose of stanozolol, administered over several years, slowed the emergence of the leukemic clone, thus explaining the appearance of the curve.

Several hypotheses might explain this unexpected result. The first of these hypotheses involved the stimulation of leukemic cells, making them more sensitive to drugs usually having little effect on AML, for example, methotrexate and vincristine. Another hypothesis involved the stimulation of normal residual clones capable of inhibiting the growth of leukemic clones. The last hypothesis involved a modification in the environment of the stem cells by the delayed effect of an androgen steroid.

A characteristic enabling the identification of patients having a survival, in remission, of greater than four years has been sought. Besides the fact that they are contained within the M-1 category of FAB classification (18), no identifying characteristic can be related to sex, age, or hematological data of blood and marrow.

However, in the absence of a control population, the true effect of stanozolol remains hypothetical. The comparison of these results with those of a similar system (19) have allowed the assessment of the true value of stanozolol. From the following tests it is proposed that the composition of the induction and reinduction chemotherapy must be given equal consideration.

SECOND TEST: STANOZOLOL IN INDUCTION PHASE

Experimental studies have led to the conclusion that testosterone and most of its derivatives act rapidly on the stem cell (20) at high doses both in vivo and in vitro (5). On this basis androgens were used for treatment of aplasias generally at doses superior to 1 mg/(kg)(day). In the initial study the role of stanozolol in effecting an improvement in the number of complete remissions must be excluded, as the improvement was low when compared with the results obtained using chemotherapies consisting of cytosine-arabinoside.

For this reason a multicentric test control was included (21) that consisted of giving 1 mg/kg of stanozolol at the beginning of treatment. This test was also used to determine the efficiency of rubidomycine and rubidazone.

The overall result of the induction treatment was unfavorable, having a level of complete remission of less than 52%. The percentage of complete remissions found in the two groups of patients receiving stanozolol was no different from that of patients not treated with stanozolol (Table 1). In a number of cases severe hepatic complications with jaundice arose, leading to the interruption of stanozolol treatment.

The study of survival of the patients showed that the administering of stanozolol during maintenance treatment (Fig. 2) gave unfavorable results with a significant decrease in the mean survival time. Although the time of surveillance was short, it was decided to abandon this protocol. The possible explanation of this failure is discussed later (see "Discussion").

THIRD TEST: STANOZOLOL AND HYDROXYUREA IN INDUCTION PHASE

Byron has shown (12) that testosterone and its derivatives have the effect of strengthening the initiation of cell cycle in stem cells in Go phase brought about with androstane. This initiation of the cell cycle brings about a large increase in the 3H Thymidine suicide level and makes the stem cells sensitive to the action

Table 1. Results of Test II[a].

	Random			
Result	With Stanozolol		Without Stanozolol	
CR	23	(57%)	22	(62%)
Failure	5		1	
PR	4		2	
Death in induction	9		10	
Total	41		35	

With permission from Cl. Jacquillat, Paris, St. Louis.

[a]Stanozolol at High Dosage has been Associated, by Randomization, with Chemotherapy/ARA-C DNR (76 patients).

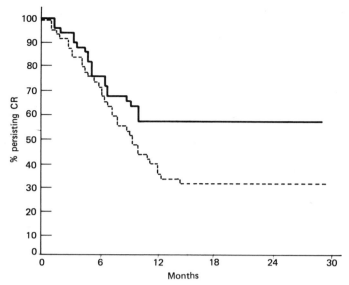

Figure 2. Actuarial curve of the duration of the first complete remission.●——● without stanozolol (85 patients); ●---● with stanozolol (65 patients). Test II (stanozolol and ARA-C).

of hydroxyurea. In one patient not responding to multiple chemotherapies, including cytosine-arabinoside, and treated with a high dose of stanozolol, it was possible to obtain a rapid and extensive decrease in circulating blasts using hydroxyurea. A protocol of stanozolol treatment—1 mg/kg daily—together with chemotherapy using rubidomycine, vincristine, and hydroxyurea (1,500 mg/m²) has been developed.

Eighteen patients were treated in a preliminary test, in the absence of a control, resulting in 62% complete remission (July 1977 to July 1978). These results led to a random study of 21 patients (July 1978 to September 1979). The results of the latter study appear to confirm the positive effect of stanozolol on the efficiency of cycle-dependent chemotherapy (Table 2). The harmful effect of hydroxyurea in the absence of androgen treatment led to the dropping of this test. From the 9 patients not treated with stanozolol at induction, 5 did not respond to chemotherapy and had a persistently dense blast infiltration in the marrow. Among those patients only one obtained complete remission under multiple chemotherapy consisting of cytosine-arabinoside.

The study of remission duration, and survival of these patients (Figs. 3 and 4) was rather short, but a negative conclusion may be made. The type of curve obtained for the first test was not found, and the mean survival time remained identical to that found by other authors, that is, approximately 12 months. It is of particular interest that:

1. A large number of patients who died were in complete remission during the first six months of surveillance. Three of these patients were in complete

Table 2. Results of Test III[a].

| | Age | | | | |
Result	< 15	15–30	31–50	51–70	Total
CR	3	3	10	2	18
Failure	0	0	2	4	6
PR	0	0	1	4	5
Total	3	3	13	10	29

Controlled Test	CR	PR	Failure	Total
With stanozolol	8	1	2	11
Without stanozolol	2	0	7	9

[a]All Patients with Stanozolol (Pilot Study and Randomized Study). CR was 62%. Results of the Controlled Trial by Randomization. (20 Patients; Total Rate of CR = 50%.)

remission but died of infection (epidemic contamination by Serratia marcescens).

2. Complete remission was obtained in six patients, with relapse at the sixth to twelfth month, using a multiple chemotherapy consisting of cytosine-arabinoside, thioguanine, and rubidomycine. In two cases the evolution persisted for more than six months, until death.

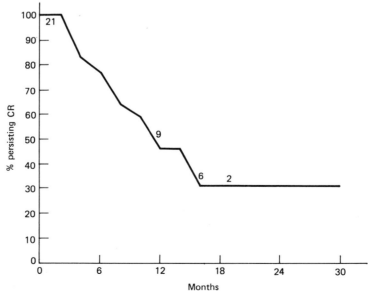

Figure 3. Test III (stanozolol + HU). Duration of the first CR.

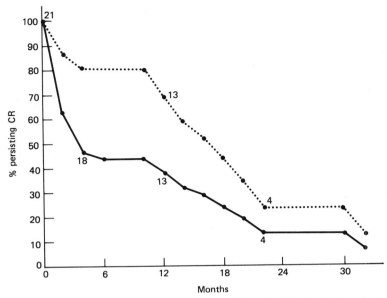

Figure 4. Test III. Actuarial survival curve. ●---● patients in CR; ●——● all patients. Median survival was 16 months for patients who achieved a CR (five months for all patients).

DISCUSSION

The analysis of the results of these three therapeutic tests lead us to two conclusions. Among the patients initially treated with a combination of rubidomycine-vincristine, 22 obtained complete remission. Among these 22 patients there appeared a large percentage with very long survival in complete stable remission, living more than five years after the beginning of complete remission. These patients may be regarded as cured. On the other hand, in the two other tests, where stanozolol was used in a high dose in association with either cytosine-arabinoside or hydroxyurea, the result was negative, and there was little possiblity of finding the same percentage of long survivors. These results, in appearance contradictory, allow further discussion of several points.

The Failure of the Combination Cytosine-Arabinoside and Stanozolol (High Dose) Treatment

The control test (test II) has confirmed that stanozolol is not effective in the induction phase (Table 1) and has a detrimental effect on survival (Fig. 2).

The problem was its toxic nature, particularly hepatic. As a result, in several cases it was necessary to stop treatment, and this toxicity has been implicated in deaths at induction. Slavin et al. (22) have shown the importance of changes, observed in the intestinal mucous during the course of chemotherapeutic induction of AML; they particularly emphasized the role of cytosine-arabinoside and showed the importance of infections lesions and the development of metastatic abscesses in the liver. Although no systematic study was carried out, it is possible to imagine that the addition of an androgenic steroid in the induction phase would increase this toxicity. In any case, the lack of favorable results obtained using stanozolol in the induction phase has led to the rapid rejection of this type of therapy.

The negative effect of stanozolol on the survival period of patients in complete remission poses a very different problem. The comparison of the two curves seems to show an adverse effect which impairs complete remission duration, and survival. No toxic factors were apparent. The significant increase in the number of relapses, compared with control subjects, deserves discussion. It has been proved that cytosine-arabinoside acts by increasing the growth of leukemic cells. Vogler (23) and Lampkin (24) have emphasized that this mechanism is a very important factor in the response of leukemic cells to this drug. Our hypothesis involves a negative cumulative effect of both stanozolol and cytosine-arabinoside. It may be supposed that both the drugs have a cytolytic effect on the normal stem cells necessary to maintain and prolong complete remission.

The Effects of Stanozolol Used in Combination with Hydroxyurea

The results obtained confirm the positive effects of the combination of rubi-domycine-vincristine-hydroxyurea-stanozolol in inducing complete remission. However, the effect is negative on the prolonging of complete remission and survival.

In the absence of stanozolol the combination of hydroxyurea with rubido-mycine and vincristine gave very unfavorable results with only two complete remissions for nine patients. On the other hand, the introduction of hydroxyurea treatment in patients having received stanozolol gave a number of complete remissions greater than 62%.

The analysis of these results, despite the low number of patients, indicates that stanozolol acts in the same way on leukemic cells as on normal stem cells, as shown by Byron (12). It was not possible to show by labeling index measurements a modification in the proliferation of the leukemic cell pool 48 hours after administering stanozolol and before the beginning cytoreducing chemotherapy.

The study of the survival curves and the duration of complete remission leads to the discussion of two further problems. The appearance of the curve during the first year of surveillance is identical to that found by many other authors. The hypothesis, for our first test, of retarded growth of the leukemic clone does not appear valid here. At the beginning of the test hydroxyurea was used in the reinduction therapy. Four patients fell quickly into relapse, and three others obtained a second complete remission longer than the first, after ceasing hydroxyurea treatment. The other problem was the percentage of long survival desired, that is, 30% of the patients in complete remission. Despite the short observation time, it would seem that this desired percentage was not obtained.

The discussion of these results leads us to three conclusions, each having various consequences:

1. The increase in the percentage of complete remission, if a result of the improvement of the efficiency of the chemotherapy, is not accompanied by an increase in the duration of complete remission or the survival of the patients. To test the effect of cytosine-arabinoside on this phenomenon, it

was decided to study the duration of complete remission and survival time as a function of the chemotherapy used in the induction phase. The first group of patients was treated in the same manner as in test I, that is, in the absence of cytosine-arabinoside. It was hoped that by bettering the supportive care, an increase in the number of complete remissions would be obtained. This test, started in November 1979, seems to confirm this. The second group received a combination of rubidomycine-thioguanine-cytosine-arabinoside, analogous with that used by some others. The maintenance treatment used for all patients was the combination of stanozolol (in low dose), 6-MP, and methotrexate. The reinduction therapy for each group consisted of the same drugs used in induction.

2. The heterogeneity of the acute myeloid leukemias is well known and recognizable by cytological methods. A study was begun to confirm the existence of an androgenic steroid receptor on the leukemic cells and to relate this to the response of these cells to testosterone in culture. The existence of steroid receptors on leukemic cells has been shown and confirmed in approximately 50% of the cases (25). It has also been shown that the behavior of leukemic cells in culture in vivo using the diffusion chamber technique (26) is not homogenous, and in one group an apparent effect of stanozolol introduced into the mouse is shown (unpublished data). Our hypothesis is that certain AML may respond readily to an androgenic steroid stimulus, and others not at all.

3. The most significant apparent result from the first experiment is in the long run a group of long-surviving patients. This result was obtained by the prolonged administering of a particular steroid, stanozolol, in low dose. The hypothesis for a specific effect of this steroid on the microenvironment of the stem cells is certainly a basis for further research.

REFERENCES

1. Sotto JJ, Hollard D, Schaerer R, et al: Androgènes et rémissions prolongées dans les leucémies aiguës non lymphoblastiques. *N Rev Fr Hemat* 15:57, 1975.

2. Hollard D, Sotto JJ, Berthier R, et al: High rate of long term survival in AML treated by chemotherapy and androgenotherapy. *Cancer* 45:1540, 1980.

3. Kennedy BJ, Gilbertsen: Increased erythropoiesis induced by androgenic hormonotherapy. *New Engl J Med* 256:720, 1957.

4. Gardner FH, Pringle JC: Androgens and erythropoiesis. Preliminary clinical observations. *Arch Int Med* 107:112, 1961.

5. Nathan DC, Gardner FH: Effects of large doses of androgens on rodent erythropoiesis and body composition. *Blood* 26:411, 1965.

6. Singer JW, Adamson J: Steroids and hematopoiesis. III. The response of granulocytes and erythroid colony forming cells to steroids of different classes. *Blood* 48:855, 1976.

7. Udupa KB, Reissmann KR: Acceleration of granulopoietic recovery by androgenic steroids in mice made neutropenic by cytotoxic drugs. *Cancer Res* 34:2517, 1974.

8. Brodsky I, Dennis LH, Kahn SB: Testosterone enanthate as a bone marrow stimulant during cancer chemotherapy. Preliminary reports. *Cancer Chem Rep* 34:59, 1964.

9. Camitta BM, Thomas ED, Nathan DG, et al: A prospective study of androgens and bone marrow transplantation for treatment of severe aplastic anemia. *Blood* 53:504, 1979.

10. Gluckman E, Devergie A: Treatment of severe aplastic anemia with antilymphocyte globulin and androgens. *Exp Haemat* 6:679, 1978.

11. Najean Y, Pecking A: Groupe commun d'étude des aplasies médullaires. *Nouv Presse Med* 6:3083, 1977.

12. Byron JW: Comparison of the action of 3H thymidine and hydroxyurea on testosterone treated hemopoietic stem cells. *Blood* 40:198, 1972.

13. Broxmeyer HE, Ralph P: In vitro regulation of a mouse myelomonocytic leukemia line adapted to culture. *Cancer Res* 37:3578, 1977.

14. Francis CE, Berney JE, Bateman SM, et al: The effect of androstanes on granulopoiesis in vitro and in vivo. *Brit J Haemat* 36:501, 1977.

15. Rosenblum AL, Carbone PP: Androgenic hormones and human granulopoiesis in vitro. *Blood* 43:351, 1974.

16. Byron JW: Analysis of receptor mechanism involved in the haemopoietic. Effects of androgens: Use of Tfm mutants. *Exp Haemat* 5:429, 1977.

17. Michallet M, Hollard D, Guignier M, et al: Parenteral nutrition in patients with leukemia and non-Hodgkin malignant lymphoma under chemotherapy. *J Parent Enter Nutr* 3:247, 1979.

18. Bennett JM, Catovsky D, Daniel TT, et al: Proposals for the classification of the acute leukemias. *Brit J Haemat* 33:451, 1976.

19. Pavlovsky S, Peñalver J, Eppinger-Helft M, et al: Induction and maintenance of remission in acute leukemia. *Cancer* 31:273, 1973.

20. Gorshein D, Hait WN, Besa EC, et al: Rapid stem cell differentiation induced by 19-nortestosterone decanoate. *Brit J Haemat* 26:215, 1974.

21. Jacquillat C: Groupe d'étude "chimiothérapie." Société française d'Hématologie (unpublished data).

22. Slavin RE, Marco AD, Saral R: Cytosine arabinoside induced gastrointestinal toxic alterations in sequential chemotherapeutic protocols. *Cancer* 42:1747, 1972.

23. Vogler WR, Cooper LE, Groth DP: Correlation of cytosine arabinoside. Induced increment in growth fraction of leukemic blast cells with clinical response. *Cancer* 33:603, 1974.

24. Lampkin BC, Nagao T, Mauer AM: Drug effect in acute leukemia. *J Clin Invest* 48:1124.

25. Marcille G, Hollard D: Androgenic steroid receptors in some AML cells (manuscript in preparation).

26. Laurent M, Clemancey-Marcille G, Hollard D: The evolution of normal and leukemic (AML and AMML) human haematopoietic cells in diffusion chamber. *Scand J Haemat*, 1980 (in press).

8

Are Androgens Useful in the Management of Hematologic Malignancies?

Santiago Pavlovsky

Androgens such as testosterone, testosterone propionate, testosterone enanthate, methyltestosterone, fluoxymesterone, oxymetholone calusterone, D1-testolactone, dromostanolone propionate, and stanozolol have been widely used in different programs to stimulate erythropoiesis in myeloid metaplasia, chronic leukemia, and multiple myeloma; to improve hematopoietic tolerance to cytotoxic drugs; and to produce tumor response in certain cases of advanced cancer of the breast, prostate, and kidney (1). They are usually given in pharmacologic doses. Side effects include hypercalcemia, hyperuricemia, fluid retention, liver dysfunction, masculinization in the female, acneiform eruptions, prostatic hypertrophy, and increased libido (1).

Androgens may stimulate the stem-cell population in bone marrow to proliferate from the G_0 resting stage into other cycle stages more responsive to erythropoietin (1,2). It has been said that in cyclic neutropenia androgens cause an increase in granulocyte count and a concomitant decrease in the monocyte count (1). In addition, Horn et al. (3) in a study of 80 patients with breast carcinoma demonstrated that calusterone may cause marked thrombocytosis.

Several uncontrolled trials report that androgens combined with chemotherapy may improve therapeutic results in multiple myeloma (4–8), the non-Hodgkin's lymphomas, Hodgkin's disease (1,9), acute myelocytic leukemia (10–14), smoldering leukemia (15–18), chronic lymphocytic leukemia (9), hairy cell leukemia (19), and myelofibrosis with myeloid metaplasia (20–22) by stimulating marrow function and therefore allowing large chemotherapeutic doses, by stimulating the immune system, or by acting as an anticoagulant (23).

In most of these uncontrolled trials several other therapies were administered concurrently, including vitamin B_{12}, folic acid, red cell transfusion, high-dose pyridoxine, corticosteroids, splenic irradiation, or splenectomy. Thus the interpretation of the reported results is difficult.

In spite of the fact that androgen therapy has been widely used in most of the hematological malignancies mentioned above with the purpose of stimulating hematopoiesis as well as preserving hematopoiesis in patients treated with cytotoxic drugs, few well-designed randomized studies have been published (Table 1).

My purpose is to review all the data published concerning androgen therapy in hematologic malignancies, in an effort to draw some conclusions about their usefulness.

ACUTE MYELOBLASTIC LEUKEMIA

Hollard et al. (10,11,13) from the Centre Hospitalier Régional de Grenoble, France, have used stanozolol 0.15 mg/day in a nonrandomized study as an adjuvant to the treatment of acute nonlymphocytic leukemia. The androgen was

Table 1. Results of Controlled Clinical Trials of Androgen Therapy in Hematologic Malignancies

Disease	Therapy	Results	Ref
Myeloma	Melphalan vs. Melphalan-prednisone vs. Melphalan-prednisone testosterone	Androgens did not increase survival or improve any parameter of response except for a slight increase of hemoglobin	30
AML	Chemotherapy alone vs. chemotherapy plus androgens during maintenance	No difference in remission or survival between the groups	28
AML	Chemotherapy alone vs. chemotherapy plus androgens during induction and maintenance therapy	No difference in complete remission rate or duration of complete remission	27
Lymphoma	MOPP vs. MOPP plus androgens	The androgen group had more anemia, leukopenia, and thrombocytopenia, and drug doses needed to be reduced more often in the androgen group	32

administered from the beginning of induction therapy with vincristine, daunorubicin, and prednisone and throughout the maintenance period with 6-mer-
captopurine and methotrexate. Twenty-two (53%) of 40 patients achieved complete remission. The median duration of survival for the patients who achieved
complete remission was 48 months. These results compared with other series
published with similar induction and maintenance therapies without androgen
therapy show a great increase in the duration of complete remission and survival
(48 versus 5 to 12 months) (13,25,26).

Poirot et al. (13), from the same group, published a series of nine children
treated with stanozolol—(0.15 mg/kg daily orally)—plus the same combination
chemotherapy. Complete remission was achieved in seven patients. Duration of
complete remission was greater than 16 months in remitting patients, and the
median duration of survival was 37 months (range 10 months to 6 years) in
those patients. Neither study had a control group.

These encouraging results led to two randomized studies in which combination
chemotherapy alone for acute myelocytic leukemia was compared with the same
drug regimen plus stanozolol. The Institut de Recherches sur les Maladies du
Sang in cooperation with other hematologic centers in France treated 195 evaluation patients with combination chemotherapy that included cytosine arabinoside (Ara-C) with rubidazone and Ara-C with daunorubicin. Stanozolol 0.1
mg/kg daily orally begun on the first day of treatment was added to one arm of
each study. Patients who received stanozolol during induction continued receiving the androgen at the same dose during three years of maintenance therapy. The control group received the same maintenance therapy consisting of
sequential series every 28 days of Ara-C plus rubidazone or daunorubicin (27)
without the androgen.

A total of 112 (57%) of 195 evaluable cases achieved complete remission with
no difference observed between the induction schedules. The median duration
of complete remission was 12 months. Fifty-two patients in complete remission
received stanozolol compared with 60 patients who did not. No statistically significant difference in duration of complete remission was observed between the
groups.

Another randomized study was carried out by our cooperative group
(GATLA) (28). This study was initiated in March 1976 and the evaluation was
done in October 1979. Two hundred and forty-five previously untreated patients
with acute myelocytic leukemia entered the study and were randomized to receive
one of two induction combination therapies. Group A received daunorubicin 45
mg/M² weekly × 3, vincristine 1.5 mg/M² weekly × 3 with prednisone 40 mg/
M² daily for 21 days followed by 5 day courses of Ara-C 100 mg/M² daily in two
daily doses plus 6-mercaptopurine 100 mg/M² daily. Two or more courses were
given until complete remission was achieved. Group B received daunorubicin
45 mg/M² daily × 3 and Ara-C 100 mg/M² daily × 7 in two daily doses. If
complete remission was not achieved, courses of 2 days of daunorubicin and 5
days of Ara-C were added. All the patients who achieved complete remission
received the same combination chemotherapy consisting of sequential courses
every 28 days of Ara-C and 6-mercaptopurine for 5 days with one dose of CCNU
75 mg/M² po, followed by one course of daunorubicin-vincristine and 7 days of
prednisone. The doses were equal to the ones of the induction period. During

the first months of complete remission five doses of intrathecal methotrexate 10 mg/M² with dexamethasone 2 mg/M² were added. All patients who achieved complete remission were randomized to receive or not receive stanozolol 30 mg/M² every 10 days IM. The randomization occurred at the start of induction therapy.

A total of 245 patients were evaluable from the study. All patients who started induction therapy without major transgression of the protocol, including those who died in the first hours or days from the beginning of therapy, were considered evaluable.

Sixty-one (40%) of 151 patients in group A and 41 (43%) of 95 patients in group B achieved complete remission. No statistical difference was observed. Of the 102 patients who achieved complete remission, 63 had received stanozolol and 39 had not received it. The median duration of complete remission was 8 and 10 months, respectively, with 18% and 29%, respectively, remaining in complete remission at 30 months (Fig. 1). The difference in complete remission between androgen and nonandrogen therapy was not significant. The median duration of survival of patients who achieved complete remission in both groups was 15 months. These figures are similar to the ones obtained by our group in previous studies, including immunotherapy with C. parvum and continuous maintenance therapy (25,26,29) (Table 2).

MULTIPLE MYELOMA

Androgen therapy has been incorporated in several protocols for the treatment of multiple myeloma in an effort to increase the hemoglobin level in anemic patients and to strengthen the skeleton (4–8). However, few of these trials have been controlled.

Costa et al. (30) in a combined study of Acute Leukemia Group B and the

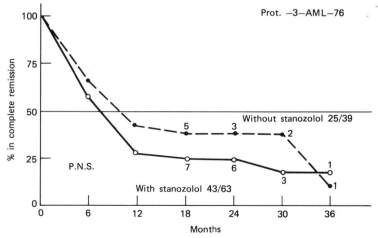

Figure 1. Duration of complete remission in AML with and without androgen therapy (GATLA study; see text for details).

Table 2. Duration of Complete Remission According to Different Maintenance Protocols in AML of Gatla

Years of Pt Accrual	Induction Therapy	Maintenance Therapy	Intensification Pulses	Total No. Pts Entered	No. CR	% CR	Median Duration CR (mo)	% in CR at 36 mo	Ref
1967–1970	DNM-VCR-PRED	6MP-MTX	DNM-VCR-PRED (every 6 mo)	86	30	35	5	3	26
1970–1973	DNM-VCR-PRED followed by Ara-C+6MP	6MP-MTX	DNM-VCR-PRED and Ara-C-6MP (sequentially every month)	143	64	45	6	13	25
1973–1976	DNM-VCR-PRED followed by Ara-C+6MP	C. parvum vs. nothing	Ara-C-6MP-CCNU and DNM-VCR-PRED (sequentially every month)	181	80	44	8 vs. 10	10 / 18	29
1976–1979	DNM-VCR-PRED + Ara-C+6MP vs. Ara-C-DNM	Stanozolol vs. nothing	Ara-C-6MP-CCNU and DNM-VCR-PRED (sequentially every month)	246	102	42	8 vs. 10	18 / 10	28

DNM = daunorubicin, VCR = vincristine, Pred = Prednisone, 6MP = 6-mercaptopurine, MTX = methotrexate, Ara-C = cytosine arabinoside, C parvum = Corynbacterium parvum immunotherapy.

Eastern Cooperative Oncology Group designed a protocol for previously untreated patients with multiple myeloma. Patients were stratified in groups of
good and poor risk and randomly allocated to one of three treatment programs.
A-melphalan, B-melphalan and prednisone, and C-melphalan, prednisone and
testosterone enanthate—10 mg/kg weekly. Good risk patients who received melphalan alone responded with a rise of hemoglobin value in 24% of cases. The
frequency of response was significantly higher following the addition of prednisone to melphalan therapy 67% ($P = .01$). Further addition of testosterone
increased the rate of response from 67% to 77%. Patients who received prednisone with or without testosterone responded faster with a rise in hemoglobin
in 4 and 5 weeks versus 19 weeks in patients treated with melphalan only.

In poor risk patients, the rise in hemoglobin was observed in 24% of the
melphalan group, 38% of the melphalan-prednisone group, and 30% in the
melphalan-prednisone-testosterone group; this difference was not statistically
significant.

The response rate of other parameters, such as marrow plasma cells or serum
paraprotein concentration, was significantly greater in good risk patients with
the addition of prednisone to melphalan, and the response rate was quicker.
Further addition of testosterone was not associated with increased frequency of
response. The benefit in poor risk patients was less.

No additional beneficial effect on azotemia, hypercalcemia, pain, or performance could be ascribed to prednisone or testosterone.

The median survival in good risk patients was 30 months for those treated
with melphalan alone, 53 months for those treated with melphalan-prednisone,
and 36 months for those who were treated with the addition of testosterone. In
poor risk patients the median survival was shortened with the addition of prednisone or testosterone and prednisone (21,9, and 4 months, respectively).

The authors concluded that in good risk patients the addition of testosterone
to the prednisone-melphalan regimen increases response rate but not survival
time.

Kiang et al. (7) report the results of 34 patients with multiple myeloma treated
with cyclophosphamide or melphalan-prednisone. Adjuvant androgen therapy
with either fluoxymesterone (10 mg bid, orally or testosterone enanthate 400
mg 2 × week × 2 to 4 weeks then 400 mg in alternate weeks or 400 mg per
month IM) was nonrandomly administered to 16 patients, and 18 received no
androgen therapy. A decrease of M-protein and increase in hemoglobin of 2 g/
100 ml or more occurred more frequently in the androgen group. Unfortunately
the group with androgen therapy received higher total doses of cyclophosphamide, and the duration of chemotherapy was longer. Both factors may have
contributed to the better response rate in the androgen group. Therefore the
result of that study is, at best, difficult to interpret.

REFRACTORY ANEMIA WITH EXCESS OF MYELOBLASTS IN THE BONE MARROW

Najean et al. (18) reported 90 patients with refractory anemia and an excess of
marrow blasts who were treated with high doses of androgens—oxymetholone
2.5 mg/kg daily, methandrosterone 1 mg/kg daily, metandrolone 2.5 mg/kg daily

or norethandrolone 1 mg/kg daily. The average survival was 13 months. Of 60 deaths in which the cause was known, 38 (64%) were associated with a change to frank acute myelocytic leukemia, and the remainder with granulocytopenia or thrombocytopenia. The androgen therapy appeared to have little if any effect on the course of the disease, but a review of the relevant literature (15–17) suggests that the development of frank acute leukemia may be accelerated with this treatment.

ANDROGEN THERAPY IN CONJUNCTION WITH COMBINATION CHEMOTHERAPY IN OTHER HEMATOLOGIC MALIGNANCIES

Keener et al. (31) reported two series of patients with depressed hematopoiesis due to chemotherapy for leukemia transformation of malignant lymphoma. Group A received repeated blood transfusions, prednisone, and a combination of antibiotics. Group B received androgens for at least two weeks. Both groups showed a significant increase in leukocytes after two weeks. This increase was somewhat higher in group B, but the difference was not statistically significant.

Zittoun et al. (32) reported the results of a randomized study of the effect of adjuvant androgen therapy on the hematologic toxicity of antineoplastic chemotherapy. Twenty-eight patients with Hodgkin's disease and 4 patients with non-Hodgkin's lymphoma were included in this study. Chemotherapy consisted of mechlorethamine, vincristine, procarbazine, and prednisone (MOPP) for six cycles at 14-day intervals. Patients were randomized into two groups: Group I (16 patients) received methanolone—2 mg/kg per day orally throughout chemotherapy, including therapy-free intervals—and group II received no androgen. The hematologic tolerance was satisfactory in 8 of 16 patients in group I and 10 of 16 in group II. Anemia and thrombocytopenia were significantly greater in group I.

The leukocyte count was lower in group I than in group II, but the difference was not significant. The greater hematologic toxicity in group I made it necessary to reduce the total drug doses compared with group II; the difference in drug tolerance between the groups was significant for procarbazine only ($69.8 \pm 30\%$ of the total theoretical dose in group I versus $94.4 \pm 17\%$ in group II). The authors suggested that the increased hematotoxicity in group I can be explained by the recruitment of hematopoietic stem cells, but this was not investigated in the study.

CONCLUSION AND SUMMARY

Androgen therapy has been widely used in combination with chemotherapy in most of the hematologic malignancies. The arguments for its use are that androgen therapy *(1)* stimulates marrow function, which allows for later doses of chemotherapy, *(2)* stimulates the immune system, and *(3)* has an anticoagulant effect.

Most of the published studies that are said to support androgen therapy are uncontrolled trials and are difficult to evaluate.

In acute myelocytic leukemia, two controlled studies were performed using stanozolol. In one study stanozolol was given orally and daily and in the other it was given IM every 10 days. The androgen was given in combination with chemotherapy in both studies. Both of these controlled studies failed to demonstrate any significant effect of androgen therapy.

In multiple myeloma the combination of melphalan-prednisone-testosterone produces a higher increase of hemoglobin value in good risk patients compared with melphalan-prednisone. However, the time to response was similar, and no difference was observed in other parameters of response such as number of marrow plasma cells, serum paraprotein concentration, azotemia, hypercalcemia, pain, or performance. Median survival was longer (53 months) in patients treated with melphalan-prednisone than in those treated with melphalan-prednisone-testosterone (36 months).

In refractory anemia with excess of myeloblasts in the bone marrow (smoldering leukemia), the use of androgen therapy has little if any effect on the anemia, and the progression to frank acute leukemia may actually be accelerated by this treatment.

Androgen therapy has been widely used for the purpose of reducing hematologic toxicity when used with intensive combination chemotherapy for solid tumor or lymphoma. However, a randomized study in lymphoma patients using methanolone in combination with MOPP showed that the group that received androgen therapy had a greater degree of anemia, thrombocytopenia, and leukopenia compared with the group that received no androgen. The greater hematologic toxicity in the androgen group made it necessary to reduce drug doses in that group rather than the control group.

The lack of effect of androgens in most of the controlled trials in hematologic malignancies in which they have been studied is clear. This fact, along with the observation from some studies that they may be harmful, suggests very strongly that androgens have no proved value in the treatment of hematologic malignancies.

REFERENCES

1. Brodsky I, Rigberg S: The role of androgens and anabolic steriods in the treatment of cancer, in Greenspan EM (ed): *Clinical Cancer Chemotherapy.* New York, Raven Press, 1975, p 349.

2. Alexanian R, Alfrey CP: Erythrokinetics and androgens in bone marrow cancer. *Cancer* 38:833, 1976.

3. Horn Y, Halden A, Gordon GS: The platelet stimulating effects of 7-β 17-α dimethyltestosterone (calusterone). *Blood* 40:684, 1972.

4. Bergsagel DE: Plasma cell neoplasms, in Greenspan EM (ed): *Clinical Cancer Chemotherapy,* New York, Raven Press, 1975, p 131.

5. Cline MJ, Berlin NI: Studies of the anemia of multiple myeloma. *Am J Med* 33:510, 1960.

6. Gardner FH: Fluorides for multiple myeloma. *N Engl J Med* 287:1252, 1972.

7. Kiang DT, Theologides A, Fortuny I, et al: Hormone therapy for malignant myeloma. *Lancet* 2:147, 1973.

8. Schilling A, Finkel HE: Ancillary measures in treatment of myeloma: Use of immune serum globulin, fluoride or androgen. *Arch Intern Med* 135:193, 1975.

9. Kennedy BJ: The use of androgens in the treatment of diseases of the hematopoietic system. *Pharmacol Ther* 2:39, 1977.

10. Hollard D, Sotto JJ, Bachelot C, et al: Essai d'androgenotherapie dans le traitement des leucemies aigues non lymphoblastiques. Premiers results. *Nouv Presse Med* 5:1289, 1976.

11. Hollard D, Berthier R, Sotto JJ: Androgens and long-term complete remission in acute granulopoietic leukemias. *Recent Results Cancer Res* 62:95, 1977.

12. Poirot P, Pouzol P, Sotto JJ, et al: Essai d'androgentherapie dans le traitement des leucemias aigues non lymphoblastiques de l'enfant. *Pediatrie* 33:89, 1978.

13. Sotto JJ, Holland D, Schaerer R, et al: Androgens et remissions prolongées dans les leucemies aigues non lymphoblastiques: Resultats d'un traitement systematique par le stanozolol associé a la chimiotherapie. *Nouv Rev Fr Hematol* 15:57, 1975.

14. Tanzer J, Desmarel ME, Frocram C, et al: High dose androgen therapy as an adjuvant in the shock therapy of acute myeloblastic leukemia: Initial results (letter to editor). *Nouv Presse Med* 5:2543, 1976.

15. Dreyfus B: Preleukemia states: I. Definition and classification. II. Refractory anemia with an excess of myeloblasts in the bone marrow (smoldering acute leukemia). *Blood Cells* 2:33, 1976.

16. Izrael V, Jacquillat C, Chartang C, et al: Les myeloblastoses partielles. *Bull Cancer* 61:341, 1974.

17. Linman JW, Bagby GC: The preleukemic syndrome clinical and laboratory features, natural courses and management. *Blood Cells* 2:11, 1976.

18. Najean Y, Pecking A: Refractory anemia with excess of myeloblasts in the bone marrow: A clinical trial of androgens in 90 patients. *Br J Haematol* 37:25, 1977.

19. Sehahoun G, Bouffette P, Flandrin G: Hairy cell leukemia. *Leuk Res* 2:187, 1978.

20. Gardner FH, Nathan DG: Androgens and erythropoiesis: III. Further evaluation of testosterone treatment of myelofibrosis. *N Engl J Med* 274:420, 1966.

21. Mulder H, Moers AM, Haanen C: Five patients suffering from myelofibrosis with myeloid metaplasia. *Ned Tijdschr Genneskd* 120:1243, 1976.

22. Silver RT, Jenkins DEJ, Engle RL Jr: Use of testosterone and busulfan in the treatment of myelofibrosis with myeloid metaplasia. *Blood* 23:341, 1964.

23. Davidson JF, Lochhead M, McDonald GA, McNichol GP: Fibrinolytic enhancement by stanozolol: A double blind trial. *Br J Haematol* 47:13, 1972.

24. Segaloff A: The use of androgens in the treatment of neoplastic disease. *Pharmacol Ther C* 2:33, 1977.

25. Eppinger-Helft M, Pavlovsky S, Suarez A, et al: Sequential therapy for induction and maintenance of remission in acute myeloblastic leukemia. *Cancer* 35:347, 1975.

26. Pavlovsky S, Penalver J, Eppinger-Helft M, et al: Induction and maintenance of remission in acute leukemia. Effectiveness of combination therapy in 227 patients. *Cancer* 31:273, 1973.

27. Jacquillat C: Personal communication.

28. Pavlovsky S, Scaglione C, Eppinger-Helft M, et al: Evaluacion de dos esquemas de induccion y empleo de estanozolol como adyuvante de la terapia de mantenimiento en leucemia mieloblastica aguda (abstract). *IV Congreso Argentino Oncologia Clinica*, Buenos Aires, 1979.

29. Eppinger-Helft M, Pavlovsky S, Hidalgo G, et al: Chemoimmunotherapy with Corynebacterium parvum in acute myelocytic leukemia. *Cancer* 45:280, 1979.

30. Costa G, Engle RL, Schilling A, et al: Melphalan and prednisone an effective combination for the treatment of multiple myeloma. *Am J Med* 54:589, 1973.

31. Klener P, Donner L, Smothachova I: Inhibition of hematopoiesis due to cytostatic therapy and its treatment. *Cas Lek Cesk* 116:117, 1977.

32. Zittoun R, Barthelemy M, Bouchard M, et al: Increased hematological toxicity of antineoplastic drugs with simultaneous androgen therapy. *Nouv Presse Med* 6:2669, 1977.

Part 2

ADJUVANT THERAPY
OF SOLID TUMORS

9

Adjuvant Radiotherapy for Breast Cancer

Florence Chu

In the treatment of operable breast cancer surgery fails to cure a significant proportion of patients, particularly those with positive axillary lymph nodes. There has always been a pressing need to improve the results by adding adjuvant treatment to surgery. For decades radiation therapy has been used either pre-operatively or postoperatively to supplement the surgical procedure.

The rationale for combining surgery and radiation therapy is easy to understand. Surgery is known to be the most effective way of removing gross disease, and radiation therapy is known to be capable of sterilizing cancer cells in local and regional areas. The most commonly performed surgical procedure, radical mastectomy or modified radical mastectomy, does not include dissection of the internal mammary and supraclavicular lymph nodes. These regional lymphatic drainage areas have a high probability of harboring metastatic cancer cells. There is also a possibility of residual disease left behind in the operative field that may serve as a source of local recurrence and distant spread. Radiation therapy sterilizes cancer cells in these areas and improves local and regional tumor control. Further, if the patient's occult lesions are confined to the local and regional areas, this approach may eradicate the disease and cure the patient.

Despite the sound rationale for combining radiation with radical surgery, controversy exists regarding the use of adjuvant radiation treatment. For many years there have been conflicting views and arguments that still continue. The issue has become even more complex since the advent of adjuvant chemotherapy. In order to facilitate our understanding of this subject, it is necessary to review some of the clinical trials and retrospective studies. After weighing all the facts, we can then judge the value of adjuvant radiation therapy in the treatment of operable breast cancer.

One of the fundamental principles of good cancer management is to achieve both local tumor control and prolonged survival. Numerous studies have demonstrated beyond any doubt that combined surgery and radiation therapy offers better local-regional tumor control than surgery alone, particularly in stage II patients. The value of radiation therapy in improving local-regional tumor control is, therefore, clear-cut. There is no dispute here.

The continuous debate regarding adjuvant radiation therapy is usually related

111

to the survival benefit or lack of survival benefit. Historically, most patients who are given pre- or postoperative radiation therapy are usually those with more advanced disease or with less favorable prognosis. This selection is responsible for the inferior survival results often associated with patients who received radiation therapy.

In an attempt to avoid biased selections, randomized clinical trials have been carried out. The first trial was by Paterson and Russell (1), which was followed by the National Surgical Adjuvant Breast Project (NASBP) trial (2). Both studies showed that routine postoperative radiation therapy did not affect the survival rate. Unfortunately, these results have been misunderstood by many as concrete evidence for the lack of the value of radiation therapy without realizing that the conclusions that can be made from these studies are limited.

Paterson and Russell's clinical trial (1) was done in the late 1940s and early 1950s during the orthovoltage era. Their study was designed to compare the efficacy of radiation therapy given prophylactically with that given therapeutically at a later date. A total of 1,461 stage I and II patients were entered into the study. One group was randomly assigned to receive postoperative radiation therapy immediately after radical mastectomy, and another group of patients were observed and treated only when local recurrence developed. Two different radiation therapy techniques were used during two different periods. First, a *quadrate technique* was used, treating the axilla and the chest wall (720 cases). The strategically important peripheral lymphatic drainage areas (internal mammary and supraclavicular nodes) were not irradiated. During the second period a *peripheral technique* was used, treating the axilla, supraclavicular area, and parasternal region (741 cases). At no time were both the chest wall and regional lymphatic areas irradiated simultaneously. The radiation dose given was modest, and the equipment used was a 250-kV x-ray machine. For the quadrate technique the dose was 3,500 to 4,000 R given over a three-week period. For the peripheral technique a dose of 3,250 R was given to the midplane of the supraclavicular and axillary regions. The given dose on the parasternal field was 4,250 R.

With each technique, there was no statistically significant difference in the mortality rate at five years between the treated and the observed groups. However, a significant reduction in recurrence rates was achieved when postoperative radiation therapy was administered. For instance, when the skin flap was irradiated, the recurrence rate in the area was lowered from approximately 20% to 11%, and when the supraclavicular area was treated, the recurrence rate in this region was reduced from 17% to 6%.

The conclusions from this study may be stated as follows: radiation therapy, even with modest doses, reduced the incidence of recurrence in the treated areas, and the postoperative radiation therapy as given did not appear to have influenced the survival rate. The survival results of patients who received prophylactic postoperative radiation therapy were similar to those patients who were observed and given therapeutic irradiation when recurrence developed.

It must be stressed that Paterson and Russell's finding of lack of survival improvement should not be extrapolated to mean no survival benefits for other patients who were treated with a different radiation therapy technique, that is, megavoltage therapy, higher radiation dose, and more adequate coverage of areas of potential disease.

The second trial was by the National Surgical Adjuvant Breast Project (2) to evaluate the efficacy of postoperative radiation therapy in patients with stages I and II disease. Radiation therapy was directed to the internal mammary and supraclavicular fields. Approximately 75% of the patients had supervoltage radiation. The radiation dosages ranged from 3,500 R in three weeks to 4,500 R in five weeks. The control patients received either placebo or thiotepa. A total of 1,882 patients were entered into this randomized study. After eliminating 779 patients for various reasons, most of which were protocol violation, 1,103 patients were available for analysis. Of these, 415 patients were used for the five-year analysis.

Fisher et al. (2) reported that the five-year disease status and survival rates were similar in both the radiation therapy group and the control groups. However, there was a significant reduction in the recurrence rates in the regional lymph node areas that were irradiated.

Fisher's study has been criticized for the exclusion of a large number of patients, a variation in radiation factors and dosage, and the inclusion of thiotepa patients in the control group (3). Again, it must be pointed out that the conclusions made by Fisher et al. are relevant only to the radiation therapy technique used in the NSABP trial. The findings should not be used to close the door to further investigation of adjuvant radiation therapy.

There have been other clinical trials, for example, studies to compare simple mastectomy plus radiation therapy with radical mastectomy and simple mastectomy and radiation therapy with extended radical mastectomy and many other schemes (4–6). The interpretations of the results of various clinical trials were confused unnecessarily by Stjernswärd, who implied that radiation therapy has a deleterious effect on survival (7–9). Stjernswärd combined the data of several clinical trials and compared the survival results of surgery alone with surgery and radiation therapy. He concluded that radiation therapy decreased the survival rate, and he further postulated that this decreased survival could be due to suppression of the host immunity by irradiation.

In the analysis of the data of several clinical trials Stjernswärd ignored important variables that existed in these trials. There were differences in patient population, the surgical procedures performed, the radiation therapy techniques used, and the other parameters that have a definitive prognostic influence. It seems unreasonable that he put all the variables together and attributed the decreased survival rate solely to radiation therapy. This type of comparison is unfair, and, therefore, his conclusions cannot be considered valid.

Stjernswärd's method of statistical analysis has been severely criticized (3,10–12). His hypothesis that radiation therapy suppresses immunity, facilitating tumor growth and metastasis, has also been challenged (13–15). To many investigators the significance of lymphopenia and depressed immune response in relation to tumor growth is largely unclear at the present time.

According to Turnbull, Turner, and Jones (15) there are reasons to believe that the radiation therapy effect on the immune response may not be important to the tumor host relationship. The results of several clinical studies, to be discussed later, tend to support this view.

In contrast to those reports which showed no survival benefits from routine postoperative radiation therapy there have been reports in the literature demonstrating direct or indirect evidence of beneficial survival effects of adjuvant radiation therapy.

RANDOMIZED STUDIES

One randomized trial was done at the Norwegian Radium Hospital, Oslo, Norway, and was reported by Høst and Brennhovd in 1977 (16). The value of postoperative radiation therapy as an adjuvant to radical mastectomy was assessed. A total of 1,090 patients were entered into the study. In the first part, orthovoltage x-rays were used, delivering modest doses to the chest wall and regional lymph node areas. In the second part, cobalt 60 was used to irradiate the internal mammary and supraclavicular areas, delivering a higher radiation dose (5,000 rad in four weeks). All patients were given radiation castration.

In stage I patients, orthovoltage or cobalt 60 postoperative irradiation did not influence the survival or the relapse rate. In stage II cases, orthovoltage radiation therapy reduced the incidence of local and regional recurrences but did not affect the survival. Cobalt 60 irradiation, however, not only significantly reduced the relapse rate but also increased the cumulative survival rate up to five years (Fig. 1). This difference in survival is statistically significant ($P = .05$).

Figure 2 shows the disease-free survival. In stage II, patients irradiated with cobalt 60 had statistically significantly higher survival rates than the control group. The patients irradiated with orthovoltage also showed a higher disease-free survival rate as compared with the control, but this difference is not statistically significant.

Further analysis by these authors showed that in patients with medial tumors and patients with four or more positive axillary nodes, cobalt 60 irradiation appeared to have produced a higher survival rate as compared with orthovoltage-irradiated patients and the controls. However, the numbers of patients in separate subgroups were too small to be statistically significant.

Høst and Brennhovd believe that radiation techniques and dosages are im-

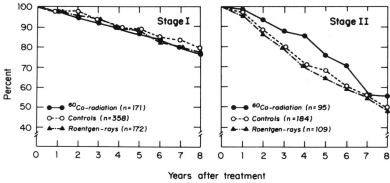

Figure 1. Survival rates according to primary treatment, surgery alone, surgery plus orthovoltage radiation therapy, and surgery plus cobalt 60 radiation therapy. From Høst and Brennhoud (16).

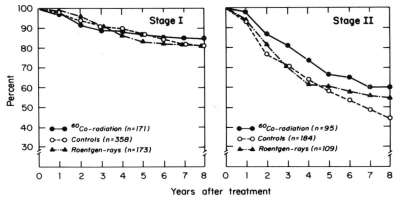

Figure 2 Disease-free survival rates according to primary treatment, surgery alone, surgery plus orthovoltage radiation therapy, and surgery plus cobalt 60 radiation therapy. From Høst and Brennhoud (16).

portant. They attributed the improved results to a higher radiation dosage achieved by cobalt 60 irradiation given to the regional lymph nodes.

Another controlled clinical trial was carried out by the Stockholm group (17–19), whose study was designed to compare the results of preoperative radiation, postoperative radiation therapy, and surgery alone. This study was started in 1971 at the Radiumhemmet in cooperation with five surgical departments. A total of 960 patients have been included in this study, which was closed to patient entry in 1976. The surgical procedure performed was modified radical mastectomy. Radiation therapy was given to the breast (preoperatively) or chest wall (postoperatively) and the internal mammary, axillary, and supraclavicular nodal regions. The radiation dose was 4,500 rad in five weeks, using cobalt 60 and electron beam therapy.

An analysis of the results of treatment showed that the number of patients with recurrent disease is significantly lower in the two groups given radiation therapy than in the group treated by surgery only. The disease-free survival rates of the three groups are shown in Figure 3. Both preoperatively and postoperatively irradiated patients had statistically significant higher disease-free survival as compared with those who had surgery alone.

The survival rates in the three treatment groups showed that the preoperatively irradiated group had a statistically significantly higher survival rate than the postoperatively irradiated group and the surgery alone group (Fig. 4).

RETROSPECTIVE STUDIES

There are retrospective studies that suggested beneficial effects of adjuvant radiation therapy. One such study (20) is the analysis of the results of treatment of 674 patients treated in the late 1940s and early 1950s at Memorial Hospital, New York City. One group of patients received no postoperative radiation therapy after radical or extended radical mastectomy, and another group received

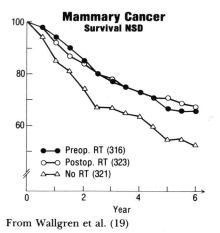

From Wallgren et al. (19)

Figure 3. Disease-free survival rates in the three treatment groups, surgery alone, surgery plus postoperative radiation therapy, and surgery plus preoperative radiation therapy.

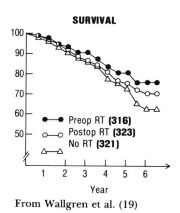

From Wallgren et al. (19)

Figure 4. Survival rates in the three treatment groups, surgery alone, surgery plus postoperative radiation therapy, and surgery plus preoperative radiation therapy.

postoperative therapy to the internal mammary and supraclavicular lymph node areas. Most patients were given 3,500 rad in about 3½ weeks, using 250 kV(p) x-rays. Some patients with a high risk of chest wall recurrence were also treated to the chest wall through tangential fields, to a dose of about 4,000 rad in four weeks. Since this was not a randomized study, selections did exist. The usual selection was to irradiate patients with more advanced disease. This was evidenced by the presence of axillary lymph node metastases in 83% of the irradiated patients and in only 46% of the nonirradiated patients. Also, the patients selected for radiation therapy had higher levels of axillary lymph node metastasis. There was apical involvement of the axilla in 52% of the irradiated patients with positive axillary nodes and in 29% of those who received no irradiation.

The results of treatment showed that although there was no significant difference in survival rates when patients were divided according to negative and positive axillary nodes between the irradiated and nonirradiated groups, radiation therapy appeared to have had beneficial influence on a subgroup of patients who had apical axillary involvement. It was found that when the axillary nodes were positive in the low and midaxilla, the survival rates of the two groups were similar. However, when the axillary nodes were positive in the apex of the axilla, those patients who received postoperative radiation treatment had a higher percentage of survival (39% versus 22%) (Table 1). This difference of 17% approaches statistical significance. Many patients with apical axillary involvement also had a large primary tumor or lymphatic permeation of the skin. These patients received radiation therapy to the chest wall, as well as to the lymph nodes. It is conceivable that there may be a subgroup of patients whose lives can be prolonged by postoperative radiation therapy. More studies are needed to identify such subgroups better.

Radiation therapy definitely reduced local and regional recurrences. For example, in patients with positive axillary lymph nodes, the incidence of supra-

Table 1. Five-Year Survival Rates According to the Levels of Axillary Lymph Node Metastasis.

	Postoperative radiation therapy			No postoperative radiation therapy		
	Total #pts.	# pts. survived	%	Total # pts.	# pts. survived	%
Low axilla	37	23	62	90	57	63
Mid axilla	40	15	38	63	29	46
Apex of axilla	89	35	39	63	14	22
Level unknown	4	2	-	3	3	-
Overall	170	75	44	219	103	47

From Chu et al. (20).

clavicular nodal recurrence at the five-year level was 23% without postoperative therapy. When patients were treated with orthovoltage irradiation, receiving a tumor dose of 3,500 rad in 3½ weeks, the incidence of supraclavicular recurrence was reduced to 10% (20). When megavoltage radiation was used and the dose delivered was 4,000 to 4,500 rad in 4 weeks, the recurrence rate was further reduced, to 6% (21). These data (Fig. 5) not only confirm the effectiveness of radiation therapy in reducing recurrence in the irradiated areas but also demonstrate that tumor control is dose-dependent. In order for adjuvant radiation therapy to be more effective, adequate radiation doses must be given.

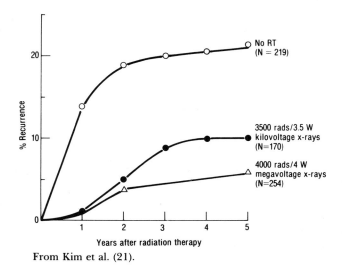

From Kim et al. (21).

Figure 5. Rates of supraclavicular metastasis in patients with positive axillary lymph nodes; no radiation therapy, 3,500 rad in 3 1/2 weeks—from Chu et al. (9)—and 4,000 to 4,500 rad in 4 weeks.

Fletcher and Montague (22), in a retrospective analysis of the M. D. Anderson Hospital data, also reported beneficial effects of adjuvant radiation therapy on survival. They compared results of radical mastectomy followed by irradiation of peripheral lymph nodes. The radiation dose given was 5,000 rad, delivered over a period of about five weeks. In the radical mastectomy group 11.5% had histologically positive axillary nodes, and the 10-year survival rate was 54%. In the combined radical mastectomy and radiation therapy group 65.7% of the patients had positive axillary lymph nodes. Despite this high percentage of axillary nodal involvement, a 10-year survival rate of 56% was achieved (Table 2). It is an established fact that the prognosis of patients correlates with the status of axillary lymph nodes. A series of cases that contain a large number of patients with positive axillary lymph nodes would certainly be expected to have lower survival rates than a series that contains fewer patients with positive axillary nodes. Although the data are not from a randomized trial, they do suggest strongly that the curative effects of irradiation are real.

Fletcher and Montague also stressed the importance of adequate radiation dosages given to the peripheral lymphatic areas. Faulty techniques may lead to geographical miss of the lymph nodes. They attributed the poor radiation therapy results from those early clinical trials to orthovoltage therapy, inadequate dose, and inadequate radiation therapy portals.

Another report that deserves more attention is the one by Berg and Robbins (23), who studied the entire population of breast cancer patients treated in 1969 in the state of Iowa. There were 1,051 patients who had definitive surgery. The five-year relative survival for all patients was 71%. An unexpected finding was the advantage found for adjuvant radiation therapy given after radical mastectomy. The five-year relative survival rate of patients treated by radical mastectomy alone was 58%, and, by radical mastectomy and radiation therapy, it was 71% (Table 3). This difference is statistically significant at the 5% level. The increased survival rate is particularly impressive in view of the fact that there was always a tendency to select cases with more axillary nodal metastases for irradiation. This selection should have produced a lower survival rate for the

Table 2. Five- and Ten-Year Survival Rate of Patients Treated at the M. D. Anderson Hospital.

Treatment Modality	No. of Pts.	Patients with Histologically Positive Nodes %	(No.)	Average Number of Involved Nodes Per Patient in the Patients with Involved Nodes	Percentage of Survival 5 Year	10 Year
Radical mastectomy only	287	11.5	(33/287)	5	71.7	54
Radical mastectomy followed by peripheral lymphatic irradiation (5000 rad in 4 weeks+ to the supraclavicular area and internal mammary chain with ^{60}Co or ^{137}Cs)	356	65.7	(234/356)	6	71.3	56

* Berkson-Gage, not age adjusted
° No elective chemotherapy
+ Presently given in 5 weeks in 25 fractions, 200 rad per fraction
From Fletcher and Montague (22).

Table 3. Five-Year Relative Survival with and without Radiation for Various Types of Surgery

| Operation | X-Ray | Stage of Disease[a] | |
		Localized	Regional
Radical	Yes	95% (41)	71% (144)
mastectomy	No	91% (336)	58% (170)
Modified	Yes	— (1)	36% (15)
radical	No	89% (37)	57% (29)
Simple	Yes	62% (21)	54% (14)
mastectomy	No	78% (113)	44% (23)

[a]Number of cases in parentheses. Difference statistically significant at the 5% level.

From Berg and Robbins (23).

irradiated patients, but the results suggested a favorable effect of irradiation on survival. Further analysis of the data showed that the improved survival was observed in patients with one positive axillary node only, with more than one positive node but less than 50% of nodes involved, or in patients with more than half of the lymph nodes involved (Table 4).

Radiation therapy parameters were also examined. It was found that the five-year relative survival rate of patients given no irradiation was 58%, in patients who received orthovoltage radiation therapy it was 64%, and in patients who received supervoltage radiation, 75%. The difference in results between orthovoltage and supervoltage radiation therapy is not statistically significant, but the difference between supervoltage irradiation and none is significant. These findings again appear to support the observation that supervoltage irradiation, delivering a higher radiation dosage, is more advantageous than orthovoltage therapy in achieving good results.

Based on these data of several studies, there appears to be sufficient evidence to suggest strongly that radiation therapy does actually cure a number of patients

Table 4. Effect on Survival Rates of Irradiation of Cases with Various Amounts of Cancer in the Axilla[a]

| Amount of Node Involvement | Relative Five-Year Survival[b] | |
	Radiation	No Radiation
One node only	89% (28)	79% (30)
> 1 node, less than half	71% (28)	58% (35)
Half or more	53% (39)	42% (30)

[a]Cases with radical mastectomy only.

[b]Number of cases in parentheses.

From Berg and Robbins (23).

whose disease is confined to the local and regional areas. Such a number would be small, and, therefore, the survival benefits are difficult to demonstrate. Even though the number of cases cured by adjuvant radiation therapy may be small, each individual patient's life is important, each life saved is worth the effort.

There is no dispute regarding the fact that radiation therapy reduces local and regional recurrences, particularly in stage II and other high risk cases. The combination of radiation therapy and surgery results in better tumor control than surgery alone. This local control aspect is also important because the patient's quality of life is improved by being free from recurrence on the chest or lymph node areas. It is preferable to prevent recurrence than to treat them when they occur. If adjuvant radiation therapy is not given immediately after surgery, the patient may miss a chance of cure at an earlier stage of breast cancer when the disease might still be confined to the chest wall and regionnal lymph node areas. Failure to eliminate this focus of cancer increases not only the risk of local and regional recurrences but also of distant spread. Further, local and regional recurrences are often symptomatic and sometimes difficult to eradicate. Opponents of routine postoperative radiation therapy argue that many patients receive radiation therapy unnecessarily. However, unnecessary treatment can be minimized by better definition of patients for adjuvant radiation therapy. Stage I cases, for instance, should be excluded from routine postoperative radiation therapy except for the group of patients with inner quadrant or central primary tumors.

In view of the reasons stated, postoperative radiation therapy should be given to patients with a high risk of harboring occult disease in the local or regional areas. Patients with inner quadrant or central primary tumors should receive postoperative radiation therapy to the internal mammary and supraclavicular regions, even though the axillary nodes are negative. This is because the chances of medial spread are high in patients with inner half or central primaries. There is no need to give postoperative therapy to stage I patients with an outer quadrant tumor and negative axillary nodes, since these patients do well with surgery alone. Patients with a large primary tumor, greater than 4 or 5 cm in diameter, extensive metastases to the axillary lymph nodes, or histological evidence of lymphatic permeation of the skin by cancer cells should receive postoperative radiation therapy to the chest wall and lymph node areas. A total dose of 4,500 rad in four weeks or 5,000 rad in five weeks is recommended.

Since many patients with seemingly early breast cancer already have occult dissemination at the time of surgery, a local form of treatment is insufficient to cure these patients. A systemic therapy is clearly needed. Bonadonna (24,25) and others (26,27) in their clinical trials have demonstrated lower relapse rates in patients who received adjuvant chemotherapy as compared with those who did not. The benefits are more evident in premenopausal women. Adjuvant chemotherapy is now being used widely with a decreased use of adjuvant radiation therapy. However, there is still a fair proportion of patients receiving postoperative radiation treatment. This is because (a) many surgical, radiation therapy, and medical oncologists firmly believe in the importance of good local-regional tumor control and the efficacy of radiation therapy in providing such control and also the possibility of a cure; (b) although recent chemotherapy results are extremely encouraging, chemotherapy has not yet reached the degree of complete effectiveness in dealing with all lesions. Our clinical experience has shown a significant number of patients who required radiation treatment for chest wall, parasternal, or supraclavicular recurrence after they have failed adjuvant chemotherapy. It would appear that adjuvant chemotherapy should use the assistance of adjuvant radiation therapy to reduce the number of cancer cells in local-regional areas so that chemotherapy may become more effective in dealing with minimal tumor burden. This concept of combining effective local agents (surgery and radiation therapy) with systemic agents (chemotherapy) offers a real possibility of curing many patients with occult disseminated disease. There is definitely a need for developing an optimal combination of surgery, radiation therapy, and chemotherapy to improve the overall results.

The combination of radiation therapy and chemotherapy requires caution and thorough investigation. At present our knowledge regarding the interactions of adjuvant radiation therapy and adjuvant chemotherapy is limited. Simultaneous use of the two agents may produce intolerable toxicities. A reasonable approach, for instance, may involve the sequential use of the two agents, with chemotherapy being administered first, to deal with systemic disease, and with radiation therapy being given in between cycles of chemotherapy, to treat the areas that have a high probability of heavy tumor burden. Well-designed, randomized studies should be carried out in order to obtain meaningful data. In our research efforts we should also attempt to delineate the kind of cases that would benefit most from this combined approach.

SUMMARY

Radiation therapy is of definite value in killing or inhibiting cancer cells. The purpose of its use as an adjuvant to surgery in the treatment of operable breast cancer is to eliminate the residual disease and occult lesions that are likely present in the operative field and lymphatic drainage areas.

Numerous studies have demonstrated the ability of radiation therapy to reduce local and regional recurrence, particularly in more advanced operable cases. Several reports have shown the possible beneficial effects of adjuvant radiation therapy on survival. The reported increased survivals are usually seen in patients who receive adequate amounts of radiation therapy to the peripheral lymph node areas or to the lymph nodes and chest wall. It is realized that small increments of increased survival are difficult to demonstrate, but our firm conviction is that each patient deserves the best chance of cure and every life saved is worthwhile. Based on the principles of good cancer management in accomplishing both local tumor control and prolonged survival, adjuvant radiation therapy should be used to treat patients with a high risk of local-regional disease. Each of the three main treatment modalities, surgery, radiation therapy, and chemotherapy, has its advantages and limitations. We must develop optimal treatment regimens, using the advantages, to offer our patients the best possible results.

The value of adjuvant radiation includes the following:

1. Preventing local-regional recurrence.
2. Providing disease-free status in the treated areas and thus improving the patients' quality of survival.
3. Offering a chance of permanent elimination of a source of cancer spread.

4. Offering a chance of cure, even though the chance may be limited.

5. Radiation therapy reduces the tumor burden, which is of particular importance in view of the fact that chemotherapy is more effective in dealing with minimal tumor burden than with gross tumors.

6. Adjuvant radiation therapy should not be used routinely in all operable cases. It should be used in those patients with a high risk of developing local or regional recurrence.

7. The radiation field and dosage should be adequate in order to achieve good results.

8. The value of radiation therapy is there. It is up to us to use it best.

REFERENCES

1. Paterson R, Russell H: Clinical trials in malignant disease. Part III: Breast cancer—evaluation of postoperative radiotherapy. *J Faculty Radiol* 10:175–180, 1959.

2. Fisher B, Slack H, Cavanaugh J, Gardner B, et al: Postoperative radiotherapy in the treatment of breast cancer: Results of the NSABP clinical trial. *Ann Surg* 172:711–732, 1970.

3. Levitt SH, McHugh RB: Radiotherapy in the postoperative treatment of operable cancer of the breast. Part I. Critique of the clinical and biometric aspects of the trials. *Cancer* 39:924–932, 1977.

4. Bruce J: Operable cancer of the breast: A controlled clinical trial. *Cancer* 28:1441–1452, 1971.

5. Cancer Research Campaign: Management of early cancer of the breast. Report on an International Multicentre Trial Supported by the Cancer Research Campaign. *Brit Med J* 1:1035–1038, 1976.

6. Kaae S, Johansen H: Simple versus radical mastectomy in primary breast cancer, in Forest APM, Kunkler PB (eds): *Prognostic Factors in Breast Cancer.* Edinburgh, Livingstone, pp 93–102, 1968.

7. Stjernswärd J: Can survival be decreased by post-operative irradiation? *Int J Radiat Oncol Biol Phys* 2:1171–1175, 1977.

8. Stjernswärd J: Decreased survival correlated to local irradiation in "early" operable breast cancer. *Lancet* 2:1285–1283, 1974.

9. Stjernswärd J, Jondal M, Vanky F, Wigzell H, et al: Lymphopenia and change in distribution of human B and T lymphocytes in peripheral blood induced by irradiation for mammary carcinoma. *Lancet* 2:1352–1356, 1972.

10. Brady LW, Fletcher GH, Levitt SH: The role of radiation therapy after mastectomy. *Cancer* 39:2868–2874, 1977.

11. Levitt SH, McHugh RB, Song CW: Radiotherapy in the postoperative treatment of operable cancer of the breast. Part II. A re-examination of Stjernsward's application of the Mantel-Haenxzel statistical method. Evaluation of the effect of the radiation on immune response and suggestions for postoperative radiotherapy. *Cancer* 39:933–940, 1976.

12. Watson T: Can survival be increased by post-operative irradiation? *Int J Radia Oncol Biol Phys* 2:1181–1183, 1977.

13. Blomgren H: Lymphopenia and breast metastasis. *Int J Radiat Oncol Biol Phys* 2:1177–1179, 1977.

14. Blomgren H, Berg R, Wasserman J, Glas U: Effect of radiotherapy on blood lymphocyte population in mammary carcinoma. *Int J Radiat Oncol Biol Phys* 1:177–188, 1976.

15. Turnbull AR, Turner DTL, Jones BM, Wright R: Radiation versus immunity in early breast cancer. *Clin Oncol* 5:237–244, 1979.

16. Høst H, Brennhoud IO: The effect of post-operative radiotherapy in breast cancer. *Int J Radiat Oncol Biol Phys* 2:1061–1067, 1977.

17. deSchryver A: The Stockholm Breast Cancer Trial: Preliminary report of a randomized study concerning the value of preoperative or postoperative radiotherapy in operable disease. *Int J Radiat Oncol Biol Phys* 1:601–609, 1976.

18. Wallgren A, Arner O, Bergstrom J, Blomstedt B, et al: Preoperative radiotherapy in breast cancer. *Cancer* 42:1120–1125, 1978.

19. Wallgren A, Arner A, Bergstrom J, Blomstedt B, et al: The value of preoperative radiotherapy in operable mammary carcinoma. *Int J Radiat Oncol Biol Phys* 6(3):287–290, 1980.

20. Chu FCH, Lucas JC, Farrow JH, Nickson JJ: Does prophylactic radiation therapy given for cancer of the breast predispose to metastasis? *Am J Roentgenol Radium Ther Nucl Med* 99:987–994, 1967.

21. Kim JH, Chu FCH, Hilaris BS: The influence of dose fractionation on acute and late reactions in patients with post-operative radiotherapy for carcinoma of the breast. *Cancer* 35:1583–1586, 1975.

22. Fletcher G, Montague ED: Does adequate irradiation of the internal mammary chain and supraclavicular nodes improve survival rates? *Int J Radiat Oncol Biol Phys* 4:481–492, 1978.

23. Berg JW, Robbins GF: Selection of treatment regimens for women with potentially curable breast carcinoma. *Am Surg* 2:86–91, 1977.

24. Bonadonna G, Brusamolino E, Valagussa P, Brugnatelli L, et al: Combination chemotherapy as an adjuvant treatment in operable breast cancer. *N Engl J Med* 294:405–410, 1976.

25. Bonadonna G, Rossi A, Valagussa P, Banfi A, et al: The CMF program for operable breast cancer with positive axillary nodes: Updated analysis on the disease-free interval, site of relapse and drug tolerance. *Cancer* 39:2904–2915, 1977.

26. Fisher B: Adjuvant chemotherapy in breast cancer. *Int J Radiat Oncol Biol Phys* 4:295–298, 1978.

27. Fisher B, Glass A, Redmond C, Fisher ER, et al: L-Phenylalanine Mustard (L-PAM) in the management of primary breast cancer: An update of earlier findings and a comparison with those utilizing L-PAM plus 5-Fluorouracil (5-FU). *Cancer* 39:2883–2903, 1977.

10

Does Adjuvant Radiotherapy Improve the Outcome of Breast Cancer Treatment?

Arvin S. Glicksman

The use of routine postoperative radiotherapy for patients with early breast cancer remains a matter of some controversy. Proponents argue that local control is enhanced and this contributes to the duration and quality of disease-free survival. Opponents argue that this local effect is probably immaterial to the long-term survival of these patients and that the treatment may actually contribute negatively in terms of survival.

Early in this century radiotherapy was found to be useful in dealing with locally advanced breast tumors, particularly the ulcerated, secondarily infected lesions that were difficult problems in local management (1). About the same time Halsted's radical mastectomy was becoming more widely recognized and accepted as the important surgical approach to localized breast cancer (2). In this historical context it must be recognized that Halsted's operation was introduced for patients with local disease that would be considered advanced by today's standards. Not surprisingly, local failure was seen frequently after radical mastectomy. Since radiotherapy had already been shown to have local beneficial affects in breast cancer, it came to be relied on more frequently in the postoperative setting to enhance the chances of local-regional control after surgical removal of the primary tumor.

Over the next 50 years, the selection of patients for whom the radical mastectomy was appropriate became more and more well-defined with terminology such as operable versus inoperable being applied to patients. Finally, there were introduced staging systems that have varied not only on both sides of the Atlantic but even both sides of Manhattan (3). During this time, surgeons were also attempting to extend the regional extirpation of tumor by internal mammary node dissection, low neck dissection, or both, as well as spending a good deal more thought in defining the surgical procedure for the axillary dissection and the care with which the skin flaps would be dissected in the standardization of the Halsted procedure (4,5).

During this same era there was a steady increase in the quality of radiotherapy. For the most part 250 kV x-ray became the standard (6). The modes of application varied to the supraclavicular fossa, internal mammary area, and the axilla with or without treatment of the chest wall. Since radiation pneumonitis could vary from 10% to 40%, depending on the technique that was being used, there was serious concern for the continued application of postoperative radiotherapy in early breast cancer as the surgical techniques improved (7,8).

In the late 1940s Ralston Paterson at the Christie Hospital in Manchester, England, designed and executed a series of prospective randomized trials to explore the usefulness of prophylactic postoperative radiotherapy in early breast cancer and at the same time to see if treatment to the node-bearing areas rather than to the chest wall made any difference. Because treatment procedures at the Christie were very carefully monitored and the organization was rigidly controlled, in the next six years this one clinic was able to complete these two studies entering 1,461 cases, 709 treated, 752 watched. There was clearly no difference in survival in these two patient populations, nor was there any difference in the quadrate versus the peripheral technique (9). In 1963 Paterson concluded that "when there is a well-established follow-up system prophylactic post-operative x-ray therapy for the case in which operation was wisely chosen and well-performed is unnecessary" (10).

From our vantage point one can argue that the radiotherapy techniques that Paterson investigated were somewhat restricted in that the quadrate technique did not adequately treat the peripheral nodes and the peripheral technique did not adquately cover the chest wall. Furthermore, the dose of the radiation would be considered somewhat low by today's standard even accounting for differences between 250 kV and megavoltage radiation. Be that as it may, in the next 15 to 20 years there has not been a prospective randomized trial that has seriously challenged the results that the Manchester study produced in the 1950s.

The appropriateness of postoperative radiotherapy when less than a radical mastectomy is performed has also been extensively investigated. In the early 1950s Professor Robert McWhirter in Edinburgh recorded the effectiveness of radical radiotherapy after a simple mastectomy (11). Controversy raged around this report in terms of the comparability of the cases, particularly since the axilla was not being dissected in the patients treated by radiotherapy. This was carried in some cases even to the extent of questioning whether some of the patients actually had cancer (12). There was no doubt that the treatment produced a fair amount of morbidity, but it was associated with survival rates that appeared to be comparable with those achieved by radical surgery alone.

In 1951 Sigvard Kaae and Helge Johansen undertook a prospective randomized clinical trial in which patients with stage I and II breast cancer were assigned to either an extended radical mastectomy by the Dahl-Ivorsen procedure or a simple mastectomy plus radical radiotherapy (13). Six hundred and sixty-six patients were entered into the trial, 425 of whom were evaluable at 5, 10, and 15 years. The crude survival rates for all patients were essentially the same throughout the study (Table 1). At 10 years local-regional recurrences were 22% for those treated by the McWhirter technique (intensive radiotherapy) and 27% for those treated by the extended radical mastectomy and no postoperative radiotherapy. Distant metastases were 47% in the first group and 46% in the

Table 1. Copenhagen Trial[a]

			Percent Survival		
	Treatment Policy	Total Patients	5 yr	10 yr	15 yr
All patients	Simple mastectomy and radiotherapy	331[b]	55	36	27
	Extended radical mastectomy	335[b]	56	38	27
Operable patients	Simple mastectomy and radiotherapy	219	66	46	36
	Extended radical mastectomy	206	67	50	37
Clinical stage I	Simple mastectomy and radiotherapy	149	75	54	44
	Extended radical mastectomy	141	77	59	47
Operable minus clinical stage I	Simple mastectomy and radiotherapy	70	46	29	19
	Extended radical mastectomy	65	48	29	17

[a]Kaae and Johansen.
[b]Twenty-four percent of patients in both treatment arms were excluded from treatment as biologically inoperable, refused, or other reasons.

second group. In clinically staged I cases, local-regional recurrences were identical in both groups. In other than clinically staged I cases there was a slightly higher incidence of local-regional recurrences in the surgical cases, but the difference between the two groups did not even approach the $P = .1$ level of statistical significance.

This study indicated that radiotherapy has a role to play when less than radical surgery is performed for operable breast cancer. When a simple mastectomy plus extensive radiation is compared with an extended radical mastectomy, the two procedures offer essentially the same survival probability and local control. The next question is whether the radiation is all that necessary. The trial of the Cancer Research Campaign in England studied 2,268 patients by simple mastectomy and radiotherapy versus simple mastectomy alone (14). For early operable cases there was no difference in the overall survival in both groups. The distant metastasis rate was the same in both groups. The major and only advantage to the radiotherapy was that there was better local-regional control, but this did not contribute to survival of the patients.

There have been a number of retrospective analyses over the last 25 years with less than clear answers to the question of the merit of postoperative radiotherapy. During the years 1950 and 1951, most patients received postoperative radiotherapy at Memorial Hospital in New York. In 1952 and 1953 and again in 1954 and 1955 most patients did not receive radiotherapy. Two analyses were done and published in 1966 and 1967 (15,16). Although the numbers were modestly different, the conclusion of both papers was that routine postoperative radiotherapy did not significantly alter the survival of patients operated on at Memorial Hospital who were then treated with orthovoltage radiotherapy. The radiotherapy was directed to the supraclavicular fossa, the axilla, and the internal mammary chain. Only a small number of patients received chest wall irradiation as well. Dr. Chu has concluded that only those patients with high axillary nodes may have benefited from postoperative radiotherapy because that group alone comes close to being statistically significantly different from the group not irradiated. However, the overall result for the five-year survival of 51% for patients receiving postoperative radiotherapy and 71% for those not receiving postoperative radiotherapy is significantly different ($P = .001$). Taken at face value this would indicate a deleterious effect of the radiation. In reality, patients with negative axillary nodes comprised only 17% of the patients who received postoperative radiotherapy and 53% of those who did not. This is clearly a skewed population of patients; to compare such groups of patients is one of the hazards of retrospective analyses.

More recently Weichselbaum et al. reviewed the experience at the Harvard Joint Center using megavoltage radiation with a somewhat higher dose of radiation (17). Their policy is to deliver 4,500 rad, four fraction per week for a TDF* of 81. For stage I patients there was a 76% five-year survival, 79% for stage II, and 57% for their stage III patients. Lacour et al. reported the results of an international study of 1,580 cases treated by surgery alone (18). Their results are not appreciably different. For stage I they reported 87% five-year survival; stage II had 60%, and stage III had 49% survival.

Fisher et al. have reported the experience of the National Surgical Adjuvant Breast Project, which examined the question of postoperative radiotherapy in a number of studies. In a study initiated in 1961 (19), 1,103 women were randomly assigned to postoperative radiotherapy to the node-bearing area (470 patients) or to controls, 316 of whom received thiotepa and 317 a placebo. No significant difference in survival with or without disease could be detected at five years. In another study that the NSABP initiated in 1971 over 1,600 patients have been randomly assigned to radical mastectomy, radical mastectomy plus radiotherapy, or total mastectomy for patients with clinically negative nodes or radical mastectomy or total mastectomy plus radiation for patients with clinically positive nodes (20). At four years there is no significant difference in survival in any of the groups (Table 2). Local failures are less frequent in patients who receive radical mastectomy plus radiotherapy or total mastectomy and radiotherapy as compared with those who have had either the radical or the total mastectomy alone. However, regional recurrences are the same in the clinically negative group (all around 2.3%). For the clinically positive nodes the radical mastectomy patients had a 4.7% regional recurrence as compared with 6.7% for the total mastectomy plus radiation. Distant disease was the same in all groups.

The radiotherapy for NSABP Protocol No. 4 was designed and supervised by

*Time dose fractionation units: A system that attempts to assign a similar value to varying dosage schedules having similar biological effect. See Orton CG and Ellis F: A simplification in the use of the NSD concept in practical radiotherapy. *Brit J Rad* 46:529–537, 1973.

Table 2. NSABP Protocol No. 4

	Clinically Negative Nodes			Clinically Positive Nodes	
	RM[a]	TM and RT[b]	TM[c]	RM[d]	TM and RT[e]
Number of patients	354	282	344	277	224
% Failures	20.9	19.1	23.8	37.9	38.4
Local	3.1	0.0	4.9	5.1	1.3
Regional	2.5	2.1	2.9	4.7	6.7
Distant	12.7	14.2	2.8	20.2	24.6
Combinations	2.6	2.9	3.3	7.9	5.7
% Deaths	13.3	14.9	13.4	27.1	26.3

[a]Radical mastectomy.
[b]Total mastectomy and radiation.
[c]Total mastectomy.
[d]Radical mastectomy.
[e]Total mastectomy and radiation.
[f]Patients in each arm of study per protocol with follow-up.

Dr. Eleanor Montague. It was based on the techniques developed and in use at the M. D. Anderson Hospital (21). Initially, the compliance by the multiple institutions was only fair, with between 15% and 20% deviations from the protocol. However, for the last part of the study the deviation rate fell below 5% (22). Here we have some 34 university centers in the United States and Canada fairly uniformly applying megavoltage radiation, 4,500 to 5,000 rad, to the supraclavicular fossa, internal mammary chain, and axilla, using tangential fields to deliver a comparable dose to the chest wall. The TDF of this treatment is around 85. In her own institution in retrospective analyses, the 5- and 10-year survival for patients with radical mastectomy versus radical mastectomy plus peripheral lymphatic irradiation are not different. What is different is the number who had positive axillary nodes and therefore may have benefited from the postoperative radiotherapy. The TDF of the Anderson treatment initially was 93 and currently is 82 (23). It is not unusual for a single institution to report a treatment response rate not derived from a randomized trial that cannot be duplicated in a prospective randomized trial performed in multiple institutions. This has been true not only for studies such as this involving radiotherapy and surgery but many chemotherapy-radiotherapy studies as well. Single institutional studies can be considered pilot studies, but the group trials more closely approach what can be accomplished by the collegium of well-trained oncologists. This, in turn, still has to be translated into community-level treatment if it is to be applicable to the population as a whole.

Brady et al (24), in discussing the role of radiation after mastectomy, conceded that essentially all the clinical trials have indicated "that there was no improvement in the survival rates in the combined treatment. However, in several series diminution in the incidence of local-regional failures has been observed with combined treatment." They go on to point out, however, that the new Norwegian prospective randomized trial reports a statistically significant improved crude and disease-free survival in patients receiving postoperative radiotherapy using cobalt irradiation as compared with those who received 250-kV x-ray or not postoperative radiotherapy (25). One thousand and ninety patients were entered into this trial, 170 of whom were stage I and 95 stage II who received cobalt irradiation. Comparable numbers received 250-kV x-ray or served as surgical controls.

In the beginning there appeared to be a diminution in local-regional recurrences for stage I patients who received the cobalt irradiation, but this was not the case for stage II patients. Actually, there was no advantage associated with any of the three treatment policies for patients with stage I disease. For the patients with stage II disease who received cobalt irradiation there appears to be a significant improvement in survival at four years. However, as Brady and coauthors point out, "patients continually die of their disease up to 15 to 20 years after diagnosis." As it now turns out, the Høst study is not statistically significant at six and seven years. This may indicate a problem in the number of patients at risk at this time. This data is based on a life-table analysis, a statistical method that emphasizes early differences. Had the authors used the *log-rank* analysis method (26), the late effects rather than early differences in survival would have been appreciated.

This study suffers from other difficulties. The patients were assigned to treatment by random number without any attempt at stratification by age, tumor pathology, location, or stage. Furthermore, all patients received ovarian irradiation. The authors reported that a comparison of the two groups of patients regarding age and lymph node involvement shows no difference. A good deal more could be done statistically to validate this statement.

From the radiotherapy point of view this study was important in that the cobalt irradiation dose was approximately 10% higher than previously reported treatment policies. Since it is the contention of many defenders of postoperative radiotherapy for breast cancer that all prior studies had been based on either inappropriate treatment fields or inadequate doses, they look to this study as a major advance. The continued follow-up of these patients is extremely important. Unfortunately, the number of patients in whom these observations will be significant is rather small despite the large number of patients that were initially entered into the study (i.e., 1,090 patients, but only 95 of whom received cobalt irradiation with this higher dosage).

The Cancer Research Campaign Trial referred to earlier (14) indicated that simple mastectomy alone or simple mastectomy combined with routine postoperative radiotherapy in stage I and II disease were not significantly different in terms of overall survival. There was, however, appreciably more local recurrence in patients who had simple mastectomy, and this was especially true in the stage II patients. Logically this leads to their conclusion "this strongly suggests that local recurrences do not act as a significant nidus for subsequent distant dissemination." Of importance is that this study established that "radiotherapy on demand," that is, given at the time local recurrence is diagnosed, in no way altered the chances of survival for the patient. In this study of over 2,000 patients radiotherapy for local recurrences was successful in 75% of the cases. The major argument presented by proponents of routine postoperative radiotherapy is that this treatment significantly reduces the incidence of local recurrence and this in some way affects survivorship. The CRC study clearly showed that there is no relationship between local control and the probability of survival. This is not surprising. It has been apparent that most local-regional recurrence occurs within two years. Control of these recurrences does not impact on the overall survival of the patient as much as the appearance of local-regional recurrence three to five years after surgery (27). In the first instance, chest wall disease tends to be a local manifestation of a generalized problem, and the local control is not enough (28). These patients are candidates for systemic therapy as well as efforts to control the local problem. Despite reports by Tapley et al. (29) that local-regional control for recurrences is not usually successful, Florence Chu has shown approximately a 70% control for patients receiving chest wall irradiation for local recurrences (27). This is in keeping with the CRC study.

Thus one can present the following propositions (Table 3). (*1*) Suppose that we have 100 patients at risk and all 100 receive postoperative irradiation. In the best of all possibilities there would still be approximately a 5% local failure rate. (*2*) Suppose instead that the 100 patients who are at risk are given "radiotherapy on demand." The local-regional failure rate could be expected to be 23% for all stage I and II patients. Seventy percent of group 2 patients could be expected to respond to the radiotherapy. A 30% failure rate of the 23 patients receiving the radiotherapy would result in a total of 7 patients.

Since the control on the chest wall does not affect survivorship of the patients, it would be extremely difficult to establish a significance between the ultimate 5% failure rate for the radiotherapy patients and the ultimate 7% failure rate for the treatment "on demand" patients. How many patients would be necessary in a trial to prove that these were indeed different? In the first proposition all 100 patients would receive radiotherapy, although 77 patients had no need for it and therefore had no chance to benefit from this ministration. In the second proposition only the 23 patients who manifested a clear need for this treatment would receive treatment. Sixteen of the 23 would stand to benefit from it. The overall savings in the use of resources by the community in terms of radiotherapy equipment and personnel, which is generally in short supply and expensive, can be formidable, not to mention patients' time, effort, psychological impact, and the very low, but always present chance, of an untoward effect.

One recently completed study warrants special notice. The Stockholm Breast Cancer Trial randomly assigned 960 patients to one of three treatment plans

Table 3. Treatment of Chest Wall Recurrences

Proposition I	(routine postoperative radiotherapy)	
	100 patients at risk	
	100 patients irradiated	
	5% failure rate	= 5 patients
Proposition II	(radiation on demand)	
	100 patients at risk	
	23 patients irradiated	
	30% failure rate	= 7 patients

(30). One group was treated by a modified radical mastectomy (Patey procedure), another group received postoperative irradiation, and the third group received preoperative irradiation. The analysis of these patients dated January 1, 1977, had a mean follow-up time of 39 months. Less than 400 of these patients have been observed for four or five years. However, using the log-rank method of analysis for differences between the groups and life-table method for survival, there was no significant difference in the patients treated by surgery alone or postoperative radiotherapy. There appears to be some survival benefit for preoperative radiotherapy, which also reduced the incidence of local and regional recurrence. This was particularly important, since distant metastases appeared to be diminished as well. The postoperative radiotherapy afforded control of local and regional disease but did not diminish distant metastases or mortality. Whether the preoperative radiotherapy will remain significantly better than no radiotherapy or postoperative radiotherapy will have to be carefully assessed as this study acquires an increased number of patients at risk five and more years.

It has been argued by some that even if routine postoperative radiotherapy has not been beneficial to all patients, there are special subsets of patients for whom postoperative radiotherapy may well be a benefit. They further argue that these subgroups may be overlooked in larger studies. Patients with a medial or central lesion have a higher incidence of internal mammary node disease. High axillary node involvement is another possibility. Ackerman and Delregado (31) were concerned that internal mammary node involvement was present in approximately half the patients with axillary metastases. Therefore, not only the axilla and supraclavicular fossa but also the internal mammary node chain should be irradiated in those patients with positive axillary disease.

In the large international surgical trial (18) no significant differences in survival were noted when 746 patients treated with a standard Halsted radical mastectomy were compared with another group of 697 patients treated by extended radical mastectomy. The five-year survival rate was 69% for the first group and 72% for the second. There was a slight but not significant improvement in survival when an internal mammary node dissection was done in patients with inner and medial lesions who had positive axillary nodes. This held true only for the small lesions (T_1 and T_2). The argument could be extended, therefore, that patients with inner or medial lesions may stand to benefit from radiotherapy, particularly if an internal mammary node dissection was not performed. Donigan (32) examined the internal mammary nodes of 113 patients on whom he operated and found 22% of them had positive internal mammary node disease. Five patients were treated with radiotherapy and 20 were not. There was no difference in the survival. In this study internal mammary node involvement reflected a generalized tumor spread, and in that situation local therapy can be expected to have a negligible influence. These patients were candidates for systemic therapy rather than local treatment. In another study of patients who showed local recurrences Kagan and Nussbaum carefully analyzed whether the location of the lesion or postoperative radiotherapy had any impact on a subsequent course of events (33). They found that this was not the case. In the large prospective randomized trial of the CRC reported by Murray and Mitchell in England and the NSABP studies of Fischer and his colleagues in the United States the location of the tumor did not influence the outcome after adjuvant radiotherapy.

If the proponents of routine postoperative radiotherapy have difficulty in establishing the legitimacy of their therapy, there are some opponents to routine postoperative radiotherapy who claim an adverse effect of this treatment. Stjernsward has written a number of papers in the last decade arguing against postoperative radiotherapy on the grounds of decreased survival after such treatment (34–36). In his many papers he presents evidence that the radiotherapy diminishes the immunological status of the patient in one way or another, produces leukopenia, and changes the distribution of B and T lymphocytes and that all this has an adverse affect on survival. Although the tests that he has performed may indicate a depressed immunological state, the evidence that this is responsible for a poor host response to the tumor is yet to be established.

Provocative data concerning the late outcome of patients who receive radiotherapy can be derived from a retrospective analysis of patients treated at the Royal Marsden Hospital in London from 1935 to 1945. This study was done by Iris Hamlin, who was looking for evidence of possible host resistance in carcinoma of the breast (37). In this study the clinical stage of the patient plus the grading of the malignancy was considered along with other histological features such as sinus hysticytosis of lymph nodes, mast cell infiltration of the tumor and lymph nodes, and plasma cell populations of the germinal centers of the lymph nodes. These latter characteristics were grouped to grade the host response to the tumor. Taken all together, the grade of the tumor and the host response significantly affected outcome regardless of stage.

Approximately one-third of the patients received postoperative radiotherapy. Of those who received radiotherapy, 23.8% survived 15 years, and 53.3% of those who did not receive radiotherapy survived 15 years. When Dr. Hamlin's data were restructured in a table looking at stage of disease and whether radiotherapy was given or not, it was clear that in each clinical stage, with or without positive nodes, patients who received routine postoperative radiotherapy in the decade of 1935 to 1945 fared worse by 1960 than those who did not receive routine postoperative radiotherapy (Table 4). Clearly, this is a retrospective

Table 4. Carcinoma of the Breast: 15-Year Survival

Clinical Stage	Number of Patients	Negative Nodes		Positive Nodes	
		Postoperative Radiotherapy	No Radiotherapy	Postoperative Radiotherapy	No Radiotherapy
Stage I	59	10:14	16:18	3:16	7:11
		68%	89%	19%	64%
Stage II	76	7:12	9:10	12:39	5:15
		59%	90%	31%	33%
Stage III	137	4:13	5:10	9:90	5:24
		38%	50%	10%	21%
All patients	272	21:39	31:38	24:145	17:50
		54%	82%	17%	34%

Royal Marsden Hospital, 1935–1945.
Data from Hamlin (37).

analysis, and I have regrouped Dr. Hamlin's patients in this analysis. We do not know the selection process by which the patients came to receive radiotherapy, although it had been the practice of some surgeons at the Marsden to give postoperative radiotherapy routinely and others not to. Whether this prevailed in all instances is not certain from these data. Be that as it may, radiotherapy did not add to the chances of surviving. If anything, the irradiated patients had only about a 50% chance of surviving to 15 years as compared with the nonirradiated patients.

In the last decade surgery followed by multiple-drug chemotherapy has become established for patients with breast cancer (38), particularly in premenopausal women and possibly in postmenopausal women (39,40). Most oncologists argue that postoperative radiotherapy does not alter the frequency of distant metastases, nor does it improve the survivorship of patients. Accordingly, what is needed is improved adjuvant chemotherapy to affect the distant disease. Radiotherapy should be reserved for local-regional recurrences and given "on demand."

More recently it has become fairly well-established that patients with one or more positive nodes benefit from three- and five-drug intensive chemotherapeutic regimens (41). In this setting Holland and his coworkers have reported an adverse affect associated with radiation in those patients who were placed on a five-drug (Cooper) program (42). This may be because of diminished tolerance to chemotherapy as well as a delay in the onset of the chemotherapy during the course of postoperative radiotherapy. Nissen-Meyer and colleagues reported on a Scandinavian adjuvant chemotherapy study after mastectomy for carcinoma of the breast (43). Essentially all the patients received postoperative radiotherapy. However, 1 out of the 11 participating institutions delayed the onset of the chemotherapy for two to four weeks. This represented 110 out of a total entry of 1,136 patients. A significant improvement in survival was found in the 1,026 patients who received immediate postoperative chemotherapy but not in the small group who had the delay in the onset of the chemotherapy because of the radiotherapy.

On the other hand, in a study performed by the Cancer and Leukemia Group B (Protocol 7581) and recently reported by Chu et al. a three-week delay in the onset of multiple-drug chemotherapy was not associated with an adverse outcome (44). In that study approximately 50 patients had received routine postoperative radiotherapy and 450 had not. As a group, the patients who had received postoperative radiotherapy fared less well than those women who had not received postoperative radiotherapy. They tolerated significantly less chemotherapy. In the entire group those who received less than 75% of cyclophosphamide fared significantly worse than those who received more than 75% of the required dose, and this may account for their poor showing.

There may have been other reasons for the poor outcome of these women. For instance, to a greater extent the patients who received radiotherapy had larger tumors and more positive axillary nodes, and a higher percentage were postmenopausal than the nonirradiated patients in the study. However, when matched controls were used, the differences in survival did not disappear, although these differences never reached statistically significant levels. In a study reported from the Massachusetts General Hospital Carey and his colleagues were not able to show a difference in survival for irradiated or nonirradiated patients who received either three-drug or five-drug chemotherapy (45).

It is far from clear what influence routine postoperative radiotherapy will have on women who are given adjuvant chemotherapy. In the sequence of surgery, radiotherapy, and then chemotherapy, the delay and diminished dose of chemotherapy tolerated may adversely affect the chances of response. In some other sequence this might not be so. However, since it has been difficult to establish a place for routine postoperative radiotherapy and since adjuvant chemotherapy, particularly for the premenopausal woman with one or more positive nodes, appears to be an important factor in improving prognosis, it is difficult to support the continued use of postoperative radiotherapy in those patients. To the extent that we are still somewhat uncertain about the postmenopausal woman, trials of radiotherapy in different sequences might be indicated; but even in this case it is only a tenuous possibility, particularly since modification of drug dosage and further analysis of the data may indicate a benefit for the postmenopausal woman as well from chemotherapy alone (46).

In the light of the accumulating evidence, how much of a controversy really remains? Stjernswärd polled 32 centers around the world asking whether they used routine postoperative irradiation (47). Of the 26 responses, 25 did not give routine postoperative radiotherapy in patients with negative axillary nodes. There was some hedging in that some would irradiate parasternal nodes for medial or centrally located tumors particularly if it was a high-grade malignancy. For patients with positive axillary nodes 16 out of 26 clinics would give postoperative radiotherapy. However, 12 of the 26 institutions are participating in ongoing studies of one kind or another to establish a better understanding of their current practice or to evolve newer approaches. This accurately reflects the uncertainty that radiotherapists have in continuing to give routine postoperative radiotherapy.

With the compilation of the numerous prospective randomized trials it is difficult to develop yet another study to try to establish the legitimacy of routine postoperative treatment. With the prospect of increasingly effective chemotherapy in an adjuvant setting, it may be more appropriate for the radiotherapist to accept a "watch and wait" policy, being prepared to step in when other treatments have failed.

REFERENCES

1. Pusey WA, Caldwell CW: *Practical Application of Roentgen Rays in Therapeutics and Diagnosis.* Philadelphia, WB Saunders, 1903.

2. Halsted WS: The results of operation for the cure of cancer of the breast performed at the Johns Hopkins Hospital from June, 1889–January 1894. *Ann Surg* 20:497–555, 1894.

3. Harmer MD: Classification and staging, in Hayward JL, Bulbrook RD (eds): *Clinical Evaluation of Breast Cancer.* London, Academic Press, 1966, pp 109–123.

4. Auchinshlos H Jr: The nature of local recurrence following radical mastectomy. *Cancer* 11:611–619, 1958.

5. Urban JA: Role of super-radical operations for breast cancer, in *Sixth National Cancer Conference Proceedings.* Philadelphia, JB Lippincott, 1970, pp 145–151.

6. Lenz M: Tumor dosage and results of roentgen therapy of breast cancer. *Am J Roent Rad Ther* 56:67–74, 1946.

7. Chu FCH, Phillips R, Nickson JJ, McPhee JG: Pneumonitis following radiation therapy of cancer of the breast by tangential technic. *Radiology* 64:642–54, 1955.

8. Meurk ML, Chu FCH: Dose distributions with four radiation technics for carcinoma of the breast. *Radiology* 73:607–617, 1959.

9. Paterson R, Russell MH: Clinical trials in malignant disease. Part III—Breast cancer and evaluation of post-operative radiotherapy. *J Fac Radiol* 10:175–180, 1959.

10. Paterson R: *The Treatment of Malignant Disease by Radiotherapy*, ed 2. Baltimore, Williams & Wilkins, 1963, p 316.

11. McWhirter R: Single mastectomy and radiotherapy in the treatment of breast cancer. *Br J Radiol* 28:128–139, 1955.

12. Johnson RE: Breast cancer. Measurement of effects of treatment. *Cancer* 5:267–270, 1952.

13. Kaae S, Johansen H: Does single mastectomy followed by irradiation offer survival comparable to radical procedures? *Int J Radiat Oncol Biol Phys* 2:1163–1166, 1977.

14. Cancer Research Campaign Report. Management of early cancer of the breast. *Br Med J* 1:1035–1038, 1976.

15. Robbins GF, Lucas JC, Franklin AA, Farrow JH, et al: An evaluation of post-operative prophylactic radiation therapy in breast cancer. *SGO* 122:979–982, 1966.

16. Chu FCH, Lucas JC, Farrow JH, Nickson JJ: Does prophylactic radiation therapy given for cancer of the breast predispose to metastases? *Am J Roent* 99:987–994, 1967.

17. Weichselbaum R, Marck A, Hellman S: The role of post-operative irradiation in carcinoma of the breast. *Cancer* 37:2682–2690, 1976.

18. Lacour J, Bucalossi P, Cacers E, Jacobelli G, et al: Radical mastectomy vs. radical mastectomy plus internal mammary dissection. *Cancer* 37:206–214, 1976.

19. Fisher B, Slack NH, Cavanaugh PJ, Gardner B, et al: Post-operative radiotherapy in the treatment of breast cancer: Results of the NSABP Clinical Trial. *Ann Surg* 172:711–732, 1970.

20. Fisher B, Montague E, Redmond C, Barton B, et al: Comparison of radical mastectomy with alternative treatments for primary breast cancer. *Cancer* 39:2827–2839, 1977.

21. Fletcher GH: *Textbook of Radiotherapy*, ed 2. Chapter 6, in collaboration with Tapley NduV, Montague ED, Brown GR. Philadelphia, Lea and Febiger, 1973, pp 457–496.

22. Hanson W: Personal communication.

23. Fletcher GH, Montague ED: Does adequate irradiation of the internal mammary chain and supraclavicular nodes improve survival rates? *Int J Radiat Oncol Biol Phys* 4:481–492, 1978.

24. Brady LW, Fletcher GH, Levitt SH: Cancer of the breast: The role of radiotherapy after mastectomy. *Cancer* 39:2868–2874, 1977.

25. Høst H, Brennhovd IO: The effect of post-operative radiotherapy in breast cancer. *Int J Radiat Oncol Biol Phys* 2:1061–1067, 1977.

26. Peto R, Pike MC, Armitage P, Breslow NE, et al: Design and analysis of randomized clinical trials requiring prolonged observation of each patient. II. Analysis and examples. *Br J Cancer* 35:1–39, 1977.

27. Chu FCH, Lin FJ, Kim JH, Huh SH, et al: Locally recurrent carcinoma of the breast. *Cancer* 37:2677–2681, 1976.

28. Donigan WL, Perez-Mesa CM, Watson FR: A biostatistical study of locally recurrent breast cancer. *SGO* 122:529–540, 1966.

29. Tapley NduV, in collaboration with Fletcher G, Montague ED: The breast, in Tapley NduV (ed): *Clinical Applications of Electron Beams*, New York, John Wiley & Sons, 1976, pp 219–220.

30. Wallgren A: A controlled study: Pre-operative versus post-operative irradiation. *Int J Radiat Oncol Biol Phys* 2:1167–1169, 1977.

31. Ackerman LV, DelRegardo JA: *Cancer: Diagnosis, Treatment and Prognosis*, ed 3. St. Louis, CV Mosby, 1962, p 1111.

32. Donigan WL: The influence of untreated internal mammary metastases upon the course of mammary cancer. *Cancer* 39:533–538, 1977.

33. Kagan AR, Nussbaum H: Cancer of the breast: Is post-operative irradiation indicated? *Cancer* 29:561–565, 1972.

34. Stjernswärd J, Jondae M, Vanky F, Wigzell H, et al: Lymphopenia and change in distribution of human B and T lymphocytes in peripheral blood induced by irradiation for mammary carcinoma. *Lancet* 2:1352–1356, 1976.

35. Stjernswärd J: Decreased survival correlated to local irradiation in "early" operable breast cancer. *Lancet* 2:1285–1286, 1974.

36. Stjernswärd J: Re-evaluation of the role of routine use of post-operative radiotherapy in operable breast cancer, in Montague ACW, Stonesifer GL, Luvison EF (eds): *Breast Cancer*. New York, AR Liss, Oncology, 1977, pp 405–424.

37. Hamlin IME: Possible host resistance in carcinoma of the breast: A histological study. *Br J Cancer* 22:383–401, 1968.

38. Schabel FM Jr: Rationale for adjuvant chemotherapy. *Cancer* 39:2875–2882, 1977.

39. Bonadonna G, Brusomolino E, Valagussa P, Rossi A, et al: Combination chemotherapy as an adjuvant treatment in operable breast cancer. *New Engl J Med* 294:405–410, 1976.

40. Bonadonna G, Rossi A, Valagussa P, Banfi A, et al: The CMF program for operable breast cancer with positive axillary nodes. *Cancer* 39:2904–2915, 1977.

41. Cooper RG, Holland JF, Glidewell O: Adjuvant chemotherapy of breast cancer. *Cancer* 44:793–798, 1979.

42. Holland JF, Glidewell O, Cooper RG: Adverse effect of radiotherapy on adjuvant chemotherapy of breast cancer. *SGO* (in press).

43. Nissen-Meyer R, Kjellgren K, Malmio K, Mänsson B, et al: Surgical adjuvant chemotherapy results with one short course with Cyclophosphamide after mastectomy in breast cancer. *Cancer* 41:2088–2098, 1978.

44. Chu FCH, Weinberg V, Glicksman AS, Holland JF, et al: The long term effect of post-operative radiation therapy given prior to adjuvant chemotherapy in patients with early stage breast cancer. Presented at the 21st meeting of the American Society of Therapeutic Radiologists, New Orleans, May 1979.

45. Carey RW, Sohier WD, Kaufman S, Weitzman SA, et al: Five drug adjuvant chemotherapy for breast cancer. *Cancer* 44:35–41, 1979.

46. Holland JF: Personal communication.

47. Stjernswärd J: Adjuvant radiotherapy trials in breast cancer. *Cancer* 39:2846–2867, 1977.

11

Combined Modality Treatment of Small Cell Carcinoma of the Lung

James D. Cox

INTRODUCTION

Small cell carcinoma of the lung (SCCL) has been recognized as a distinct entity since 1926, when it was described as "oat-celled sarcoma" or "medullary carcinoma of the mediastinum" (1). The Committee of Pathologists, chaired by Kreyberg, who drafted the World Health Organization classification, placed small cell carcinoma as the second of four major types of carcinoma of the lung (2). They subclassified small cell carcinoma into fusiform, polygonal, and lymphocyte-like, which included "oat-cell" carcinoma. There is, as yet, no general agreement that this subclassification of SCCL has clinical significance. Therefore, for the purposes of this discussion, small cell carcinoma is considered a single entity.

The Veterans Administration Lung Group (VALG) initiated systematic studies of patients with carcinoma of the lung in 1958. Careful histopathologic review by a three-member panel, using the proposed WHO classification, was an integral part of these studies from their inception. The VALG found SCCL to be the most rapid to disseminate and kill of all the types of bronchopulmonary cancer. Patients who received only supportive care had a median survival of less than three months (3). In patients with *limited disease*, defined as tumor confined to one hemithorax and the ipsilateral supraclavicular nodes, the median survival was about four months. Survival was not improved by irradiation of the thoracic disease in such patients (4). However, it must be noted that even with limited disease, the tumor burden was often massive, the pretreatment evaluation of these patients for metastasis was not rigorous by contemporary standards, and the irradiation was administered with conventional x-ray generators in over 90% of the Veterans Administration hospitals. With very careful selection, a few patients with localized SCCL can be cured by surgical resection (5). However, Matthews et al. reported autopsy findings from 19 patients with SCCL who died within 30 days of curative resection and found that 13 (68%) of patients had demonstrable residual disease (6).

Britain's Medical Research Council conducted a trial that compared surgical resection with thoracic irradiation for patients with operable SCCL. Of 144 evaluable patients, 73 were to receive irradiation and 71 were assigned to the thoracotomy group. Only 48% of the latter group actually had a complete resection; 85% of the irradiated group completed the planned course of treatment. Ten years after completion of this study, 3 patients were free of disease in the group assigned to radiotherapy. Only 4% of patients in the thoracotomy group survived 2 years, and the only long-term survivor had refused thoracotomy and had been treated successfully with irradiation (7). The irradiated patients received total doses ranging from 2,000 rad in 10 days to 6,600 rad in 42 days (8), which indicates the lack of agreement and, indeed, the lack of information about the dose-time relationships required for local control of SCCL.

PATTERNS OF FAILURE AFTER TREATMENT

Since there is such a high failure rate after treatment with either surgery or irradiation, it is important to assess the patterns of treatment failure. Such an analysis is undertaken with the expectation that different approaches to therapy will be suggested.

A prospective randomized trial by the VALG compared thoracic irradiation (5,000 to 6,000 rad in four to six weeks) with the same irradiation plus CCNU* and hydroxyurea. All patients had limited disease and a performance status on the Karnofsky scale (9) of 30 or higher. The patients with SCCL who received combined irradiation and chemotherapy had a median survival of 38 weeks compared with a median of 29 weeks for those who received only thoracic irradiation. However, survival beyond the median was identical for the two groups (10). The first site of failure was also similar for the two groups, although the median time to failure was somewhat longer for the patients who received chemotherapy (11).

The first sites of clinical failure are shown in Table 1 for 17 patients with SCCL treated only by thoracic irradiation and the 14 patients who received irradiation plus CCNU and hydroxyurea. Of the 28 patients who failed, 25% first showed progressive disease within the field of irradiation. The large proportion of patients who died without clinical evidence of disease progression usually had some complication from the tumor in the lung or mediastinum. It is notable that no patient failed first in the brain. As we shall see, the frequency of clinically apparent intracranial metastasis increases with improved systemic therapy and prolonged survival.

Another approach to patterns of failure is the evaluation of the causes of death based on autopsy findings. Since survival is the most common end point of clinical trials with SCCL, it is important to understand the lethal events. Of 300 consecutive autopsies of VALG patients treated with one or two chemotherapeutic agents, with or without thoracic irradiation, 57 pateints had small

---

*1-(2-Chloroethyl)-3-cyclohexyl-1-nitrosourea.

Table 1. Small Cell Carcinoma—Limited Disease

First Site of Failure after Irradiation ± CCNU and Hydroxyurea	
Local	7 (25%)
Lungs	5 (18%)
Bone	1 (3.5%)
Brain	0
Liver	1 (3.5%)
Other distant	2 (7.0%)
Death without progression	12 (43%)
	28 100%
No failure	3

cell carcinoma (11). The causes of death are listed in Table 2. If a patient had any metastasis beyond the thorax, carcinomatosis was listed as the cause of death. No patient had brain metastasis alone, that is, without other metastasis. Deaths from infection, hemorrhage, and respiratory failure, and perhaps cardiac failure represent complications of the primary tumor and involved mediastinal lymph nodes. It is clear that local failure is a major problem, but wide dissemination is found in most patients.

The brain is an important site of metastasis in SCCL because of both the frequency and the grave prognostic import of this site of involvement. As has been shown convincingly in acute lymphocytic leukemia, the central nervous system (CNS) is a *sanctuary* region, which chemotherapeutic agents do not reach with sufficient concentration to be effective with administered systemically.

At autopsy, 40% to 50% of patients with SCCL have brain metastasis. Four hundred autopsies between 1969 and 1978 that included brain examination revealed 82 patients with SCCL; 37 (45%) had brain metastasis (12). An extensive review of the literature reported by Bunn et al. (13) showed that 11% (33:292) of patients with SCCL had brain metastasis and 22% (73:325) had clinical evidence of intracranial disease after chemotherapy. It was thought that the lipid soluble nitrosoureas, especially CCNU, which is active and widely used for SCCL, might decrease the occurrence of brain metastasis. However, chemotherapy trials

Table 2. Small Cell Carcinoma of Lung

Causes of Death	
Carcinomatosis	40 (70%)
CNS	—
Infection	6 (11%)
Hemorrhage	4 (7%)
Respiratory failure	2 (3%)
Heart failure	5 (9%)
	57 100%

that included a nitrosourea also yielded a 22% (55:253) CNS failure rate (14). CNS metastases were found at autopsy in 42% (309:740) of patients with SCCL. In more recent chemotherapy series without prophylactic treatment of the CNS, 63% (60:95) of patients who came to autopsy had CNS metastasis. Furthermore, the metastases involved the leptomeninges, the spinal canal, and the spinal cord. As patients with SCCL live longer, metastasis to the central nervous system has been found more frequently. Nugent et al. reviewed the records of 209 patients with SCCL treated at the National Cancer Institute–Veterans Administration Medical Oncology Branch between 1969 and 1977. Prolonged survival was associated with increased frequency of CNS metastasis. They found that the cumulative actuarial probability of developing CNS metastasis rose to 80% for patients who survived two years (15).

DEVELOPMENT OF CHEMOTHERAPY

The unusual responsiveness to chemotherapy of small cell carcinoma, in comparison with the other histologic types of carcinoma of the lung, has been recognized for at least 30 years. An extensive review in 1977 (16) summarized the response rates to a large number of cytotoxic drugs used as single agents. Responses to nitrogen mustard were published as early as 1949. With response rates of 20% to 40% for at least 15 different drugs, the development of combination chemotherapy was predictable. A recent survey of this development (13) showed a definite superiority of the multiagent combinations over chemotherapy with single drugs.

The high response rates and improved median survivals with combination chemotherapy have led many to conclude that irradiation plays little or no role except for palliation of patients with extensive disease. It is assumed that control of intrathoracic disease is no more important than control at any other site, and control even of bulky disease can be accomplished with chemotherapy alone. To relegate radiotherapy only to a palliative role, it also must be assumed that patients who develop brain metastases can be salvaged with therapeutic cranial irradiation, thus making prophylactic irradiation unnecessary. There are sufficient data to show that these assumptions are false.

A word must be said about staging and restaging procedures. All investigators acknowledge that SCCL is, for all practical purposes, disseminated at the time of diagnosis. However, much has been made of the differences in median survival between limited and extensive disease. As will be seen, some patients with limited disease, perhaps 15% to 20% are alive and well for rather long periods after aggressive treatment; some may be cured (17). However, one must be certain that improved survival is not simply the result of a process of rigorous selection. As more extensive pretreatment evaluations are carried out, including computed tomography of the brain, thorax, and upper abdomen, peritoneoscopy with directed hepatic biopsies, multiple bone marrow biopsies, and so on, smaller proportions of patients are found to have limited disease. These patients may have a more favorable prognosis regardless of treatment. For example, the median survival of 33 patients with limited disease SCCL who were treated in VALG protocol 13 L (1971 to 1974) was 22 weeks. In protocol 15 (1974 to 1978), patients with limited disease who were only irradiated survived a median of 31 weeks. The improvement in median survival in the more recent study was due to selection of patients with higher performance status and more thorough studies to eliminate patients with dissemination.

To determine if progress is actually being made with SCCL, it is important to avoid reporting only selected, favorable subgroups such as limited disease patients (after very aggressive staging) and complete responders (after very aggressive restaging). It is also important to evaluate survival beyond the median in all patients. Two treatment programs can differ in median survival but can have the same long-term survival (10). Conversely, median survival may be the same with different regimens, but long-term survival rates may be strikingly different. The real test of improved treatment is a better long-term survival for the entire group of patients.

LOCAL-REGIONAL CONTROL WITH IRRADIATION

The rapid clinical and roentgenographic response of SCCL to irradiation was appreciated many years ago. In the first edition of their classic text, Ackerman and del Regato noted that some tumors "... show a definite, often marked radiosensitivity." They further observed that "in more undifferentiated tumors, in spite of greater radiosensitivity, the difficulty lies in the metastatic spread ..." (18).

The rate and degree of response of SCCL to irradiation led many to conclude that total doses lower than those used with other carcinomas of the lung were sufficient. Other investigators were impressed that rapid regrowth followed the rapid response of these tumors if total doses were not carried to high levels. A review of existing prospective trials for SCCL revealed a range of dose-fractionation regimens from 3,000 rad in 2 weeks to 7,500 rad in 11 weeks (19). To define more precisely the dose required to control SCCL, 35 patients who received local-regional irradiation without concomitant chemotherapy at The Medical College of Wisconsin (MCW) were analyzed retrospectively (19). Variations of total dose, fractionation, and time were reduced to the nominal standard dose (NSD) of Ellis (20) by the formula

$$\text{NSD} = \frac{D}{N^{0.24}T^{0.11}}$$

where D is the total dose (rad), N is the number of fractions, and T is the number of days for the course of treatment. The NSDs ranged from 1,165 to 2,055 with a median of 1,647 (approximately 5,500 rad in 5½ weeks, five fractions per week). Sixteen patients (46%) failed within the field of irradiation; seven patients (20%) failed to respond completely, and nine (26%) recurred after initial disappearance of tumor. Below the median NSD of 1,647, 67% (12:18) of tumors persisted or recurred. Above the median NSD, only 24% (4:17) recurred [Fig. 1 ($P = .01$)].

Since chemotherapy is essential in the management of patients with SCCL, it is important to appreciate the dose-time relationships for irradiation combined with cytotoxic drugs. Figure 1 shows a high local control rate in the MCW

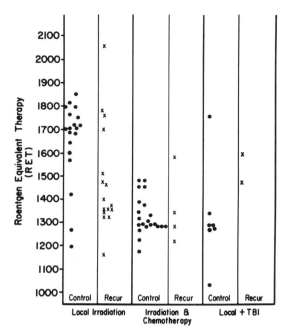

Figure 1. Control of thoracic tumor by treatment group and biologic dose.

experience when low doses of irradiation—NSD of approximately 1,300 (3,000 rad in 10 fractions in two weeks)—are combined with effective chemotherapy. Most of these patients were entered in a randomized, prospective study that compared total body irradiation (TBI) with chemotherapy as systemic adjuvants to local-regional irradiation (21). Patients who failed after TBI were immediately treated with chemotherapy. There was no evidence that TBI prolonged the time to progression, nor did it decrease bone marrow tolerance to the chemotherapy, which consisted of cyclophosphamide, 600 mg/m²; doxorubicin (Adriamycin), 25 mg/m²; and vincristine, 1.4 mg/m², IV on days 1 and 8 repeated every 28 days for eight cycles. Local control was achieved in 82% (28:34) of patients in spite of the very modest doses of irradiation.

The dose of irradiation and the efficacy of the chemotherapy regimen are critical to the achievement of permanent control in the intrathoracic tumor. Lyman et al. (22) used the same chemotherapy but limited the dose of irradiation to 3,000 rad in 20 fractions in four weeks (NSD ≅ 1,110); 36% (8:22) patients failed in the chest. Williams et al. (23) used 3,000 rad in two weeks (NSD ≅ 1,300) with a combination of cyclophosphamide, vincristine, procarbazine, and CCNU and observed a 62% (8:13) thoracic failure rate. It is important to minimize the dose of irradiation to the chest in order to minimize short- and long-term morbidity, but any reduction in biologic dose is dependent on a highly effective chemotherapy regimen.

A further word should be said about total body irradiation as a systemic form of therapy. TBI was used as adjuvant therapy in nine patients who received 3,000 rad in two weeks to the primary and mediastinal disease. Eight patients were included in the randomized study noted above (21), and one patient received TBI after she refused chemotherapy. All patients had limited disease or had a positive bone marrow biopsy as the only evidence of dissemination. The TBI consisted of 10 fractions of 10 rad, five days per week, for a total of 100 rad in two weeks. Two patients recurred locally, and all developed distant metastases. Chemotherapy with CAV was started as soon as failure was documented. The survival of these patients ranged from 17 to 112 weeks with a median of 43 weeks. We concluded that TBI, in the dose used, could not control micrometastasis from SCCL, and we could not justify a trial of higher dose TBI, since it would almost certainly interfere with subsequent chemotherapy.

LOCAL CONTROL AND SURVIVAL

At this point, the question must be asked whether local control of the tumor has any effect on survival of patients with SCCL, especially those with extensive disease. The initial report from MCW indicated there was no difference in median survival for patients whose thoracic disease was controlled compared with those who failed in the chest (19). However, evaluation of long-term survival gave quite a different picture (24).

Of the 35 patients whose initial treatment was only thoracic irradiation (26 limited disease, 9 extensive disease), 19 (54%) remained free of recurrence within the field of irradiation. A comparison of those controlled with those failing locally showed identical median survivals, but survival beyond the median was much better for the patients who had local control (Fig. 2). Although there were few local failures among the 34 patients in later studies who received local-regional irradiation and chemotherapy, the effect of local control on long-term survival was even more striking (Fig. 3). As more effective chemotherapy has prolonged survival, control of the usually bulky intrathoracic disease has increased in importance. It is an axiom that local control is essential for cure, that is, long-term survival free of disease.

LOCAL CONTROL WITH CHEMOTHERAPY ALONE

The marked improvement in the ability of combination chemotherapy to render patients with SCCL free, at least temporarily, of all clinical evidence of disease raises the question whether irradiation of the chest is necessary. Many if not most chemotherapists assume there is no role for thoracic irradiation of patients with extensive disease, since only a part of the known disease can be treated and the irradiation might interfere with aggressive chemotherapy. A randomized study of combination chemotherapy with or without irradiation for patients with extensive disease showed no difference in rates of response, sites of failure, or survival (23). As noted before, the dose of irradiation used in that study (3,000 rad in two weeks), combined with effective chemotherapy, has yielded a high local control rate at MCW.

The argument against radiation therapy of patients with limited disease contends that complete response rates are so high that irradiation adds little to

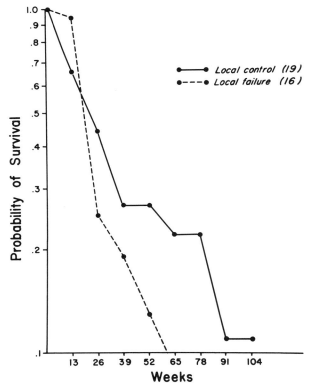

Figure 2. Effect of local control on survival after irradiation.

response, may increase morbidity, and certainly compromises bone marrow tolerance. An extensive review of the literature led Bunn et al. to conclude that radiotherapy might be unnecessary and could conceivably be deleterious when used with appropriate combination chemotherapy (13).

The most recently completed study at the MCW was designed specifically to address the question of the necessity of thoracic irradiation. Patients were entered on Study III if they had a Performance Status of 50 or more and histologic or cytologic confirmation of SCCL. All patients received immediate prophylactic brain irradiation to a dose of 2,500 rad (measured at the midsagittal plane) in 10 fractions in two weeks. Patients were begun simultaneously on combination chemotherapy with cyclophosphamide, 900 mg/m^2; doxorubicin (Adriamycin), 60 mg/m^2; and vincristine, 2 mg/m^2, administered intravenously every three weeks for six cycles. Irradiation to the local-regional disease was withheld until (*1*) there was failure of continued response during the six cycles of chemotherapy, (*2*) there was any evidence by chest roentgenogram, tomogram, or CT scan of residual thoracic disease at the end of six cycles, or (*3*) there was evidence of progression or recurrence at any time. If a complete response was found after thorough reevaluation following six cycles of chemotherapy (restaging included all studies that were initially abnormal except repeat bronchoscopy), treatment was stopped and the patients were followed. Table 3 shows the complete response

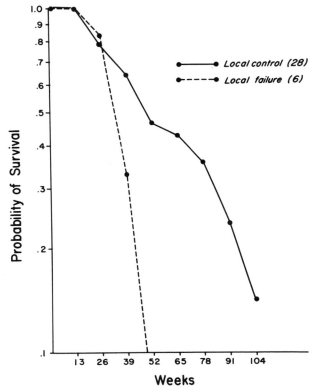

Figure 3. Effect of local control on survival after irradiation plus chemotherapy.

rate with this chemotherapy regimen was 70% (21:30). Seven patients with extensive disease had partial response (≥ 50% reduction of all evident tumor) for an overall response rate of 93% (28:30). However, Table 4 shows the fate of the 21 patients with complete responses. Nine failed at the site of the primary or nodal disease between 2 and 10 months after the last cycle of chemotherapy. When it was apparent that the thoracic failure rate was unacceptably high, the last 5 patients entered in the study actually received chest irradiation as a departure from the protocol. Four of these 5 patients are free of disease 6 to 12 months after the start of treatment. Two additional patients are undergoing reevaluation after completing their sixth cycle of chemotherapy. They will also

Table 3. Small Cell Carcinoma of Lung MCW Study III Rates of Complete Response

Number patients	30	
Limited: extensive	11:19	
Complete response: limited	11:11	100%
Complete response: extensive	10:19	53%
Complete response: total	21:30	70%

Table 4. Small Cell Carcinoma of the Lung MCW Study III Thoracic Failure after Complete Response

Number patients	21
Thoracic failure alone	6
Thoracic failure + metastases	3
Elective thoracic irradiation	5
Thoracic failure rate	56% (9 of 16)

receive thoracic irradiation, but they have been included among the 7 patients who are still free of disease with chemotherapy alone. Nonetheless, the thoracic failure rate of 56% (9:16) in the face of such high response rates from this particular chemotherapy program indicates clearly that thoracic irradiation is essential for control of the primary and mediastinal disease. Of the 9 patients who had local failure, 4 are dead (median survival 55 weeks), 4 are alive with disease (median survival 67 weeks), and 1 is free of disease at 46 weeks (10 weeks after chest irradiation for recurrence). These experiences coupled with the analysis that demonstrated the importance of local control on survival even for patients with extensive disease (24) lead us to conclude that thoracic irradiation is essential for all patients with SCCL, regardless of extent of disease. The irradiation must be timed so as not to compromise the chemotherapy. In our present study (IV), local-regional irradiation is administered after restaging following the sixth cycle of chemotherapy. Irradiation encompasses the original sites of gross disease to a minimum tumor dose of 3,750 rad in 10 fractions in three weeks.

Reports of treatment programs that have consistently included both thoracic and prophylactic brain irradiation, plus highly effective combination chemotherapy, have documented long-term survival free of disease. Three studies have used such irradiation combined with cyclophosphamide, doxorubicin, and vincristine. The study from the National Cancer Institute, most recently reported by Brereton et al. (25), used several different fractionation schedules for the thoracic irradiation, ranging from 3,000 rad in 30 fractions, 1 fraction per day, to 3,000 rad in five consecutive days (200 rad per fraction × 3 each day). They had a 66% (33:50) complete response rate, but 13 patients (26%) failed in the chest, and 10 patients (20%) died of treatment related complications. Many complications resulted from the very intensive fractionation schemes and the simultaneous administration of doxorubicin. Nonetheless, their 29 patients with limited disease have an actuarial disease-free survival of 36% at two years. None of the patients with extrathoracic metastases remains free of disease.

Lyman et al. (22) used the same drugs, but they systematically delivered 3,000 rad in 20 fractions in four weeks, both to the local-regional tumor and the entire brain. The irradiation was administered after the first two cycles of chemotherapy. Complete responses were achieved in 40% of 35 patients (13 limited, 22 extensive). Six patients were alive and free of disease more than 12 months.

Greco et al. (26) used a similar regimen in 32 patients with disease limited to the thorax. They reported complete responses in 29 patients (91%). Fourteen patients were free of disease 8 to 28 months after the start of treatment, with 10 followed more than 12 months, and 3 followed more than 24 months.

These studies all show a survival advantage for the responders over those who fail to respond and the necessity of complete response for long-term survival. Most patients who respond completely have limited disease and successfully complete the treatment program. It is impossible to compare results from one study with another, however, since the survival curves are based on selected subgroups instead of the total number of patients treated with a given regimen.

PROPHYLACTIC IRRADIATION OF THE BRAIN

As already noted, justification for prophylactic brain irradiation is derived from the recognition that at least 20% of patients with SCCL develop clinical evidence of brain metastasis, and, at autopsy, the rate is two or three times higher. Komaki et al. (27) reported the clinical sites of metastasis in patients with inoperable carcinoma of the lung of all cell types, with a view toward the potential for prophylactic irradiation. A summary of the ongoing prospective studies showed, with one exception, only patients with SCCL were being treated prophylactically, and cranial irradiation was the major point of focus. A collection of 11 studies, most of which were not randomized, found clinical failure in the brain in only 8% (29:355) of patients who had prophylactic treatment (14).

The VALG studied prophylactic brain irradiation in patients with carcinoma of the lung of all cell types who had limited disease. All patients were required to have negative radionuclide brain scans before entry into the study. The patients received local-regional irradiation but did not receive chemotherapy. Half the patients received prophylactic brain irradiation to 2,000 rad in two weeks. A preliminary report showed a much higher rate of brain metastasis in patients with small cell carcinoma of the lung than with the other cell types but did not demonstrate any effectiveness of brain irradiation with the dose used (28). More recent data from this study for the 42 patients with SCCL showed that 33% of patients without and 22% of patients with prophylactic cranial irradiation developed brain metastasis. This was not a significant difference ($P = .24$).

The Radiation Therapy Oncology Group (RTOG) and the Eastern Cooperative Oncology Group (ECOG) entered patients with SCCL in a randomized trial to investigate prophylactic brain irradiation. All patients received local-regional irradiation and were randomized to immediate or delayed chemotherapy with cyclophosphamide and CCNU (29). The most recent data show that the difference between the chemotherapy approaches did not significantly alter the median survival or the failure pattern or rate. However, 3 of 99 patients (3%) who received cranial irradiation to 3,000 rad in two weeks developed brain metastasis, compared with 18 of 101 patients (18%) who had no brain irradiation ($P < .01$).

Three additional randomized trials were summarized by Bunn et al. (14). Of 127 patients without cranial irradiation, 35 (28%) failed in the brain. Only 6% (6:103) of patients with prophylactic irradiation developed brain metastases, and 4 of these were not found until autopsy.

It is not yet clear whether survival is altered by prophylactic cranial irradiation. Metastases in patients with SCCL rarely occur exclusively in the brain (11,12). As we have seen with assessment of the effectiveness of local tumor control on survival, it is quite possible that median survival is not altered but there is an impact on long-term survival. Again, it is axiomatic that cure of patients with SCCL necessarily demands effective prevention or control of the CNS disease.

It might be argued, indeed, that prevention is unnecessary. If only 25 of every 100 patients with SCCL develop clinical brain metastases, and 5 to 8 will fail in spite of prophylactic treatment, 80+ patients would uselessly be irradiated. Furthermore, if irradiation for established metastases could be delivered promptly and were very effective, therapeutic irradiation would be more reasonable than prophylactic treatment.

In order to evaluate the effectiveness of therapeutic brain irradiation, we reviewed our recent experience with patients having SCCL who developed brain metastasis. From 1974 to mid-1979, 40 of 188 patients (21%) seen at MCW with SCCL had clinical evidence of brain metastasis. Twenty-three patients (12%) had brain metastases, and 17 (9%) developed brain metastasis after treatment with thoracic irradiation and chemotherapy. (The low clinical failure rate is due to the consistent use of prophylactic irradiation in the past two years.) Seven patients manifested intracranial failure 12 months or more after the initial treatment, and the longest interval was 23 months.

These patients were treated to the entire brain with doses of 3,000 rad in two weeks to 4,000 rad in three weeks. Fifteen patients (38%) had complete response (CR) with return to normal neurologic function; 15 (38%) had partial response (PR) with improvement, but definite neurologic sequelae; 10 patients (25%) had little or no response or had progression. Survival did not correlate with the initial degree of neurologic impairment but was affected by the response to irradiation. Median survivals were 52 weeks for patients with CR, 17 weeks for those with PR, and 3 weeks for those with no change or deterioration of neurologic function. The corresponding six-month survivals were 58%, 34% and 0% respectively.

There was no difference in survival between the 23 patients with initial and the 17 patients with delayed brain metastasis when survival was calculated from the diagnosis of intracranial involvement. Table 5 shows the current status of the patients in this study. Half the patients have died as a direct result of CNS disease, and two of the four survivors have recurred and required retreatment. Only one patient is free of disease. He did not have any neurologic symptoms or signs but was found to have an abnormal radionuclide brain scan during the

Table 5. Current Status of Patients with Brain Metastasis from Small Cell Carcinoma of the Lung

Dead from brain metastasis	18
Dead from extracranial metastasis	18
Alive with disease[a]	3
Alive and well	1
	40

[a]2 patients recurred in brain and reirradiated.

initial evaluation. He is well 11 months after cranial and thoracic irradiation and systemic chemotherapy with cyclophosphamide, doxorubicin, and vincristine.

If these response and survival experiences are representative of what can be expected from therapeutic brain irradiation in the setting of effective control of extracranial metastases, it must be concluded that prophylactic brain irradiation is essential to assure the greatest possibility for long-term disease-free survival. As noted previously, more effective systemic therapy is associated with a higher clinical CNS failure rate, a rate that may eventually reach 80% if patients live 24 months or more (15). Using the most current data available, it must be assumed that 80 of every 100 patients with SCCL are at risk for the development of brain metastasis, and no more than half of them could be controlled with irradiation. Even if 5 patients develop brain metastasis after prophylactic irradiation, some 35 patients will still benefit from such treatment.

CONCLUSIONS

Small cell carcinoma is the most aggressive and, historically, the most lethal form of bronchopulmonary cancer. It responds rapidly and often completely to irradiation or chemotherapy. There is a striking interaction with effective chemotherapy such that a high tumor control probability can be achieved with quite modest doses of irradiation. Even the most highly effective chemotherapeutic regimens are unable to eradicate bulky disease with sufficient consistency to preclude local-regional irradiation. Local control improves survival and is a *sine qua non* for cure of patients with SCCL.

Chemotherapy is unable to control subclinical disease within the CNS. However, combination chemotherapy is now so effective against extracranial metastases that most patients with SCCL eventually fail in the brain. Therapeutic brain irradiation salvages only half the patients with clinical intracranial metastases, and this proportion might decrease as survival is further prolonged with more effective drug combinations. Therefore, prophylactic brain irradiation is required for maximum disease control.

The changing patterns of failure after treatment of SCCL may well indicate future needs for radiation therapy. CNS failures outside the brain may justify the use of craniospinal irradiation. It might also be fruitful to irradiate other sites of bulky disease beyond the chest after an initial regression is achieved with chemotherapy. It will continue to be important to search for optimal use of both irradiation and cytotoxic drug combinations to overcome this fascinating but dread disease.

REFERENCES

1. Barnard WG: The nature of the "oat-celled sarcoma:" of the mediastinum. *J Pathol Bacteriol* 29:241–244, 1926.
2. Kreyberg L, Liebow AA, Uehlinger EA: *Histological Typing of Lung Tumors.* Geneva, World Health Organization, 1967.
3. Hyde L, Yee J, Wilson R, Patno ME: Cell type and the natural history of lung cancer. *JAMA* 193:52–54, 1965.

4. Wolf J, Patno ME, Roswit B, D'Esopo N: Controlled study of survival of patients with clinically inoperable lung cancer treated with radiation therapy. *Am J Med* 4:360–367, 1966.

5. Higgins GA, Shields TW, Keehn RJ: The solitary pulmonary nodule: Ten-year follow-up of Veterans Administration–Armed Forces Cooperative Study. *Arch Surg* 110:570–575, 1975.

6. Matthews MJ, Kanhouwa S, Pickren J, Robinette D: Frequency of residual and metastatic tumor in patients undergoing curative surgical resection for lung cancer. *Cancer Chemother Rep* (pt 3)4:63–67, 1973.

7. Fox W, Scadding JG: Medical Research Council Comparative trial of surgery and radiotherapy for primary treatment of small-celled or oat-celled carcinoma of bronchus: Ten year follow-up. *Lancet* 2:63–65, 1973.

8. Scadding JG: Comparative trial of surgery and radiotherapy for the primary treatment of small-celled carcinoma of the bronchus. *Lancet* 2:979–986, 1966.

9. Karnofsky DA, Burchenal JH: The clinical evaluation of chemotherapeutic agents in cancer, in MacLeod CM (ed): *Evaluation of Chemotherapeutic Agents.* New York, Columbia University Press, 1949, pp 191–205.

10. Petrovich Z, Ohanian M, Cox J: Clinical research in the treatment of locally advanced lung cancer: Final report of VALG Protocol 13 Limited. *Cancer* 42:1129–1134, 1978.

11. Cox JD, Yesner R, Mietlowski W, Petrovich Z: Influence of cell type on failure pattern after irradiation for locally advanced carcinoma of the lung. *Cancer* 44:94–98, 1979.

12. Cox JD, Yesner R: Adenocarcinoma of the lung: Recent results from the Veterans Administration Lung Group. *Am Rev Respir Dis* 120:1025–1029, 1979.

13. Bunn PA Jr, Cohen MH, Ihde DC, Shackney SE, et al: Review of therapeutic trials in small cell bronchogenic carcinoma of the lung, in Muggia F, Rozencweig M (eds): *Lung Cancer (Progress in Therapeutic Research,* vol 11). New York, Raven Press, 1979, pp 549–558.

14. Bunn PA Jr, Nugent JL, Matthews MJ: Central nervous system metastases in small cell bronchogenic carcinoma. *Semin Oncol* 5:314–322, 1978.

15. Nugent JL, Bunn PA Jr, Matthews MJ, Ihde DC, et al: Central nervous system metastases in small cell bronchogenic carcinoma: Increasing frequency and changing pattern with lengthening survival. *Cancer* 44:1885–1893, 1979.

16. Broder LE, Cohen MH, Selawry OS: Treatment of bronchogenic carcinoma: II. Small cell. *Cancer Treat Rev* 4:219–260, 1977.

17. Minna JD, Brereton HD, Cohen MH, Ihde DC, et al: The Treatment of small cell carcinoma of the lung: Prospects for cure, in Muggia F, Rozencweig M (eds): *Lung Cancer (Progress in Therapeutic Research,* vol 11). New York, Raven Press, 1979, pp 593–599.

18. Ackerman LV, del Regato JA: *Cancer: Diagnosis, Treatment and Prognosis,* ed 1. St. Louis, The CV Mosby Company, 1947, p 461.

19. Cox JD, Byhardt RW, Wilson JF, Komaki R, et al: Dose-time relationships and the local control of small cell carcinoma of the lung. *Radiology* 128:205–208, 1978.

20. Ellis F: The relationship of biologic effect of dose-time-fractionation factors in radiotherapy, in Ebert M, Howard A (eds): *Current Topics in Radiation Research.* Amsterdam, North Holland Publishing Co, 1968, pp 357–397.

21. Byhardt RW, Cox JD, Wilson JF, et al: Total body irradiation versus chemotherapy as a systemic adjuvant for small cell carcinoma of the lung. *Int J Radiat Oncol Biol Phys* 5:2043, 1979.

22. Lyman GH, Hartmann RC, Saba HI, Preston D, et al: Combination chemotherapy and radiation therapy of undifferentiated small cell bronchogenic carcinoma. *South Med J* 71:519–525, 1978.

23. Williams C, Alexander M, Glatstein EJ, Daniels JR: Role of radiation therapy in combination with chemotherapy in extensive oat cell cancer of the lung. *Cancer Treat Rep* 61:1427–1431, 1977.

24. Cox JD, Byhardt R, Komaki R, Wilson JF, et al: Interaction of thoracic irradiation and chemotherapy on local control and survival in small cell carcinoma of the lung. *Cancer Treat Rep* 63:1251–1255, 1979.

25. Brereton HD, Kent CH, Johnson RE: Chemotherapy and radiation therapy for small cell car-

cinoma of the lung: A remedy for past therapeutic failure, in Muggia F, Rozencweig M (eds): *Lung Cancer (Progress in Therapeutic Research*, vol 11). New York, Raven Press, 1979, pp 575–586.

26. Greco FA, Richardson RL, Snell JD, Stroup SL, et al: Small cell lung cancer: Complete remission and improved survival. *Am J Med* 66:625–630, 1979.

27. Komaki R, Cox JD, Eisert DR: Irradiation for bronchial carcinoma. II. Pattern of spread and potential for prophylactic irradiation. *Int J Radiat Oncol Biol Phys* 2:441–446, 1977.

28. Cox JD, Petrovich A, Paig C, Stanley K: Prophylactic cranial irradiation in patients with inoperable carcinoma of the lung: Preliminary report of cooperative trial. *Cancer* 42:1135–1140, 1978.

29. Seydel HG, Creech RH, Mietlowski WL, Perez CA: Preliminary report of a cooperative randomized study for the treatment of localized small cell lung carcinoma. *Int J Radiat Oncol Biol Phys* 5:1445, 1979.

12

Is Combined Modality Treatment of Small Cell Carcinoma of the Lung Necessary?

Joseph Aisner

INTRODUCTION

Small cell undifferentiated carcinoma of the lung accounts for approximately 20% of all lung cancer (1). It is now recognized as a distinct clinical pathologic entity (2) with unique biological behavior including rapid tumor proliferation, high labeling index, short doubling time, and large proliferative fraction (3). These features are seen clinically as a short symptomatic period with abrupt presentation, early tumor dissemination, and a short median survival of six to eight weeks in untreated patients (4–6). Although it has been recognized for some time that this tumor is sensitive to both radiation and chemotherapy (7), in the past such therapies have generally been palliative. Recently aggressive treatments using either combination chemotherapy alone or combination chemotherapy and radiotherapy have resulted in significant prolongation of median survival and occasional long-term disease-free survival (7–14). Clearly this suggests the potential for cure, and this has created an enthusiasm for treatment. Many treatment programs use various combinations of the active drugs with and without radiotherapy delivered either concomitantly or sandwiched between courses of chemotherapy. It has been argued that both treatment modalities are necessary—radiotherapy to control the local disease and chemotherapy to treat the disseminated disease (15–18). It is currently unclear however, whether chemotherapy alone might achieve similar results. The purpose of this chapter is to examine the relative contributions of each treatment modality.

SMALL CELL BRONCHOGENIC CARCINOMA IS A DISSEMINATED DISEASE

Until recently there were essentially no long-term survivors of this disease (19,20). Large surgical series showed five-year survivals of less than 1% in patients undergoing complete resection (19,20) and less than 5% in patients undergoing

155

radiotherapy (20). Radiotherapy alone results in a short median survival of less than four months (21), and most patients die with metastatic disease. The American Joint Committee for Cancer Staging and End Results Reporting concluded for lung cancer "stage grouping . . . is significant for all cell types except undifferentiated small cell (oat cell) carcinoma in which there is no significant relationship between stage and survival rates" (19). In one necropsy series of patients undergoing apparent complete resection distant metastases were documented in nearly 70% (22). These data have led to the recognition that even if the tumor is technically resectable, surgery has essentially no role in the treatment of small cell carcinoma of the lung. (What about the very occasional long-term survivors reported in the literature with only regional therapy? (20,23). Although one may find small cell carcinoma in an apparently localized form, the majority of these patients develop recurrence and die of disease.) In a study of asymptomatic solitary pulmonary nodules where undifferentiated small cell carcinoma represented only 4% of the tumors (contrasted to the usual proportion of 20% further showing the rarity of this presentation) the five-year survival was only 36% (23). This strongly suggests that isolated small cell carcinoma is distinctly unusual and that even when it appears to be isolated there usually are widespread micrometastases. Early dissemination of this disease is therefore the rule and the majority of the patients have disease outside the thorax with metastases involving bone marrow, liver, and brain as well as other organs (2,14,-24,25). Nearly all patients have regional metastases with involvement of the hilar or mediastinal nodes (2,25). When these patients are not treated with systemic therapy (e.g., when patients with thoracic disease are treated with only regional treatment such as surgery or radiotherapy) the extrathoracic disease becomes rapidly manifest, and the patients die of metastatic disease (28). When radiotherapy is given to patients with apparently limited disease, 80% have manifest metastatic disease within one year (29). Thus, regardless of our ability to document the metastases, this disease should be, and is now, considered a systemic process with at least micrometastases involving multiple organs.

WHAT IS THE PRIMARY TREATMENT MODALITY?

When all lung cancers were approached as a single disease and small cell carcinoma of the lung was approached surgically, the postoperative morbidity and mortality exceeded the five-year survival rate (25). Radiotherapy for small cell carcinoma became "standard therapy" when it was recognized that surgical resection did not favorably alter the natural history of the disease and radiotherapy provided some local regression with a modest prolongation of survival for patients with limited disease (20,30). Patients with extensive disease, however, achieved no improvement in survival with the use of radiotherapy alone (7,9). During the time in which radiotherapy is administered, the micrometastases grow and may become clinically evident, converting the patient's status to disseminated disease. Highly optimistic projections of a survival rate of more than two years for patients having disease confined to the thorax treated with radiotherapy alone would be approximately 4%. Thus, although local "control" may be important for local symptoms, such control is of secondary importance to the overall treatment strategy if long-term disease-free survival is the goal. Radiotherapy alone can therefore no longer be considered the principal therapy for small cell carcinoma.

Many chemotherapeutic agents have also been shown to produce tumor regression in small cell carcinoma of the lung (7,31,32). Single-agent chemotherapy has, however, produced only transient incomplete tumor regressions with only modest palliation. Complete responses were infrequent, and median duration of survival from the time of chemotherapy was usually less than 20 weeks (7,33). With the success of combination chemotherapy in a variety of other human neoplasms (34) it was logical that combinations of active drugs should be applied to small cell carcinoma of the lung. It was the application of such combination chemotherapy regimens that provided for a much higher complete remission rate and the very pronounced prolongation of median survival in this disease (5,7–14). Since small cell carcinoma of the lung must now be considered a systemic disease in all circumstances and since combination chemotherapy is the currently available form of systemic therapy, combination chemotherapy must be considered the primary treatment modality for small cell carcinoma of the lung. Irradiation of the primary disease, if necessary, should be considered an adjunct to the primary treatment modality; that is, radiotherapy is an adjunct to combination chemotherapy. In many centers, irradiation of the primary and some metastatic sites is included in the treatment program. Is the radiotherapy still administered because it was the first palliative therapy? In view of the response to chemotherapy, is there a need for radiotherapy?

STAGING AND RESTAGING

The most important prognostic factor in small cell carcinoma of the lung is the extent of clinically evident disease. Patients are staged according to gross extent as either having limited disease—all disease confined to one hemithorax exclusive of pleura but possibly including mediastinal and ipsilateral scalene and lower cervical nodes—or extensive disease—any disease beyond the confines of the definition of limited disease. This limited-extensive staging system was introduced primarily for its suitability to radiotherapy, the principal modality of nonsurgical therapy available at the time of introduction of the staging system. Limited disease is thus that extent of tumor which can be encompassed by a single radiotherapy port. This staging system has proved to be of prognostic importance. Patients with limited disease are more likely to respond to therapy and achieve complete remissions, and they have longer durations of survival than patients with extensive disease (5,28). Recently it has been further recognized that certain patients with extensive disease do less well than others (35).

The therapeutic implications of the staging system are less clear. Limited-extensive staging might have important therapeutic value if different treatment modalities were applied to different stages. If, however, all stages were treated similarly (e.g., with combination chemotherapy alone) or if certain isolated extrathoracic sites (e.g., bone or bone marrow) did not carry similar prognostic information (35), the staging system might need to be reconsidered in terms of site of involvement or total tumor burden. Currently, most studies use aggressive staging procedures in order to stratify the patients for therapy carefully according to extent of disease. These staging procedures include bronchoscopy, chest roentgenography (plain roentgenograms and whole lung tomograms), liver scans, bone scans, bilateral iliac crest bone marrow aspirates and biopsies, and computerized tomographic brain scans (24). Some studies, in addition, do peritoneoscopy and liver biopsies (24). Although many studies carefully stage the patients before treatment, it is unclear whether all studies restaged the patients as carefully once there was an alleged change of status. Thus, in many studies, complete remission (complete disappearance of all signs and symptoms of disease) may have been documented simply by chest roentgenography and not by bronchoscopy, tomograms, scans, and repeat biopsies. This is of particular importance among the patients who received radiotherapy to the primary site because the irradiation may have produced tumor shrinkage with associated normal tissue fibrosis. This could potentially lead to some confusion between residual disease and fibrosis and muddles the classification of complete response.

COMPLETE REMISSIONS

The importance of achieving complete remission in human cancers has already been emphasized (34). Many investigators have established that patients with small cell lung cancer who achieve complete remission survive significantly longer and with a better quality of life than those who do not achieve complete remission (5,8,10–14,28,36,37). In the studies at the Baltimore Cancer Research Program (BCRP) all the patients who have achieved long-term (> 2 years) disease-free survival are those patients with limited disease who have achieved complete remission (8,36). This is a common finding in other recent studies (9–13,37) and strongly suggests that the potential for cure in this disease rests on the ability to achieve eradication of demonstrable disease. The question that arises is whether combination chemotherapy can produce as high (or higher) complete remission rates as high as or higher than those produced by combined modality therapy (combination chemotherapy plus radiotherapy).

If one were to review much of the earlier chemotherapy studies which used single agents or combinations of only two drugs, one would certainly find a low complete remission rate (5,7,28,33), and one might infer from the combined modality studies performed at that time that local irradiation enhanced the remission rate. It has subsequently been demonstrated that three drugs in combination are superior to two drugs, and four drugs (depending on the combination) may be superior to three (5,7,38). Thus in the current era—combination chemotherapy using three or more drugs in combination administered aggressively to maximum tolerated doses—the complete remission rate is much higher and comparable with that seen with combined modality therapy. Tables 1 to 4 review the therapeutic experience in a selected group of recent studies using chemotherapy alone (Tables 1 and 3) or combined modality treatment (Tables 2 and 4) for limited (Tables 1 and 2) and extensive disease (Tables 3 and 4). One must consider that for each category these are a heterogenous group of reported studies. However, if one looks only at the range of total response in

Table 1. Chemotherapy Alone in Limited Disease Small Cell Carcinoma of the Lung

Combination	Number of Patients	Response %		Median Survival (Weeks)
		CR	Total	
CYC, ADR, VP16 ± MER[8,36]	30	>63[a]	87	58+
CYC, ADR, VP16 + CCNU, VCR, MTX, PROC[36]	20	>60	90	46+
CYC, CCNU, MTX + ADR, VCR, PROC[13]	19	74	100	58
CYC, ADR, VCR, BLEO[39]	4	100	100	56
CYC, ADR, VCR[40]b	18	50	75	50+
CYC, CCNU, MTX[41]b	69	NS	92	58
	164	64[c]	90	[d]

CR = complete remission; NS = not stated; CYC = Cyclophosphamide; ADR = Doxorubicin; VP16 = VP16–213; MER = methanol extracted residue of BCG; VCR = Vincristine; MTX = Methotrexate; PROC = Procarbazine; BLEO = Bleomycin.

[a]Part of an ongoing study with patients still improving.

[b]Part of a prospectively randomized trial comparing chemotherapy alone with combined modality therapy.

[c]Percent CR based on denominator of 91 patients (total of all stated values).

[d]Range 46+ to 58+ weeks.

general, complete remission (where stated in the reports) and the duration of survival, there are remarkable similarities between chemotherapy alone and combined modality therapy. These treatments are similar when one compares limited disease treatments (Tables 1 and 2) or extensive disease treatments (Tables 3 and 4). Certainly, the combined modality treatments are not any better. (It might be argued that such comparisons are not entirely valid, since there are a wide variety of selection factors as well as the degrees of staging and restaging.) However, the large number of patients should override this concern. Furthermore, in each of the categories there are prospectively randomized studies that compare chemotherapy alone with combined modality treatments (40,41,50). In each of these randomized studies, there is no difference in the groups with respect to response rates or survival. Overall the ranges of survival achieved with chemotherapy alone are comparable with the ranges seen with combined modality. Several recent reports of combined modality treatment project a slightly higher percentage of long-term survival than other studies (11,12). The projected survival in one of these studies, however, has shown progressive deterioration on sequential analyses (11,52) so that the final percent of long-term survivors has not yet been determined. Comparing the projected survival curves in these recent studies with the survival of patients with limited disease seen at the Baltimore Cancer Research Center (Fig. 1), one sees that the curves are remarkably similar except for the tail end of the curve. In the BCRP curve there

Table 2. Combined Modality Therapy in Limited Disease Small Cell Carcinoma of the Lung

Drug Combinations	Radiation (Rad)	Number of Patients	Response %		Median Survival (Weeks)
			CR	Total	
CYC, ADR, VCR[40]a	3,500 sandwich[a]	14	71	100	56
CYC, MTX, CCNU[41]a	4,000 split sandwich[a]	65	NS	87	45
CYC, ADR, VCR[11]	Variable concurrent	29	80	83	NS
CYC, ADR, VCR + VP16, HMM[12]	3,000 concurrent	32	90	100	64+
CYC, ADR, VCR[9]	4,500 sandwich	108	41	75	52
CYC, ADR, VCR[42]	6,000 split sandwich	20	55	70	38
CYC, ADR, VCR, BCG[10]	4,500 split sandwich	16	31	70	52
CYC, CCNU, VCR, PROC[43]	3–5,000 sandwich	12	40	70	58
CYC, VCR, MTX[43]	3–5,000 sandwich	11	40	70	42
CYC, ADR, VCR, MTX, PRED[44]	4–5,000 sandwich or concurrent	24	NS	65	NS
CYC, ADR, VCR + VP16 DDP[45]	4,500 sandwich or concurrent	17	65	95	NS
CYC, ADR, VCR, BCG[46]	3,600 split sandwich	19	79	100	78
CYC, ADR, VCR + CCNU, MTX, PROC[47]	2,500 sandwich	66 / 433	24 / 50[b]	83 / 82	47 / c

SPLIT = split course technique; NS = not stated in publication; sandwich = RT given between courses of chemotherapy; concurrent = RT started together with first course of chemotherapy; CYC = Cyclophosphamide; MTX = Methotrexate; ADR = Doxorubicin; VCR = Vincristine; VP16 = VP16–213; HMM = Hexamethylmelamine; PROC = Procarbazine; PRED = Prednisone.

[a]Part of a prospectively randomized trial comparing chemotherapy alone with combined modality therapy.
[b]CR rate based on denominator of 354 patients (total of literature stated numbers).
[c]Range = 38 to 78 weeks and 3 without stated medians.

Table 3. Chemotherapy Alone in Extensive Disease Small Cell Carcinoma of the Lung

Combination	Number of Patients	Response %		Median Survival (Weeks)
		CR	Total	
CYC, ADR, VP16 ± MER[8,35]	44	40[a]	86	32 +
CYC, ADR, VP16 + CCNU, VCR, MTX, PROC[36]	23	30[a]	79	31 +
CYC, MTX, CCNU[38]	52	NS	75	25
CYC, MTX, CCNU, VCR[38]	53	NS	78	33
CYC, MTX, CCNU + ADR, VCR, PROC[13]	42	36	91	38
CYC, ADR, VCR, BLEO[39]	25	8	72	39
CYC, ADR, VP16 + BCNU, VCR, MTX, PROC[48]	15	20	87	35 +
CYC, MTX, CCNU[49]	73	NS	81	37
CYC, MTX, CCNU, VCR + ADR, VP16[49]	73	NS	90	37
CYC, CCNU, VCR, PROC[50]b	12	42	82	44
	412	31[c]	83	d

CR = complete remission; NS = not stated; CYC = Cyclophosphamide; ADR = Adriamycin; VP16 = VP16-213; MER = methanol extracted residue of BCG; VCR = Vincristinens; MTX = Methotrexate; PROC = Procarbazine; BLEO = Bleomycin.

[a]Part of an ongoing study with patients still improving.

[b]Part of a prospectively randomized trial comparing chemo alone with combined modality therapy.

[c]Percent CR based on denomintor of 149 (total, NS).

[d]Range 25 to 44.

are 50 patients from two consecutive studies (8,36) and the total follow-up is longer so that the final survivals in the other studies will probably be similar.

Based on the data above, particularly the prospectively randomized studies (40,41,50), radiotherapy as an adjuvant apparently does not add to survival when the radiotherapy is sandwiched between chemotherapy courses. Some of the combined modality studies in which radiotherapy was begun concurrently with aggressive combination chemotherapy have projected survivals that appear superior to other published reports (11,12). One must remember, however, that these are projected survival data and that the final survival data are necessary before one may conclude that concurrent irradiation is of benefit. One study in which concurrent irradiation was compared with sandwiched radiotherapy concluded that there was no difference in response or survival attributable to the timing of the radiotherapy (44). Therefore, although it is unlikely that the timing of the radiotherapy will change the situation, we must still await definitive prospective studies before we will be able to evaluate the role of radiotherapy begun concurrently with chemotherapy.

Table 4. Combined Modality Therapy in Extensive Disease Small Cell Carcinoma of the Lung

Drug Combinations	Radiation	Number of Patients	Response % CR	Response % Total	Median Survival (Weeks)
CYC, CCNU, VCR, PROC[50]a	2,500 chest sandwich 2,000 liver sandwich 2,000 lungs sandwich	13	38	70	36
CYC, ADR, VCR[11]	Variable	21	48	62	45
CYC, ADR, VCR[9]	3,000 chest sandwich	258	14	56	25
CYC, ADR, VCR, MTX, PRED[44]	4,500 Chest concurrent or sandwich	37	NS	48	NS
CYC, MTX, CCNU[51]	4,000 chest sandwich	53	NS	86	47
CYC, MTX, CCNU[51]	4,000 chest sandwich 4,000 abdomen sandwich	51	NS	88	43
CYC, ADR, VCR[46]	3,600 chest split sandwich	39	20	80	36
CYC, ADR, VCR + CCNU, MTX, PROC[47]	2,500 chest sandwich	81	10	65	36
		553	16[b]	65	c

MED = median; SURV = survival; NS = not stated in publications; SPLIT = split course technique; SAND = RT given between courses of chemotherapy; concurrent = RT started together with first course of chemotherapy; CYC = Cyclophosphamide; PROC = Procarbazine; ADR = Adriamycin; MTX = Methotrexate; PRED = Prednisone.

aPart of a randomized trial comparing chemotherapy alone to combined modality therapy.

bCR rate based on denominator of 412 patients (total, NS).

cRange = 25 to 47 weeks.

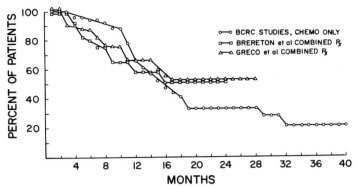

Figure 1. A comparison of published actuarial survivals from combined modality studies—Brereton et al. (11) and Greco et al. (12)—with the actuarial survival of patients at the BCRC on two consecutive chemotherapy alone studies. Although there appears to be a lower plateau on the BCRC, studies there has been a longer follow-up. Two patients without cranial irradiation relapsed with CNS only disease, proved at necropsy.

THE ISSUE OF LOCAL CONTROL

One of the strongest arguments used for the application of adjuvant radiotherapy to the primary and possibly other sites of disease has been that of local control. It is argued that without attaining "adequate" local control, long-term disease-free survival or cure cannot be obtained. This is only part of the issue. If local control were the determining factor in long-term survival, local disease progression would be the causal factor in death. Instead, distant metastases are the causal factor in the patient's demise in the majority of cases, regardless of the original extent of disease. Therefore, it is not local control that determines long-term survival but rather attainment of complete remission. Furthermore, local control, whether defined by disappearance of the primary tumor or sites or recurrence, can also be achieved with combination chemotherapy. The determination of the adequacy of local control can only be measured by the local recurrence rate (see below).

Another argument in favor of local irradiation is the special circumstance in which patients have superior vena cava syndrome. This clinical situation can progress rapidly and may require immediate treatment (53–55). There is a feeling among some that radiotherapy is the treatment of choice for this complication (53,54). Nevertheless, even in patients with limited disease, survival following radiotherapy is short (53), and there is general agreement that the superior vena cava syndrome is a poor prognostic factor even with aggressive radiotherapy (55). Superior vena cava obstruction from small cell lung cancer is, however, highly responsive to chemotherapy so that it is possible to achieve rapid tumor lysis with systemic combination chemotherapy (56). At the BCRC, patients who had superior vena cava obstruction were all treated with immediate combination chemotherapy alone, and all achieved complete disappearance of the signs and symptoms of the superior vena cava syndrome. The survival for these patients is similar to the survival for all the other patients treated on two consecutive protocols (8,36). This type of data has led to the recognition that chemotherapy alone is appropriate initial therapy for superior vena cava obstruction from small cell lung cancer (56,57). Combination chemotherapy can thus produce local regressions to produce local control. The percentage of local regressions and local control achieved by chemotherapy alone is very likely a function of the drugs and dosage used, as in radiotherapy, where within limits there appears to be a dose response relationship (15). To determine adequacy of local control, however, one must examine the sites of relapse.

SITES OF RECURRENCE

If patients who received irradiation to the primary site (thoracic site) failed only in extrathoracic sites and if patients who received only combination chemotherapy tended to fail primarily in the thoracic site, this would be a strong and cogent argument for the addition of radiotherapy to the primary site and the delivery of combined modality treatment. Tables 5 and 6 review some of the recurrence data for chemotherapy and combined modality treatments, respectively. This information is very heterogenous, with some authors reporting local relapses for the entire study group and other reporting the data only for those achieving a complete remission. In general, failures in the thoracic site occur between one-fourth ($\frac{1}{4}$) and one-half ($\frac{1}{2}$) of all cases irrespective of the treatment modalities applied. In the studies at the Baltimore Cancer Research Center, less than one-fourth of the patients analyzed for recurrence recurred or progressed in the thoracic site alone, and more than 75% of the patients, irrespective of the extent of disease, recurred in the extrathoracic sites (8,36). The range of failure rate in the thoracic site is similar for chemotherapy alone and combined modality therapy. Thus, one could argue that irradiation to the primary site does not afford much more local control than does combination chemotherapy. One might argue that the radiotherapy delivered in these combined modality therapies was not of sufficient dose to sterilize the primary site and thus the recurrence rate is similar for both chemotherapy alone and combined modality treatments. There is surprisingly little information on dose response considerations in small cell carcinoma of the lung, although and one study suggests a dose response phenomenon with local control being achieved at doses 4,500 rad (15). However, local failures were seen at high doses ($\geq$ 4,500 rad) of local irradiation, (9,11,43,58), further suggesting that even such high dose radiotherapy does not entirely sterilize the treatment field.

In one prospectively randomized study in extensive disease, the addition of radiotherapy to combination chemotherapy neither improved survival nor changed the patterns of relapse (50). These data have led many investigators to suggest that, except for cranial irradiation, radiotherapy has no role in the management of extensive disease small cell carcinoma of the lung. Such a posture is logical, since patients with extensive disease must have extrathoracic disease control to achieve any survival benefit. If there is little advantage in adding radiotherapy to combination chemotherapy for extensive disease in terms of survival or local control, one must question the benefit of using this treatment

Table 5. Relapse in Thoracic Site Following Chemotherapy for Small Cell Carcinoma of the Lung

Treatment	Patients with Extent of Disease			Patients Analyzed for Recurrence			No. with Chest Only Recurrence		
	Lim	*Ext*	*NS*	*Lim*	*Ext*	*NS*	*Lim*	*Ext*	*NS*
CYC, ADR, VP16 ± MER ± CCNU, VCR, MTX, PROC[8,36]	50	67		37	58		9	10	
CYC, CCNU, MTX + VCR, ADR, PROC[13]	19	42		14 CR	15 CR		5	5	
CYC, CCNU, VCR, PROC[48]a		12			12			7	
CYC, ADR, VP16 + BCNU, VCR, MTX, PROC[46]		15			15			1	
CYC, CCNU, MTX[37]			32			24			10
	69	136	32	51	100	24	14	23	10
		237			175			47	

NS = extent of disease not specified; CR = complete remissions; CYC = Cyclophosphamide; ADR = Doxorubicin; VP16 = VP16–213; MER = methanol extracted residue of BCG; VCR = Vincristine; MTX = Methotrexate; PROC = Procarbazine.

aPart of a prospectively randomized trial comparing chemotherapy alone with combined modality treatment.

Table 6. Relapses in Thoracic Sites Following Combined Modality Treatment Small Cell Carcinoma of the Lung

Chemotherapy	Radiation	Patients with Extent of Disease			Number Analyzed For Recurrence			No with Chest only Recurrence			Comment
		Lim	Ext	NS	Lim	Ext	NS	Lim	Ext	NS	
CYC, ADR[58]	3,000 sand or split / 4–5,000 sand			27			19			12	No differences in recurrence rate, although rad dose delayed chest recurrence
CYC, CCNU, VCR, PROC[48]a	2,500 chest sand										
CYC, ADR, VCR[12]	3,000 conc	32	13		11	13		2	8		
CYC, ADR, VCR[9]	4,500 sand	108			28			9			258 patients with ext disease nearly all failures in areas previously involved
CYC, CCNU, VCR, PROC[43]	3–5,000 sand	23			23			8			Relapses in 5/8 in CR: 2 at 5,000 R; 2 at 4,000 R; 1 at 3000 R
CYC, ADR, VCR[11]	Variable up to 6,000 R conc	29	21		8 CR	10 CR		6	4		
CYC, ADR, VCR + CCNU[47], MTX, PROC	2,500 sand			147			74			14	
Total		192	34	174	70	23	93	25	12	26	
		420			186			63			

NS = not specified; Sand = radiation delivered between courses of chemotherapy; Split = Split course technique; Conc = irradiation started together with first course of chemotherapy; CYC = Cyclophosphamide; ADR = Doxorubicin; VCR = Vincristine; PROC = Procarbazine; MTX = Methotrexate.

aPart of a prospectively randomized trial comparing chemotherapy alone with combined modality treatment.

modality in limited disease. Limited disease is, after all, a widely disseminated process whereby the extrathoracic metastases cannot be clinically documented. Thus, it is not surprising that the comparative trials failed to show a survival benefit for patients given adjuvant irradiation. Since most patients eventually recur or fail in distal sites, the current problem to be addressed is adequate total (rather than local) control. When and if combination chemotherapy produces better control of the distal disease, the issue of local control may become important. Currently the problem would appear to rest with more or better chemotherapy.

THE COMPLICATIONS OF COMBINED MODALITY TREATMENT

Since it is unclear whether radiotherapy adds to either local control or survival, why not just "hedge" and add the radiotherapy anyway? Are there specific side effects or toxicities that could make the use of radiotherapy counterproductive? There are recent reports that suggest that large doses of radiotherapy are needed to treat the intrathoracic disease (15,16,18). Thus, radiotherapy in the doses and field sizes necessary to produce regressions of "bulk disease" at the primary site may be associated with severe complications, including severe life-threatening and lethal radiation pneumonitis (9,11,12,16,59,60) and esophagitis with severe dysphagia and occasional strictures (9,11,12,16,60–62). In addition, other complications may be seen such as radiation pericarditis (16), radiation myelitis (16), and other radiotherapy complications that have been seen as a result of aggressive irradiation of the mediastinum in lung cancer (16) and Hodgkin's disease (63), such as coronary heart disease and hypothyroidism. These have important implications for long-term management. When radiation and chemotherapy are given concurrently, the possibility for enhanced radiation skin reactions and severe esophagitis occurs (64,65), and these may be of such severity as to require nasogastric or parenteral tube feeding. In one report, 5,000 rad was given concurrently with chemotherapy, and the rate of esophageal, skin, and other toxicities was unexceptably high. The toxicity continued at a high rate despite reduction of the dose to 4,400 rad and finally necessitated separating the treatment modalities (64). These complications are in addition to the complications that are associated with combination chemotherapy, are unavoidable in view of the necessity of the drug treatment, and may be potentiated by the irradiation. Perhaps of greater consequence is the fact that the radiation field sizes may be of significant magnitude as to produce some further compromise of marrow function. This is of importance, since, as discussed above, the primary treatment modality is combination chemotherapy that is limited in most cases by myeloid toxicity. Thus any treatment that has the potential for compromising the ability to deliver the primary treatment modality, that is, systemic combination chemotherapy, must be viewed with some consideration before being applied on a generalized basis. Furthermore, in view of the success with combination chemotherapy in achieving a few long-term disease-free survivors, it is possible that even more aggressive combination chemotherapy will be attempted in order to ascertain if a larger proportion of patients can be rendered free of disease in the long term.

RADIOTHERAPY AS A SYSTEMIC FORM OF TREATMENT

Other potential approaches to the use of radiotherapy in this disease include either hemibody irradiation or total body irradiation (66). In these approaches, radiotherapy is administered as a systemic form of therapy and is used to treat the entire body as an organ. This conceptually attacks the disease as a systemic process and has shown some evidence of promise in diseases such as non-Hodgkin's lymphoma (67). Unfortunately, the major toxicity from this approach is myeloid toxicity with severe dose-limiting toxicity for subsequent chemotherapy (68). At the BCRP chemotherapy was very difficult to administer after total body irradiation (in lymphomas), with decrease or delays in dosage and premature discontinuation of chemotherapy (68). Further studies using such an approach with radiotherapy are certainly warranted and deserve consideration as part of combined modality therapy. These studies must, however, be investigated with the understanding that they may well impair the ability to deliver any further chemotherapy. If it can be demonstrated that hemibody or total body irradiation alone or combined with combination chemotherapy can significantly alter the long-term disease-free survival, this would certainly be a welcome addition to the therapeutic armamentarium.

WHOLE BRAIN IRRADIATION

Radiotherapy has an unquestionable role in small cell carcinoma of the lung as the treatment modality for brain metastases. Intracranial metastases occur in approximately 10% to 15% of all patients at presentation (4,24,69–71) and can occur during the course of the illness in greater than 33% of the cases (24,70–72). Necropsy series suggest that the incidence of intracranial metastases is significantly higher and may approach as high as 80% (70,71). Once intracranial metastases become clinically evident, they can produce significant neurologic dysfunction with clinical morbidity. On this basis, many studies have added "prophylactic" radiotherapy to treat the micrometastases and avert the clinical complications of the metastatic disease. This has been done on both a randomized and nonrandomized basis, producing somewhat conflicting results (5,11,16,-18,36,43,46,50,51,69–76). All studies suggest that prophylactic cranial irradiation does not significantly alter the survival. This, however, may be a function of the poor overall survival and the small fraction that achieves long-term disease control. At the BCRP among patients not receiving brain irradiation, we have seen at least four patients who relapsed in the CNS after long disease-free intervals, and two of these patients were found to have only CNS involvement at necropsy. In most studies, prophylactic cranial irradiation is effective in reducing the clinical incidence of brain metastases. There are, however, reports of brain metastases occurring in spite of prophylactic irradiation (75). However, in this study not all patients were in complete remission and therefore may have reseeded the CNS. In one large study the incidence of brain metastases was similar in both irradiated and nonirradiated groups (51). Here again, however, it is not clear that the peripheral disease was in control before the brain irradiation. Thus, it appears that prophylactic whole brain irradiation reduces but does not totally prevent brain metastases. It is conceiveable, however, that this could be improved by altering the timing, for example, giving the whole brain irradiation after the peripheral disease is in control.

There are recent reports of leptomeningeal carcinomatosis occurring in a proportion (9% to 12%) of the patient population, some in spite of prophylactic cranial irradiation (70,71,77–80). This is seen as a consequence of increasing survival. In general, meningeal carcinomatosis (as with brain metastases) tends to occur in association with systemic relapse (86), but we have seen patients who have relapsed only in the leptomeninges and died.

At the present time, radiotherapy must remain the principal treatment modality for central nervous system metastases, since none of the chemotherapeutic agents tested (including those known to cross the blood-brain barrier) has been effective in treating or preventing the occurrence of brain metastases. On the other hand, cranial irradiation has been insufficient to stop leptomeningeal metastases. Cranial spinal irradiation with sufficiently wide ports to cover all the nerve roots involved would likely obliterate the marrow reserve, and therefore alternative approaches may be needed when there is an improvement in the number of patients achieving long-term disease control.

SUMMARY

Small cell carcinoma of the lung is a disseminated disease regardless of our ability in documenting the micrometastases. Recent advances in this disease have clearly demonstrated that combination chemotherapy is the primary treatment modality. Any treatment form that may potentially compromise the primary treatment modality should be applied if and only if it can be clearly demonstrated to improve both the quality of life and disease-free survival. Analyses of recent multiple studies using state-of-the-art chemotherapy suggest that the complete remission rate from combination chemotherapy alone is at least similar to that from combined modality therapy and that the recurrence rate within the thorax is similar for both combination chemotherapy alone and combined modality treatment. Recent prospectively randomized studies show that radiotherapy when sandwiched between aggressive combination chemotherapy courses adds to neither local control nor overall survival. Most patients fail or recur in distal extrathoracic sites regardless of treatment so that disease progression is a manifestation of inadequate systemic control. What is needed is better control of systemic metastases whether overt or subclinical, and the proper approach to this problem is likely systemic, not local treatment. Aggressive radiotherapy in sufficient doses and field sizes to control local bulky disease is likely to produce the complications of esophagitis and pericarditis especially when coupled with chemotherapy. Furthermore, such field sizes and doses are likely to impair the ability to give more or better combination chemotherapy. Radiotherapy applied as a systemic modality of treatment, that is, as total body irradiation or hemibody irradiation, is an area for further study but must be done cautiously in view of its potential to limit the use of combination chemotherapy. CNS metastases remain a significant clinical problem, and it has been previously predicted that with improvement in survival it becomes a progressively larger clinical problem

(69). Cranial irradiation given to treat the micrometastases before they become clinically overt has become the standard of treatment, but further studies of timing are needed to maximize the effect. Leptomeningeal carcinomatosis is being seen despite prophylactic CNS irradiation and may pose a potential problem if a larger fraction of the patients survive for prolonged periods.

There has been dramatically increased interest in small cell lung cancer, attributable in part to the fact that a large number of studies have demonstrated that small cell carcinoma of the lung is a highly treatable disease. Many of the studies now have long-term disease-free survivors, and some of these have been off all chemotherapy for impressive lengths of time. Although the number of such patients at the present time is small, these studies all suggest the potential for cure. Further exploration of therapeutic alternatives is clearly necessary to improve the percentage of patients who achieve long-term disease-free survival. One avenue of exploration for this purpose will be to add more drugs to established combination chemotherapy. Under these circumstances, it will be necessary to reserve the bone marrow function for the combination chemotherapy, and clearly one can justify the use of combination chemotherapy alone to treat the systemic disease process.

REFERENCES

1. Yesner R, Gelfman NA, Feinstein AR: A reappraisal of histopathology in lung cancer and correlation of cell types with antecedent cigarette smoking. *Am Rev Resp Dis* 107:790–797, 1973.
2. Cohen MH, Matthews MJ: Small cell bronchogenic carcinoma: A distinct clinicopathologic entity. *Sem Oncol* 5:234–243, 1978.
3. Muggia FM, Krezoski SK, Hansen HH: Cell kinetic studies in patients with small cell carcinoma of the lung. *Cancer* 34:1683–1690, 1974.
4. Kato Y, Fergusson TB, Bennett DE, et al: Oat cell carcinoma of the lung. A review of 138 cases. *Cancer* 23:517–524, 1969.
5. Bunn PA, Cohen MH, Ihde DC, et al: Advances in small cell brochogenic carcinoma. *Cancer Treat Rep* 61:333–342, 1977.
6. Cohen MH: Signs and symptoms of bronchogenic carcinoma. *Sem Oncol* 1:183–189, 1974.
7. Broder LE, Cohen MH, Selawry OS: Treatment of bronchogenic carcinoma: II. Small cell. *Cancer Treat Rev* 4:219–260, 1977.
8. Aisner J, Wiernik PH: Chemotherapy versus chemoimmunotherapy for small cell undifferentiated carcinoma of the lung. *Cancer* 46:2543–2549, 1980.
9. Livingston RB, Moore TN, Heilbrun L, et al: Small cell carcinoma of the lung: combined chemotherapy and radiation. *Ann Intern Med* 88:194–199, 1978.
10. Holoye PY, Samuels ML, Smith T, et al: Chemoimmunotherapy of small cell bronchogenic carcinoma. *Cancer* 42:34–40, 1978.
11. Brereton HD, Kent CH, Johnson RE: Chemotherapy and radiation therapy for small cell carcinoma of the lung: A remedy for post therapeutic failure in lung cancer, in Muggia FM, Rozencweig M (eds): *Progress in Therapeutic Research.* New York, Raven Press, 1979, pp 575–586.
12. Greco FA, Chardson RL, Snell JN, et al: Small cell lung cancer: Complete remission and improved survival. *Am J Med* 66:625–630, 1979.
13. Cohen MH, Ihde DC, Bunn PA Jr, et al: Cyclic alternating combination chemotherapy for small cell brochogenic carcinoma. *Cancer Treat Rep* 63:163–170, 1979.
14. Ginsberg SJ, Comis RL, Gottlieb AJ, et al: Long term survivorship in small cell anaplastic lung carcinoma. *Cancer Treat Rep* 63:1347–1349, 1979.

15. Cox JD, Byhardt RW, Wilson JF, et al: Dose-time relationships and the local control of small cell carcinoma of the lung. *Radiology* 128:205–207, 1978.

16. Seydel HG, Creech RH, Mietrowski W, et al: Radiation therapy in small cell lung cancer. *Sem Oncol* 5:288–298, 1978.

17. Ajaikumar BS, Barkley T Jr: The role of radiation therapy in the treatment of small cell undifferentiated bronchogenic cancer. *Int J Rad Oncol Biol Phys* 5:977–982, 1979.

18. Choi CH, Carey RW: Small cell anaplastic carcinoma of the lung: Reappraisal of current management. *Cancer* 37:2651–2657, 1976.

19. Mountain CF: Clinical biology of small cell carcinoma: Relationship to surgical therapy. *Sem Oncol* 5:272–279, 1978.

20. Fox W, Scadding JG: Medical research council comparative trial of surgery and radiotherapy for primary treatment of small celled or oat-celled carcinoma of the bronchus. *Lancet* 2:63–65, 1973.

21. Roswit B, Patno ME, Rapp R, et al: The survival of patients with inoperable lung cancer: A large scale randomized study of radiation therapy vs placebo. *Radiology* 90:688–697, 1968.

22. Matthews MJ, Kanhouwa S, Pickern J, et al: Frequency of residual and metastatic tumor in patients undergoing curative surgical resection for lung cancer. *Cancer Chemother Rep* Part III 4:63–67, 1973.

23. Higgins GA, Shields TW, Keehn RJ: The solitary pulmonary nodule ten year follow-up of Veterans Administration–Armed Forces Cooperative Study. *Arch Surg* 110:570–575, 1975.

24. Hansen HH, Dombernowsky P, Hirsch FR: Staging procedures and prognostic features in small cell anaplastic bronchogenic carcinoma. *Sem Oncol* 5:280–287, 1978.

25. Matthews MJ: Problems in morphology and behavior of bronchopulmonary malignant disease, in Israel L, Chahinian AP (eds): *Lung Cancer: Natural History Prognosis and Therapy*. New York, Academic Press, 1976.

26. Mountain CF: Surgical therapy in lung cancer: Biologic, physiologic and technical determinants. *Sem Oncol* 3:253–258, 1974.

27. Laing AH, Berry RJ, Newman CR, et al: Treatment of small cell carcinoma of the bronchus. *Lancet* 1:129–132, 1975.

28. Greco FA, Einhorn LH, Richardson RL, et al: Small cell lung cancer: Progress and perspectives. *Sem Oncol* 5:323–335, 1978.

29. Medical Research Council Lung Cancer Working Party: Radiotherapy alone or with chemotherapy in the treatment of small-cell carcinoma of the lung. *Br J Cancer* 40:1–10, 1979.

30. Carr DT, Childs DS, Lee RE: Radiotherapy plus 5 FU compared to radiotherapy alone for inoperable and unresectable bronchogenic carcinoma. *Cancer* 29:375–381, 1972.

31. Selawry OS: The role of chemotherapy in the treatment of lung cancer. *Sem Oncol* 1:259–272, 1974.

32. Wasserman TH, Comis RL, Goldsmith M, et al: Tabular analysis of the clinical chemotherapy of solid tumors. *Cancer Chemother Rep III* 6:399–419, 1975.

33. Esterhay RJ Jr: Current concepts in the management of small cell carcinoma of the lung. *Am J Med Sci* 274:232–246, 1977.

34. DeVita VT, Schein PS: The use of drugs in combination for the treatment of cancer. *New Engl J Med* 288:998–1006, 1973.

35. Ihde DC, Makuch RW, Cohen MH, et al: Prognostic implications of sites of metastases in patients with small cell carcinoma of the lung given intensive chemotherapy. *Proc ASCO/AACR* 20:264, 1979.

36. Aisner J, Whitacre M, Van Echo DA, et al: Alternating non-cross resistant combination chemotherapy for small cell carcinoma of the lung (SCCL). *Proc ASCO/AACR* 21 (in press).

37. Cohen MH, Creaven PJ, Fossieck BE Jr, et al: Intensive chemotherapy of small cell bronchogenic carcinoma. *Cancer Treat Rep* 61:349–354, 1977.

38. Hansen HH, Dombernowsky P, Hansen M, et al: Chemotherapy of advanced small cell anaplastic carcinoma: Superiority of a four-drug combination to a three-drug combination. *Ann Int Med* 89:177–181, 1978.

39. Einhorn LH, Fee WH, Farber MD, et al: Improved chemotherapy for small-cell undifferentiated lung cancer. *J Am Med Assoc* 235:1225–1229, 1976.

40. Stevens E, Einhorn L, Rohn R: Treatment of limited small cell lung cancer. *Proc Am Assoc Clinical Oncol* 20:435, 1979.

41. Hansen HH, Dombernowsky P, Hansen HS, et al: Chemotherapy versus chemotherapy plus radiotherapy in regional small-cell carcinoma of the lung: A randomized trial. *Proc Am Assoc Cancer Research* 20:277, 1979.

42. Holoye PY, Samuels ML, Lanzotti VJ, et al: Combination chemotherapy and radiation therapy for small cell carcinoma. *JAMA* 237:1221–1224, 1977.

43. Alexander M, Glatstein EJ, Gordon DS, et al: Combined modality treatment for oat cell carcinoma of the lung: A randomized trial. *Cancer Treat Rep* 61:1–6, 1977.

44. Gilbey ED, Bondy PK, Morgan RL, et al: Combination chemotherapy for small cell carcinoma of the lung. *Cancer* 39:1959–1966, 1977.

45. Natale R, Hilaris B, Golbey R, et al: Induction chemotherapy in small cell carcinoma of the lung. *Proc Am Soc Clin Oncol* 20:343, 1979.

46. Einhorn LH, Bond WH, Hornbach N, et al: Long term results in combined modality treatment of small cell carcinoma of the lung. *Sem Oncol* 5:309–313, 1978.

47. Feld R, Pringle J, Evans WK, et al: Combined modality treatment of small cell carcinoma of the lung. *Proc Am Soc Clin Oncol* 20:312, 1979.

48. Abeloff MD, Ettinger DS, Khouri NF, et al: Intensive induction therapy for small cell carcinoma of the lung. *Cancer Treat Rep* 63:519–524, 1979.

49. Dombernowsky P, Hansen HH, Sorensen S, et al: Sequential versus nonsequential combination chemotherapy using 6 drugs in advanced small cell carcinoma: A comparative trial including 146 patients. *Proc Am Assoc Cancer Res* 20:277, 1979.

50. Williams C, Alexander M, Glatstein EJ, et al: Role of radiation therapy in combination with chemotherapy in extensive oat cell cancer of the lung: A randomized study. *Cancer Treat Rep* 61:1427–1431, 1977.

51. Hansen HH, Dombernowsky P, Hirsch F, et al: Intensive combination chemotherapy plus localized or extensive radiotherapy in small cell anaplastic bronchogenic carcinoma: A randomized trial. *Proc Am Soc Clin Oncol* 18:350, 1977.

52. Johnson RE, Brereton HD, Kent CH: Small-cell carcinoma of the lung: Attempt to remedy causes of past therapeutic failures. *Lancet* 2:289–291, 1976.

53. Davenport D, Feree C, Blake D, et al: Response of superior vena cave syndrome to radiation therapy. *Cancer* 38:1577–1580, 1976.

54. Lokich JJ, Goodman R: Superior vena cava syndrome *JAMA* 231:58–61, 1975.

55. Aristizabal SA, Caldwell WL: Radical irradiation with the split-course technique in carcinoma of the lung. *Cancer* 37:2630–2635, 1976.

56. Dombernowsky P, Hansen HH: Combination chemotherapy in the management of superior vena caval obstruction in small cell anaplastic carcinoma of the lung. *Acta Med Scand* 204:513–516, 1978.

57. Greco FA, Oldham RK: Current concepts in cancer: small cell lung cancer. *N Engl J Med* 301:355–358, 1979.

58. McMahon LJ, Herman TS, Manning MR, et al: Patterns of relapse in patients with small cell carcinoma of the lung treated with adriamycin-cyclophosphamide and radiation therapy. *Cancer Treat Rep* 63:359–362, 1979.

59. McKeown J, Bradbury C, Chaudrey A, et al: Pulmonary toxicity probably due to adriamycin-radiation interaction in combined modality therapy for oat cell carcinoma. *Proc Am Soc Clin Oncol* 19:295, 1977.

60. Moore TN, Livingston R, Heilbrun L, et al: An acceptable rate of complications in combined doxorubicin-irradiation for small cell carcinoma of the lung: A Southwest Oncology Group study. *Int J Rad Oncol Biol Phys* 4:675–680, 1978.

61. Chabora BM, Hopfan S, Wittes R: Esophageal complications in the treatment of oat cell carcinoma with combined irradiation and chemotherapy. *Radiology* 123:185–187, 1977.

62. Wittes RE, Hopfan S, Hilaris B, et al: Oat cell carcinoma of the lung: Combination treatment with radiotherapy and cyclophosphamide, adriamycin, vincristine and methotrexate. *Cancer* 40:653–659, 1977.

63. Wiernik PH: Current issues in the management of patients with Hodgkin's disease, in Aisner J, Chang P (eds): *Advances in Cancer Treatment Research.* The Hague, Martinus Nijhoff Publishers, 1980, pp 53–64.

64. Mayer EG, Poneter CA, Aristizabal SA: Complications of irradiation related to apparent drug potentiation by adriamycin. *Int J Rad Oncol Biol Phys* 1:1179–1188, 1976.

65. Aristizabal SA: Complications from combination chemotherapy and irradiation in oat cell lung cancer. *JAMA* 237:1824, 1977.

66. Byhardt RW, Cox JD, Wilson JF, et al: Total body irradiation vs. chemotherapy as a systemic adjuvant for small cell carcinoma of the lung. *Int J Rad Oncol Biol Phys* 5:2043–2048, 1979.

67. Johnson RE: Total body irradiation (TBI) as primary therapy for advanced lymphosarcoma. *Cancer* 35:242–246, 1975.

68. Brace K, O'Connell MJ, Vogel V, et al: Total body radiation therapy for disseminated lymphosarcoma: results of a pilot study. *Cancer Chemother Rep* 58:401–405, 1974.

69. Hansen HH: Should initial treatment of small cell carcinoma include systemic chemotherapy and brain irradiation? *Cancer Chemother Rep* Part II 4:239–241, 1973.

70. Bunn PA, Nugent JL, Matthews MJ: Central nervous system metastases in small cell bronchogenic carcinoma. *Sem Oncol* 5:314–322, 1978.

71. Nugent JL, Bunn PA Jr, Matthews MJ, et al: CNS metastases in small cell bronchogenic carcinoma: Increasing frequency and changing pattern with lengthening survival. *Cancer* 44:1885–1893, 1979.

72. Jackson DV, Richards F II, Cooper R, et al: Prophylactic cranial irradiation in small cell carcinoma of the lung: A randomized study. *JAMA* 237:2730–2733, 1977.

73. Tulloh M, Mourer L, Forcier RT: A randomized trial of prophylactic whole brain irradiation in small cell carcinoma of the lung. *Proc Am Soc Clin Oncol* 18:268, 1977.

74. Matthews MJ: Effects of therapy on the morophology and behavior of small cell carcinoma of the lung a clinico pathologic study, in Muggia F, Rozencweig M (eds): *Lung Cancer: Progress in Therapeutic Research.* New York, Raven Press, 1979, pp 155–165.

75. Levitt M, Meikle A, Murray N, et al: Oat cell carcinoma of the lung: CNS metastases in spite of prophylactic brain irradiation. *Cancer Treat Rep* 62:131–133, 1978.

76. Moore TN, Livingston R, Heilbrun L, et al: The effectiveness of prophylactic brain irradiation in small cell carcinoma of the lung. *Cancer* 41:2149–2153, 1978.

77. Greco FA, Fer MF: Oat cell carcinoma of the lung with carcinomatosis meningitis. *N Engl J Med* 298:1146, 1978.

78. Brereton HD, O'Donnell JF, Kent CH, et al: Spinal meningeal carcinomatosis in small cell carcinoma of the lung. *Ann Int Med* 88:517–519, 1978.

79. Aisner J, Aisner SC, Ostrow S, et al: Meningeal carcinomatosis from small cell carcinoma of the lung: Consequence of improved survival. *Acta Cytolog* (Baltimore) 23:292–296, 1979

80. Aisner J, Ostrow S, Govindan S, et al: Leptomeningeal carcinomatosis in small cell carcinoma of the lung. *Med Pediatr Oncol* 9:47–59, 1981.

13

Adjuvant Chemotherapy for Osteosarcoma

Robert S. Benjamin

Osteosarcoma is a disease most commonly affecting patients in the 10- to 25-year age group (1). The prognosis for patients with clinically localized disease treated by amputation of the involved extremity has been considered to be extremely poor, with less than 25% five-year survival, development of pulmonary metastases in less than one year, and death within an additional six months to one year (1–4). With the discovery of the responsiveness of osteosarcoma to adriamycin (5), and high-dose methotrexate followed by citrovorum factor (6), a regimen referred to hereafter as HDMTX, a number of investigators initiated trials of adjuvant chemotherapy for osteosarcoma. Initial reports (3,7) appeared extremely positive, stimulating further studies. More recently, however, a pessimistic attitude regarding the value of adjuvant chemotherapy was expressed at the Osteosarcoma Study Group Meeting (8).

The reasons for this change in attitude are based on several findings: almost all patients on the initial adjuvant studies were not cured by the initial adjuvant chemotherapy studies. The initial results could not always be confirmed by other groups. Disease-free survival at the Mayo Clinic appeared to improve with time in patients treated by surgery alone. Overall survival was influenced by salvage therapy, particularly resection of pulmonary metastases. The chemotherapy used in many adjuvant trials had not been tested adequately in patients with advanced disease. The positive studies did not use a randomized, prospective control group of patients treated only with surgery. Prognostic factors were not totally defined and were rarely reported. Let us examine these factors together with current data on patients treated with and without adjuvant chemotherapy to put its role in perspective.

HIGH INITIAL CURE RATE

In November 1974, companion papers appearing in the *New England Journal of Medicine* suggested a dramatic effect of adjuvant chemotherapy on patients with this almost uniformly fatal disease (3,7). In the first paper, Jaffe et al. described

12 patients with typical osteosarcoma of an extremity treated with HDMTX (3). Follow-up ranged from 2 months to 2 years (median, 7 months). Actuarial disease-free survival at 18 months was 89% compared with 19% of a historical control group. A recent update of that study with 46 months' median follow-up reveals disease-free survival of 42% at 5 years, only half that projected in the original report (9). Two patients relapsed after 18 months. Cortes et al., using adriamycin, projected 45% disease-free survival in 21 patients followed from 1 to 32 months (10). In 13 patients who fulfilled the treatment requirements of their protocol, disease-free survival at 18 months was estimated at 89%. Both were superior to a historical control series (2). Update of this report at 5 years with 88 patients showed a projected 39% disease-free survival in the entire group and a 51% disease-free survival in those adhering to the protocol (10). Further update with an additional year of follow-up, that is, more than 2 years follow-up after closure of the protocol, reveals a 53% disease-free survival in 46 patients treated according to the protocol requirements (11). These results are somewhat closer to those in the initial reports of this series than are the long-term follow-up results from the HDMTX study. Nonetheless, the decline from almost 90% disease-free survival (and by inference, cure) to 53% disease-free survival is, at the least, discouraging.

Please note that cure, although inferred by many readers of these papers, was never implied by the authors of the preliminary reports, both of whom note that further follow-up in more patients would be needed to confirm that relapse had been prevented rather than simply delayed. Why did disease-free survival decline with further follow-up? One reason may be the extremely small sample size adequately studied in these preliminary reports. Jaffe reported on only 12 patients in whom adequate surgical control had been obtained (3), and Cortes reported on 21 patients, only 13 of whom were treated precisely according to the protocol (7). Precise details about the patients in Cortes' series are lacking. Four of the 12 patients in Jaffe's series may have been selected for relatively favorable prognosis by virtue of the fact that they received radiotherapy followed three to five months later by amputation. During that three- to five-month period, 20% to 35% of Jaffe's historical controls would have developed pulmonary metastases and therefore would have been ineligible for the study. Perhaps the major defect of the early reports was inadequate follow-up time. Almost all the patients were on treatment at the time of the report. Since chemotherapy might cause only partial destruction of residual tumor, one might expect some delay in development of metastases in partially responsive patients, thus requiring longer follow-up than in the historical control group. It is noteworthy that Cortes' initial report on all 21 treated patients had more patients, a six-month longer follow-up, a lower disease-free survival, and a better estimate of the overall disease-free survival at five years.

CONFIRMATION OF INITIAL RESULTS

Results of 15 adjuvant chemotherapy trials in 565 patients with at least 18 months follow-up are shown in Table 1 (9,10,12–24). The table is organized by drug regimen, first showing those regimens with adriamycin alone (10,12), then ad-

Table 1. Results of Adjuvant Chemotherapy Trials with at Least 18 Months' Follow-up

Author	Reference	Acronym/ Regimen[a]	No Patients	Median Follow-up (Months)	Percent Disease-Free Survival	Reference Time (Years)
Cortes	10	A	88	>18	39	5
Fossati-Bellani	12	A	15	23	40	2
Sutow	13	COMPADRI-I	44	37	55	5
Murphy	14	CYVADIC	31	24	51	3
Pouillart	15	CYVADIC	11	49	45	4
Ettinger	16	A-Pl	20	19	63	3
Jaffe	9	VM	12	46	42	5
Rosenberg	17	M ± V ± BCG	39	27	38	2
Pouillart	15	VM	15	36	36	3
Sutow	13	COMPADRI-II	60	22	51	2
Pratt	18	CA→M	24	18	52	2
Jasmin	19	CAM	15	c22	33	2
Jasmin	19	A→mCP	13	c22	50	2
Kotz	20	V-M→A or C	6	22	83	2
Goorin	21	V-M→A	22	>36	59	3
Goorin	21	V-M q week→A	25	19	78	2
Eilber	22	V-M→A	15	18	50	2
Eilber	22	IA-A- XRT→VM→A	26	22	62	2
Etchubanas	23	M→AV→AC	29	21	47	2
Campanacci	24	VA→Vm	55	36	45	4

[a]Key Abbreviations:
A or ADRI—Adriamycin
M—high dose Methotrexate with Citrovorum factor; m—standard Methotrexate
V, O, or ON—Vincristine
P—L-Phenylalanine mustard
DIC—Dimethyltriazenoimidazolecarboxamide
Pl—cis-Platinum
C—Cyclophosphamide

riamycin combinations (13–16), HDMTX (9,15,17), and, finally, combinations of adriamycin, and HDMTX (13,18–24). Disease-free survival is reported for reference times varying from two to five years in the various publications. Five studies have follow-up sufficient to report disease-free survival at four to five years (9,10,13,15,24). Median disease-free survival on these studies is 45% (range 39 to 55). Four studies have three-year disease-free survival data (14–16,21). The median is 55% with a range of 36 to 63. The remaining 11 studies (12,-13,18–23) have two-year disease-free survival ranging from 33% to 83% with a median of 50. The median disease-free survival at two years or longer is 50%.

Since there does not appear to be a major difference between disease-free survival at two and five years, it seems reasonable to combine these figures in the present analysis with the realization that the five-year figures are likely to be more accurate than the two-year figures. The two studies using adriamycin alone have a 39% to 40% disease-free survival, and the three studies using HDMTX have a median 38% disease-free survival (range 36 to 42). The adriamycin combination studies, which do not include HDMTX, or *cis*-platinum (13–15) show a median 51% disease-free survival with a range of 45 to 55 and follow-up projected to at least three years. The one study using adriamycin and platinum projects disease-free survival of 63% at three years (16). By far, the majority of the studies use, logically, the combination of adriamycin and HDMTX. Median disease-free survival of 51% (range 33 to 83) is similar to that of the other adriamycin combination studies. Notably, however, the combination studies appear to have superior disease-free survival to those using either adriamycin or HDMTX as single agents.

Much of the concern about the reproducibility of the adjuvant chemotherapy studies centers on the initial report of Jaffe's studies with HDMTX (3), rather than updated reports (9,21). One attempt at confirming Jaffe's study is that by Rosenberg et al. (17). That study reported a 38% two-year disease-free survival in 39 patients, significantly superior to the 17% two-year disease-free survival in 19 historical control patients ($P <.05$). Analysis of the patients under study revealed that only 33 of the 39 study patients had high-grade osteosarcoma, compared with 18 of the 19 controls. When disease-free survival of those with high-grade lesions was compared, 32% of treated patients were free of disease at two years, versus 16% for the control series. These differences were not considered statistically significant ($P = .11$). It is possible that unknown factors may have influenced the difference. The P value reflects the fact that differences of this magnitude might be expected by chance alone 11% of the time. The converse of this, of course, is that 89% of the time the reasons for the difference would not be due to chance alone, and the most likely explanation is benefit in the treated group due to the treatment performed. Although this isolated example certainly does not prove the value of HDMTX, it does support the fact that patients may well benefit from such therapy.

Further questions regarding the value of adjuvant chemotherapy in general and HDMTX in particular are raised by studies shown in Table 2, all of which

Table 2. Results of Adjuvant Chemotherapy Trials with Less than 18 Months' Follow-up

Author	Reference	Regimen Acronym[a]	No Patients	Median Follow-up (Months)	Percent Disease-Free Survival	Reference Time (Years)
Cortes	25	A	c.31	12	c.50	2
Cortes	25	A→MTX	c.31	12	c.50	2
Sutow	13	COMPADRI-III	44	14.5	42	2
Pritchard	26	Transfer factor	30	<18	41	2
Pritchard	26	MAO	18	<18	26	2

[a]See key for Table 1.

were premature at the time of their publication (13,25,26). Disease-free survival of 26% to 50% at two years is reported. The first two studies suggest that HDMTX may not add to the benefit already achieved with adjuvant adriamycin. In one case, a randomized comparison by Cortes and associates from Cancer and Leukemia Group B has shown about a 50% disease-free survival projected at two years, with one year median follow-up in groups of about 31 patients each. The study design, alternating two courses of adriamycin with two courses of HDMTX, will not make optimal use of either drug, however, since cells sensitive to one and not the other may regrow during the prolonged periods off the effective drug. A similar criticism may be made of the COMPADRI-III regimen of Sutow et al. (13), as well as their COMPADRI-II regimen, which has adequate follow-up (Table 1). Neither COMPADRI-II nor COMPADRI-III, which added HDMTX to a previous adriamycin-based combination, but with spaced sequential administration of the drugs, has improved disease-free survival over that achieved on the initial COMPADRI-I study, an adriamycin-based comparison not including HDMTX. Perhaps the most controversial of these studies is that reported by Pritchard et al. from the Mayo Clinic (26). Patients were randomized to receive MAO, a three-drug regimen combining HDMTX (with Vincristine) and adriamycin, or transfer factor. Seventeen patients were randomized to receive transfer factor, and 18 were randomized to receive MAO. An additional 13 patients were treated with transfer factor without randomization. Of the 30 transfer-factor-treated patients, 15 showed evidence of transfer of delayed type of hypersensitivity to at least one antigen, whereas 15 did not. The death rate and rate of metastases was more than four times higher ($P <$ .05) in patients not accepting transfer of delayed hypersensitivity or so-called nonconverters. Since this prognostic factor is of major importance, but could not be tested in the group randomized to chemotherapy, it is quite possible with the small number of patients involved that a high fraction of poor prognosis patients was included in the MAO group. No differences between treatment groups were statistically significant, patients numbers are small, and follow-up, short.

Further strong support for the value of adjuvant chemotherapy comes from the studies of Rosen et al. at the Memorial Sloan Kettering Cancer Center (27). These are shown together with those of Jenkin et al. (28) in Table 3. They are separated from the other studies reported, since continuous disease-free actuarial survival is not specified in the publications. Survival of 52% to 77% of patients in Rosen's studies at four years is most likely due to adjuvant chemotherapy but reflects as well the contribution of salvage therapy. It should be noted, however, that 68% of the patients entered on the T-5 protocol and 88% of those entered on the T-7 protocol remain free of disease, although actuarial disease-free survival, which reflects the time at which failure occurs, is not noted in the publication.

NATURAL HISTORY AND PROGNOSIS

Twelve control series of patients with osteosarcoma who were not treated with modern adjuvant chemotherapy have recently been published (1,4,20,24,29–31,33,34). Results are shown in Table 4. Five-year survival varied from 0% (35)

Table 3. Results of Adjuvant Chemotherapy Trials Whose Continuous Disease-Free Actuarial Survival Is Not Specified

Author	Reference	Regimen Acronym[a]	No Patients	Follow-up (Months)	Percent Survival	Reference Time (Years)
Rosen	27	VM→A→Surgery→ VM→A→C (T-5)	31	30–52	77	4
Rosen	27	VM→A→C (T-4)	23	30–52	52	4
Rosen	27	BCD[b]VM→A→VM (T-7)	61	9–38	88[c]	2
Jenkin	28	A or M	16	9–36	81	2

[a]See key for Tables 1 and 2.
[b]Bleomycin—B; Dactinomycin—D.
[c]Disease-free survival—not actuarial.

Table 4. Survival of Patients with Osteosarcoma Not Treated with Modern Adjuvant Therapy

Author	Reference	No of Patients	Percent Survival	Reference Time (Years)
Machinani	29	50	25	5
Larson	30	109	22	5
Cohen	31	170	30	3
			22	5
Dissing	32	49	45	2
Berg	33	50	36	2
			22	5
Weiss	34	35	12	5
Uribe-Botero	1	243	22	3
			13	5
Gehan	4	89	34	2
			23	3
			20	5
Jenkin	28	38	16	2
Campanacci	24	90	18	1.5
			6	5
Kotz	20	36	19	5
Eilber	35	14	0	4

to 25% (29) with a median of 20%. Absolute survival, therefore, was less than disease-free survival achieved with chemotherapy, even in those studies where absolute disease-free survival at five years has been reached (Table 1). The studies shown in Table 4 suggest a monotonous, dismal outlook for patients with this disease in the absence of modern chemotherapy. Disease-free survival is rarely reported, although it is noted in the studies shown in Table 5. Two-year survival ranged from 15% (4,37) to 41% (37) with a median of 19%. At the Mayo Clinic, improving survival with time had been noted (38). The data suggested a steady improvement in survival with time from about 25% to 50% (38). When disease-free survival is analyzed, as shown in Table 5, the increase in disease-free survival at two years is noted only when groups are combined. Since only disease-free survival reflects the natural history of the disease plus the effects of its initial management, the initial survival increase noted most likely reflects secondary therapy. Although the disease-free survival increased from 15% in 1963 to 1965 and 19% in 1966 to 1968 to 31% in 1969 to 1971, it decreased again to 27% in 1972 to 1974. In addition, five-year disease-free survival in the best subgroup of 43 patients seen between 1969 and 1971 was only 36%. This is lower than the four- to five-year disease-free survival rate of 45% previously noted on five adjuvant chemotherapy studies.

If, in fact, prognosis was improving with time, one would expect a similar finding in other studies. Miké et al. (36) and Gehan et al. (4) specifically looked at their series for similar trends for increase in survival with time. No such trend was noted. Miké commented on variation in survival over the time limits of her study, but none of these differences was statistically significant. If, in fact, osteosarcoma was becoming an increasingly benign disease with time, if only at

Table 5. Disease-Free Survival of Patients with Osteosarcoma Not Treated with Modern Adjuvant Chemotherapy

Author	Reference	No of Patients		Percent Disease-Free Survival	Reference Time (Years)
Berg	33	50		16	5
Rosenberg	17	23		17	2
Gehan	4	89		15	2
				12	5
Miké	36	210		21	2
				18	5
Eilber	35	14		0	3
Taylor	37	29	(1963–1965)	15	2–5
		36	(1966–1968)	19	2–5
		43	(1969–1971)	41	2
				36	5
		41	(1972–1974)	27	2
				20	4

the Mayo Clinic, one would expect a steady increase in disease-free survival within the three-year subgroups chosen. Again, in fact, this was not the case, since disease-free survival fell over the last two periods of the study.

SALVAGE THERAPY

One reason for the poor overall survival of patients with osteosarcoma treated by surgery alone is the rapid development of pulmonary metastases and their rapid progression to a fatal outcome (1–4). There are two basic approaches which can be used to treat advanced disease, the most common of which is systemic chemotherapy. The other approach involves surgical resection of pulmonary metastases. The concept of surgical excision of pulmonary metastases is not new, nor is it an infrequently performed procedure. Six-hundred twenty-two thoracotomies were performed for resection of pulmonary metastases in 409 patients with a variety of diagnoses at the Memorial Sloan Kettering Cancer Center between 1960 and 1976 (39). Twenty-nine of these patients had osteosarcoma, and it was possible to remove grossly palpable disease in 22. Sixteen patients required multiple resections, and bilateral thoracotomies were necessary in some instances. Twenty-seven percent were alive after five or more years. Although many of these patients received chemotherapy in addition, surgery clearly contributed to their longevity. At the Mayo Clinic, 13 of 28 patients are free of disease with median follow-up of 6 to 48 months and actuarial four-year survival of 57% (40).

Although these reports demonstrate the contribution of surgery to the survival of treated patients, there is only a single reported study in which surgery for metastatic disease was incorporated into the study design: the report of Rosenberg et al. (41) of the patients on their HDMTX adjuvant chemotherapy study (17). In 20 of 22 patients who relapsed from chemotherapy on that study, the first known site of metastases was the lung, and thoracotomy was performed in 18 with a resection of all known disease in 11, or half (41). All but two received additional chemotherapy, and four required repeat thoracotomy. Eight patients remain NED for more than 12 months.

A planned salvage approach for patients not treated with adjuvant chemotherapy as well as those treated with adjuvant chemotherapy is built into the current Mayo Clinic study, which does not yet show any differences in survival or disease-free survival between patients treated with adjuvant chemotherapy initially and only salvage therapy (42). Two-year disease-free survival is estimated at 52% and overall two-year survival at 74% with a median follow-up of about two years, and no differences are yet observed between the two groups. The high projected disease-free survival in this group of patients may not be compared with that of previous studies, since computerized tomography was used to screen all patients before entry.

The approach to salvage therapy without adjuvant chemotherapy may not be so successful as in the presence of adjuvant chemotherapy. Jaffe et al. compared 14 patients treated with adjuvant chemotherapy who developed pulmonary metastases with matched historical controls (43). The new number of pulmonary metastases per patient in the treated group was 3.6 versus 10.4 for the historical controls. In addition, time to recurrence was prolonged from 7.2 months in the control group to 18.6 months in the treated group. If in fact, chemotherapy is delaying the growth of pulmonary metastases or eradicating some while leaving others intact, some patients may not be surgical candidates in the absence of effective adjuvant chemotherapy who would have been salvaged had they been treated initially with adjuvant chemotherapy.

CHEMOTHERAPY

There have been few systematic studies of the effects of chemotherapy on metastatic osteosarcoma. The initial studies of Cortes (5) and Jaffe (6) demonstrated the effectiveness of adriamycin and HDMTX, respectively, in a fraction of patients. Jaffe's study showed two complete and two partial remissions in 10 patients treated with HDMTX. Calculation of the response rate is further confused by the acceptance of 25% regression as a partial response. Assuming that both patients had greater than 50% regression when considered in partial remission, the overall response rate was 40%. But estimates of the true response rate cannot be made accurately with only 10 patients. Cortes et al. updated their initial report of a 31% remission rate (5) to a 41% remission rate in 17 patients (44). In that study, a steep dose response for adriamycin was noted with one of six patients responding at doses of 20 mg/M^2 daily for four days or less, three of seven at 30 mg/M^2 daily for three days, and three of four at 35 mg/M^2 daily for three days. The Southwest Oncology Group experience was reviewed by Benjamin et al. (45). A 27% response rate was seen in 11 patients treated with adriamycin as a single agent. There were 3 complete remissions and 13 partial remissions among 46 patients treated with adriamycin in combination with DTIC with or without vincristine for a response rate of 35%. The addition of cyclophosphamide to this regimen and a decrease in the adriamycin dose of 60 mg/M^2 single dose to 50 mg/M^2 resulted in a decreased remission rate of only 24% in 29 patients. A similar response rate of 25% was seen in 20 patients treated with cyclophosphamide, vincristine, adriamycin, and actinomycin-D. Activity of cis-platinum was initially reported by Ochs et al. with one complete and four partial remissions in eight patients (46). In five other series, a 14% response rate has been noted among 49 patients (47–51).

Just as there is a dose-response curve for adriamycin, one has been demonstrated for HDMTX. Jaffe reported an increased response rate of 82% when HDMTX was given weekly (52). The number of patients is again too small for a meaningful evaluation of response rate and until recently had not been confirmed. Rosen et al. had recently reported a 75% in 41 patients, evaluated for the effect of HDMTX on their primary tumor preoperatively (53). In 10 patients with evaluable pulmonary nodules, 7 had a greater than 75% decrease. Higher doses of chemotherapy were required for prepubescent children (12 g/M^2) than for older adolescents and adults (8 g/M^2). Rosen has used the same approach of preoperative therapy to expand his preliminary series on the three-drug combination of bleomycin, cyclophosphamide, and Dactinomycin from 62% in

13 patients (54) to 82% in 22 patients (53). Clearly, then, chemotherapy has demonstrable effects on osteosarcoma that would be expected to be beneficial in the adjuvant situation.

VALUE OF ADJUVANT CHEMOTHERAPY, A REASSESSMENT

The concept of adjuvant chemotherapy need not be justified, as it is proved in experimental tumors and human tumors, for example, Wilms' tumor, Ewing's sarcoma, rhabdomyosarcoma of childhood, and breast cancer. There are two criteria that must be met for the use of chemotherapy in the adjuvant situation: first, the chemotherapy must have proved efficacy, and, second, the disease must not be highly curable in its advanced state by chemotherapy. Osteosarcoma clearly fits these two criteria. Only about one-quarter of the patients who relapse can be expected to be salvaged by surgery alone, and although this may increase with surgery plus adjuvant chemotherapy, if the adjuvant chemotherapy is effective in the treatment of salvage patients, it must be effective in the treatment of those with primary disease. Chemotherapy of osteosarcoma is clearly effective in a fraction of patients but far from curative as a sole modality in the majority of patients with advanced disease. The fact that patients receiving more intensive chemotherapy with adriamycin have done better in the adjuvant situation than patients whose doses were lowered emphasizes the fact that adriamycin must be contributing to their prolonged survival. Those patients treated with more intensive high-dose methotrexate regimens have also done better than those in whom the dose was lower.

The best argument for the beneficial effects of adjuvant chemotherapy for osteosarcoma comes from the studies of Rosen et al., which used, rather than adjuvant chemotherapy, adjuvant surgery (27,53). Patients with primary osteosarcoma were treated with chemotherapy on the T-5 or T-7 protocols. They then underwent tumor resection followed by continued adjuvant chemotherapy. Of 31 patients treated on the T-5 protocol, 15 demonstrated major tumor destruction at the time of surgery, and 16 had little or no response. All 15 responders are continuously disease-free compared with 39% of the nonresponders. On an update adding 38 patients on the T-7 protocol, there are 43 responders, all disease-free survivors, versus 33% of the 26 nonresponders (53).

Clearly, chemotherapeutic response is the critical determinant of disease-free survival. When used in the adjuvant situation, there is no way to differentiate responders from nonresponders; however, it is also clear that a substantial fraction of patients may be cured by chemotherapy, some of whom may not be salvageable if relapse is awaited. Since the majority of patients will relapse and probably die in the absence of some benefit from chemotherapy, it seems wise to use adjuvant chemotherapy in an attempt to cure the curable. The incurable will die anyway.

Preoperative chemotherapy should be used whenever possible to assess response and segregate responding from nonresponding patients. New chemotherapeutic strategies should be devised for the nonresponders. An additional potential benefit to responding patients may be increased potential for limb salvage. Soft-tissue masses often preclude limited surgery, and if they can be eliminated by preoperative chemotherapy, patients considered candidates only for amputation may be converted to limb salvage candidates.

The goal in the treatment of primary osteosarcoma is the cure of all patients with the least mutilating surgery possible. By directing research efforts toward improvement of therapeutic results from those currently attainable, rather than the retrogressive approach of trying to prove or disprove results that have been previously reported from outmoded, less than perfect studies, patients with this rare tumor should be treated in the context of clinical trials directed at this goal.

REFERENCES

1. Uribe-Botero G, Russell WO, Sutow WW, et al: A clinico-pathologic investigation of 243 cases, with necropsy studies in 54. *Am J Clin Pathol* 67(5):427–435, 1977.

2. Marcove RC, Mike V, Hajek JV, et al: Osteogenic sarcoma under the age of twenty-one. A review of 145 operative cases. *J Bone Joint Surg* 52-A:411–423, 1970.

3. Jaffe N, Frei E III, Traggis D, et al: Adjuvant methotrexate and citrovorum-factor treatment of osteogenic sarcoma. *New Engl J Med* 291(19):994–997, 1974.

4. Gehan EA, Sutow WW, Uribe-Botero G, et al: Osteosarcoma: The M. D. Anderson experience, 1950–1974, in Terry WD, Windhorst D (eds): *Immunotherapy of Cancer: Present Status of Trials in Man. Progress in Cancer Research and Therapy*, vol 6. New York, Raven Press, 1978, p 271.

5. Cortes EP, Holland JF, Wang JJ, et al: Doxorubicin in disseminated osteosarcoma. *JAMA* 221(10):1132–1138, 1972.

6. Jaffe N: Recent advances in the chemotherapy of metastatic osteogenic sarcoma. *Cancer* 30(6):1627–1631, 1972.

7. Cortes EP, Holland JF, Wang JJ, et al: Amputation and adriamycin in primary osteosarcoma. *New Engl J Med* 291:998–1000, 1974.

8. Muggia FM, Handelsman H: Introduction: Treatment of osteogenic sarcoma. *Cancer Treat Rep* 62(2):187–188, 1978.

9. Jaffe N, Frei E III, Watts H, et al: High-dose methotrexate in osteogenic sarcoma: A 5-year experience. *Cancer Treat Rep* 62:(2)259–264, 1978.

10. Cortes EP, Holland JF, Glidewell O: Amputation and adriamycin in primary operable osteosarcoma. *Cancer Treat Rep* 62(2):271–278, 1978.

11. Cortes EP, Glidewell O: Adjuvant therapy of operable primary osteosarcoma: Cancer and Leukemia Group B experience. *Recent Results Cancer Res* 68:16–24, 1979.

12. Fossati-Bellani F, Gasparini M, Bonadonna G: Adriamycin in the adjuvant treatment of operable osteosarcoma. *Recent Results Cancer Res* 68:25–27, 1979.

13. Sutow WW, Gehan WA, Dyment PG, et al: Multidrug adjuvant chemotherapy for osteosarcoma: Interim report of the Southwest Oncology Group Studies. *Cancer Treat Rep* 62:265–270, 1978.

14. Murphy WK, Benjamin RS, Eyre HJ, et al: Southwest Oncology Group study, in Jones SE, Salmon SE (eds): *Adjuvant Therapy of Cancer II*. New York, Grune & Stratton, Inc, 1979, p 365.

15. Pouillart P, Langlois A, Dumont J, et al: Combination chemotherapy for osteosarcoma (meeting abstract). *Abstract of the 4th Annual Meeting of the Medical Oncology Society and the Bi-Annual Meeting of the Immunology and Immunotherapy Group*, Nice, France, December 2–4, 1978. New York, Springer-Verlag, 29:23, 1978.

16. Ettinger LJ, Douglass HO Jr, Higby DJ, et al: Adriamycin (ADR) and cis-diamminedichloroplatinum (DDP) as adjuvant therapy in osteosarcoma of the extremities. Meeting Abstract presented at the Sixteenth Annual Meeting of the American Society of Clinical Oncology, May 26–27, 1980, San Diego, California. Vol 21, C292, p 392.

17. Rosenbergy SA, Chabner BA, Young RC, et al: Treatment of osteogenic sarcoma: I. Effect of adjuvant high-dose methotrexate after amputation. *Cancer Treat Rep* 63(5):739–751, 1979.

18. Pratt CB, Rivera G, Shanks E, et al: Combination chemotherapy for osteosarcoma. *Cancer Treat Rep* 62(2):251–258, 1978.

19. Muggia F, Catane R, Lee YJ, et al: Factors responsible for therapeutic success in osteosarcoma: A critical analysis of adjuvant trial results, in Jones SE, Salmon SE (eds): *Adjuvant Therapy of Cancer II.* New York, Grune & Stratton, Inc, 1979, p 375.

20. Kotz R: Osteosarcoma 1978: The change in prognosis through adequate surgery and adjuvant chemotherapy. *Wien Klin Wochenschr (Suppl)* 90(93):2–25, 1978.

21. Goorin A, Link M, Jaffe N, et al: Adjuvant chemotherapy (chemo) and limb salvage procedures for osteosarcoma: A seven year experience. *Abstract of the Sixteenth Annual Meeting of the American Society of Clinical Oncology,* May 26–27, 1980, San Diego, California. Vol 21, Abstract C604, p 472.

22. Eilber FR, Grant TT, Weisenburger T, et al: Limb salvage for osteosarcoma (meeting abstract). *Proc Am Assoc Cancer Res* 20:330, 1979.

23. Etcubanas E, Wilbur JR: Adjuvant chemotherapy for osteogenic sarcoma. *Cancer Treat Rep* 62(2):283–288, 1978.

24. Campanacci M, Pagani PA, Giunti A: System postoperative chemotherapy of osteosarcomas of the extremities (letter to editor). *Nouv Presse Med* 7(38):3462, 1978.

25. Cortes EP, Necheles TF, Holland JF, et al: Adriamycin (ADM) alone versus ADM and high dose methotrexate citrovorum factor rescue (HDMTX-CF) as adjuvant to operable primary osteosarcoma (OS): A randomized study by Cancer and Leukemia Group B (CALGB) (meeting abstract). *Proc Am Assoc Cancer Res* 20:412, 1979.

26. Pritchard DJ, Ritts ER, Gilchrist GS, et al: Transfer factor (TF) in the management of osteosarcoma (OGS) (meeting abstract). *Proc Am Assoc Cancer Res* 19:147, 1978.

27. Rosen G, Marcove RC, Caparros B, et al: Primary osteogenic sarcoma: The rationale for preoperative chemotherapy and delayed surgery. *Cancer* 43(6):2163–2177, 1979.

28. Jenkin RD: Radiation treatment of Ewing's sarcoma and osteogenic sarcoma. *Can J Surg* 20(6):530–536, 1977.

29. Machinami R, Imamura T, Takeyama S, et al: Typical and atypical osteosarcomas: A clinicopathologic study of sixty-two cases. *Gan* 70(5):621–638, 1979.

30. Larsson SE, Lorentzon R, Bjedren H, et al: Osteosarcoma: A multifactorial clinical and histopathological study with special regard to therapy and survival. *Acta Orthop Scand* 49(6):571–581, 1978.

31. Cohen P: Osteosarcoma of the long bones: Clinical observations and experiences in the Netherlands. *Eur J Cancer* 14(10):995–1004, 1978.

32. Dissin I, Heerfordt J, Schiodt T, et al: Osteosarcoma: An assessment of prognosis on the basis of 49 cases. *Ugeskr Laeger* 140(27):1605–1608, 1978.

33. Berg NO, Hakansson CH, Lovdahl R, et al: Radiotherapy and surgery in 50 cases of osteosarcoma treated without adjuvant chemotherapy. *Acta Ophthalmol (Copenh)* 48(6):580–585, 1977.

34. Weiss AB, Adams G, Brackin B, et al: Osteosarcoma: A review of 50 patients treated at the University of Alabama in Birmingham Medical Center between 1944 and 1975. *Clin Orthop* 135:137–147, 1978.

35. Eilber FR, Townsend CM, Morton DL: Adjuvant immunotherapy of osteosarcoma with BCG and allogeneic tumor cells, in *Immunotherapy of Cancer: Present Status of Trials in Man. Progress in Cancer Research and Therapy,* vol 6. New York, Raven Press, 1978, p 299.

36. Miké V, Marcove RC: Osteogenic sarcoma under the age of 21: Experience at Memorial Sloan-Kettering Cancer Center, in *Immunotherapy of Cancer: Present Status of Trials in Man. Progress in Cancer Research and Therapy,* vol 6. New York, Raven Press, 1978, p 283.

37. Taylor WF, Ivins JC, Dahlin DC, et al: Osteogenic sarcoma experience at the Mayo Clinic 1963–1974, in *Immunotherapy of Cancer: Present Status of Trials in Man. Progress in Cancer Research and Therapy,* vol 6. New York, Raven Press, 1978, p 257.

38. Taylor WF, Ivins JC, Dahlin DC, et al: Trends and variability in survival from osteosarcoma. *Mayo Clin Proc* 53(11):695–700, 1978.

39. Martini N, McCormack PM, Bains MS: Surgery for solitary and multiple pulmonary metastases. *NY State J Med* 78(1):1711–1714, 1978.

40. Telander RL, Pairolero PC, Pritchard DJ, et al: Resection of pulmonary metastatic osteogenic sarcoma in children. *Surgery* 84(3):335–341, 1978.

41. Rosenberg SA, Flye MW, Conkle D, et al: Treatment of osteogenic sarcoma: II. Aggressive resection of pulmonary metastases. *Cancer Treat Rep* 63(5):753–756, 1979.

42. Edmonson JH, Green SJ, Ivins JC, et al: Methotrexate as adjuvant treatment for primary osteosarcoma. *New Engl J Med* 303(11):642–643, 1980.

43. Jaffe N, Frei E III, Smith E, et al: A hypothesis for the pattern of pulmonary metastases in osteogenic sarcoma: Impact of adjuvant therapy. Abstract presented at *Proc Am Assoc Cancer Res* 19:400, 1978.

44. Cortes EP, Holland JF, Wang JJ, et al: Chemotherapy of advanced osteosarcoma, Colston Paper No. 24: Bone-certain aspects of neoplasia. Edited by CHG Price, FGM Ross, London, Buttersworth and Company, 1972, pp 265–280.

45. Benjamin RS, Baker LH, O'Bryan RM, et al: Chemotherapy for metastatic osteosarcoma: Studies by the M. D. Anderson Hospital and the Southwest Oncology Group. *Cancer Treat Rep* 62(2):237–238, 1978.

46. Ochs J, Freeman AJ, Douglass HO, et al: Cis-dichlorodiammine-platinum(II) in advanced osteogenic sarcoma. *Cancer Treat Rep* 62:239–245, 1978.

47. Rosen G, Niremberg A, Juergens H, et al: Phase-II trial of cis-platinum in osteogenic sarcoma. *Proc Am Assoc Cancer Res and Am Soc Clin Oncol* 20:363, abstract C299, 1979.

48. Baum E, Greenberg L, Gaynon P, et al: Use of cis-platinum diammine dichloride (CDDP) in osteogenic sarcoma (OS) in children. *Proc Am Assoc Cancer Res and Am Soc Clin Oncol* 19:385, abstract C315, 1978.

49. Higby DJ, Wallace HJ, Holland JF: Cis-diamminedichloroplatinum (NSC-119875): A phase I study. *Cancer Chemother Rep.* 57:459–463, 1973.

50. Samson MK, Baker LH, Benjamin RS, et al: Cis-diamminedichloroplatinum (NSC-119875, DDP) in advanced soft tissue and bony sarcomas: A Southwest Oncology Group Study. *Cancer Treat Rep* 63:2027–2029, 1979.

51. Nitschke R, Starling KA, Vats T, et al: Cis-diamminedichloroplatinum (NSC-119875) in childhood malignancies: A Southwest Oncology Group Study. *Med Pediatr Oncol* 4:127–132, 1978.

52. Jaffe N, Frei E III, Traggis D, et al: Weekly high-dose methotrexate-citrovorum factor in osteogenic sarcoma: Pre-surgical treatment of primary tumor and of overt pulmonary metastases. *Cancer* 39:45–50, 1977.

53. Rosen G, Caparros B, Nirenberg A, et al: The successful management of metastatic osteogenic sarcoma: A model for the treatment of primary osteogenic sarcoma, in van Oosterom AT, Muggia FM, Cleton FJ (eds): *Therapeutic Progress in Ovarian Cancer, Testicular Cancer and the Sarcomas.* Leiden University Press, The Netherlands, 1979, vol 16, pp 349–366.

54. Mosende C, Gutierrez M, Caparros B, et al: Combination chemotherapy with bleomycin, cyclophosphamide, and dactinomycin for the treatment of osteogenic sarcoma. *Cancer* 40(6): 2779–2786, 1977.

14

Is Adjuvant Chemotherapy of Osteosarcoma of Proved Value?

Douglas J. Pritchard

For several reasons, the concept of adjuvant chemotherapy seems particularly suitable for osteosarcoma. The primary tumor can usually be completely eliminated, by either block resection or amputation. The tumor usually involves young people who are suitable candidates for chemotherapy. In addition, the tumor tends to be predictable in the sense that when metastases occur they usually do so in the peripheral lung fields. Hence, it is relatively easy to monitor these patients and to establish well-defined disease free intervals. Although it is hoped by all concerned that one or more chemotherapeutic regimens will prove to be efficacious in the management of patients with osteosarcoma, this has not yet been proved.

There have been a variety of new developments in the diagnosis and treatment of osteosarcoma over the past decade that have changed both disease-free and actual survival statistics. In 1967 Drs. Coventry and Dahlin published a retrospective series from the Mayo Clinic. This study showed that approximately 20% of patients with osteosarcoma survived for five years or longer after amputation surgery (1). This report was initially received with skepticism, almost all believing that very few persons survived with this tumor. However, as others reviewed their experience, the 20% survival figure became an established standard. This figure was subsequently used as a benchmark against which all new forms of treatment were measured (2,3).

The population considered to have primary localized classical high-grade osteosarcoma has changed over the past decade. Part of the problem lies in the definition of what constitutes classical osteosarcoma. The histologic criteria for the diagnosis of osteogenic sarcoma are generally agreed on by almost all expert bone pathologists (4). However, there probably remain minor variations in the histologic criteria for acceptance of patients on a clinical protocol. There are now at least 12 recognized variants of osteosarcoma that must be considered in the classification of this tumor (5). For example, parosteal osteosarcoma is usually cured by surgery alone; at least 80% or 90% of patients with parosteal osteosarcoma may be cured by adequate surgery. Thus, if patients with this lesion are included in a clinical study, the results of that study will be improved regardless of the form of treatment, as long as the initial surgical treatment is adequate. Another entity, osteosarcoma of the jaw, is histiologically similar to classical osteosarcoma but has a distinctly different clinical behavior; distant metastases are relatively unusual. Again, if the study is weighted by inclusion of patients with this disorder, the results will appear to be improved. Several of the initial enthusiastic reports did, in fact, include patients with these two variants (6,7). Some of the variants of osteosarcoma are quite rare, and it is unlikely that any one study will be significantly skewed if the number of patients treated is large enough. However, most published series do not include large numbers of cases. It is essential that the histologic criteria for the diagnosis of osteosarcoma be as accurate as possible and that recognized variants be excluded for analysis. It would be ideal if a panel of well-recognized expert bone pathologists could review all the cases included in a study so that the results of different studies could be meaningfully compared.

Another recent major development has been the improvement in the clinical staging of patients with osteosarcoma. Whole lung tomograms were found to be significantly superior to plain chest roentgenograms for the detection of occult pulmonary metastases. Within the past several years, computerized tomography has been shown to be superior to whole lung tomography or plain chest roentgenograms for the detection of these occult metastases (8). Thus, patients who in the past might have been included in a clinical trial with primary localized disease may now be excluded because of the detection of metastases by more sophisticated techniques. It would be helpful in comparing treatment results to know which patients were excluded at the outset because of metastatic disease detected by computerized tomography not detectable by plain roentgenograms. Some institutions may see patients earlier in the course of the disease than others do; alternatively, some institutions may have patients referred with a higher proportion of already established metastatic disease.

Another factor that may affect the results of various treatment protocols is the changes in surgical technique that have taken place in recent years. In the past, nearly all extremity lesions were treated by amputation. Sometimes these amputations were performed adjacent to the tumor with inadequate surgical margins by today's standards. Patients treated in this way were in jeopardy for the development of local recurrence and subsequent metastases. Amputation surgery has improved with the recognition of the need for wider surgical margins. In addition, there seems to be a trend toward a higher percentage of patients treated by limb salvage procedures, especially for those with tumors that are favorably located. With the development of new endoprosthetic devices and the means to fix these devices adequately, as well as with other techniques such as the use of allografts or other materials for replacement of segmental defects, larger numbers of patients may now have adequate surgery without having amputations. Although it is obviously desirable to try to salvage the patient's limb as well as his life, the fact that the surgical treatment of osteosarcoma today is different from what it was in the past is another factor that makes it difficult to compare today's treatment results with those of the past.

Probably the single most important factor that obscures the evaluation of the efficacy of chemotherapy is the very rarity of osteosarcoma. Because of this rarity there have been very few controlled studies. We began to appreciate the value of a controlled study when we analyzed the results of a study in which all patients with classical localized osteosarcoma were treated by amputation surgery but half of the patients received, in addition, so-called prophylactic irradiation to the lung fields (9). In this randomized prospective study, analysis of the results indicated that there were no differences in either disease-free or actual survival for either of the two treatment groups; and, hence, the conclusion was drawn that prophylactic irradiation to the lung fields as used in this study was of no value. It was of considerable interest to us, however, that approximately 40% of patients in this study survived for five years or longer. Obviously, if we had not used a control group and if all patients had been treated by prophylactic lung radiation, we would have been led to believe that this form of treatment resulted in a doubling of the survival rate.

In a subsequent randomized prospective study, we compared the use of transfer factor in one treatment group with a combination chemotherapy regimen in the other treatment group (10). Again, all patients had primary, localized classical high-grade osteosarcoma. There were no significant differences in disease-free or actual survival when these two groups were compared. Again, survival was approximately double what we had experienced in the past. We could conclude either that both forms of adjunctive treatment were equally effective or that neither had any value.

In the more recent past, there have been numerous studies reporting two-year disease-free survival from 26% to 65% and actual survival from 35% to 82%. What is striking is the wide variety of different chemotherapeutic regimens that seem to result in approximately the same degree of efficacy. Numerous different chemotherapeutic regimens using different agents and different combinations or different dosages seem to give similar results that are improved compared with historical experience. Indeed, some of the immunotherapeutic approaches have shown similar results (10,12). With changes in the histologic criteria for the diagnosis of osteosarcoma, with changes in the clinical staging of patients with osteosarcoma, with different surgical techniques, and with numerous different adjunctive protocols, the question arises, how can we measure whether a particular adjunctive modality is beneficial and if it is, how beneficial is it? In other words, without some objective method of comparison of the treatment under study and an untreated control, how can we decide whether or not the method of treatment under study is beneficial?

Another important factor has entered into the discussion in the past decade, that is, the role of resectional surgery for pulmonary metastases. Although disease-free survival is dependent only on the initial treatment rendered, which may, of course, include adjunctive treatment, actual survival is influenced by treatment rendered after the development of metastatic disease. It seems very clear that the willingness of thoracic surgeons to resect metastatic pulmonary disease has led to improvement in actual survival (13–15). In the past, thoracic surgeons were generally unenthusiastic about resecting pulmonary metastases for patients with cancer. Sarcomas, in general, tend to metastasize to the lung periphery. With the development of new surgical techniques, it has become possible to resect these peripheral pulmonary lesions without sacrificing significant pulmonary function. In the past, when the patient developed one or more pulmonary metastases, thoracic surgeons generally advised a period of observation before considering pulmonary resection. Since the majority of patients showed steadily progressive disease, relatively few patients underwent thoracic surgery. When it became recognized that early aggressive removal of pulmonary metastatic disease could be curative, the attitude of the thoracic surgeons dramatically changed. Indeed, at present it seems best to monitor the lung fields routinely and frequently by computerized tomography, and when metastases appear, to resect them very aggressively. Since most patients with osteosarcoma are young, they tolerate the surgery very well, and there are relatively few significant complications. This aggressive approach has unquestionably improved the survival of patients with osteosarcoma. It is known that patients who develop metastatic disease either simultaneously with the recognition of the primary tumor or relatively soon after the treatment for the primary lesion have a worse prognosis than those who develop late pulmonary metastasis (13). Nevertheless, even patients with early metastatic disease have, in general, benefited from an aggressive thoracic surgery approach. Although the efficacy of any particular adjunctive treatment program can only be measured by the use of disease-free analysis, nevertheless, the overall goal obviously is the survival of the patient. If comparable survival can be achieved without the use of toxic chemotherapeutic agents but with an aggressive approach to pulmonary metastases, one can argue whether or not adjunctive chemotherapy is necessary and desirable. In other words, if the end results are the same with or without chemotherapy, we have to look more deeply into the relative merits and risks of chemotherapy and surgery.

All these considerations led us to conduct a very intensive review of our more recent experience with patients who have classical osteosarcoma treated by surgery alone (16,17). Two hundred fifty-six patients with classical high-grade osteosarcoma treated at the Mayo Clinic between 1963 and 1978 were studied (18). Although numerous variables were considered and analyzed, by far the most statistically significant variable was the date of treatment. That is, there has been steady improvement in both disease-free and actual survival throughout this period. The case histories, histologic material, and follow-up data of these patients were very extensively analyzed. Various statistical techniques were used in an effort to detect potential factors that might account for the observed improvement in survival. Regardless of the method of analysis or the factors analyzed, one fact seems very clear, that is, that there has been steady improvement in disease-free and actual survival regardless of the factors considered.

The recognition of the improvement in prognosis for patients with osteosarcoma led us to the development of a clinical protocol in which patients are randomized between adjunctive high-dose methotrexate and a group that received observation only after surgical treatment. This still on-going randomized controlled trial has been difficult because of problems in recruiting patients for the study. Many patients declined participation in the study because of concerns about the toxicity and problems associated with receiving chemotherapy. Others declined because of their belief that chemotherapy might be helpful. Thus far, however, there appear to be no significant differences in either disease-free or actual survival for patients who either receive this chemotherapy regimen or are simply observed, nor are there any differences for those patients who declined participation in the study whether or not they received any form of adjunctive treatment (19). We noted, however, that all patients who had been seen at the Mayo Clinic with the diagnosis of classical localized high-grade osteosarcoma, since the initiation of this study, have shown improvement in both disease-free and actual survival. Since all these patients were treated in the recent past, prolonged follow-up information is not available. If, however, actuarial projections are used to estimate the prognosis of these patients, results are comparable with those of other on-going studies that also use actuarial projections to estimate prognosis.

Obviously, the main question is why have we at the Mayo Clinic observed this dramatic improvement in prognosis? We have, of course, analyzed this question repeatedly and in depth. The histologic criteria for the selection of patients with classical osteosarcoma have remained constant throughout this period. The histiologic slides from these patients have been reviewed by other expert bone pathologists who agree that the diagnoses are correct. There probably has been some improvement in prognosis because of better clinical staging. This factor has had very little effect on prognosis until the past two or three years. There have been changes in the surgical treatment of the primary lesion that may, indeed, explain some of the observed improvement in survival. More aggressive use of thoracic surgery for resection of pulmonary metastases has definitely led to improvement in actual survival, but obviously it has had no effect on disease-free survival. Throughout this period the referral pattern remained unchanged. The size of the initial tumors also remained unchanged. Although there were minor variations in some of the known prognostic variables, none was of such importance to override the significance of date of treatment. We have no obvious explanation for this improvement in prognosis. It is possible, of course, that there may be subtle factors that we have not considered, which in combination may have influenced our results. In addition, it is conceivable that the biology of the tumor or the host's response to it may have changed during this time.

In any case, the main consideration is not why our results have shown improvement but whether the improvements that others have observed are attributable to the form of treatment used. The question becomes, can the advocate of a particular adjuvant regimen prove that this therapy is more efficacious than other experimental regimens or indeed better than simple observation, and if this proof can be shown, just how efficacious is the particular regimen? Difficult value judgments then can be made as to whether a particular regimen offers sufficient promise to warrant the difficulties, toxicity, and expense involved. At the present time, it would appear that such proof cannot be obtained without use of a controlled prospective and randomized study. We are all hopeful that an effective adjunctive chemotherapeutic regimen will be proved to be important in the management of patients with osteosarcoma; however, thus far the role of adjunctive treatment for this disease remains a dilemma (11).

REFERENCES

1. Dahlin DC, Coventry MB: Osteogenic sarcoma: A study of six hundred cases. *JBJS* 48A:1–26, 1967.

2. Marcove RC, Miké V, Hajek JV, et al: Osteogenic sarcoma under age of twenty-one. *JBJS* 52:411–423, 1970.

3. Friedman MA, Carter SK: The therapy of osteogenic sarcoma: Current status and thoughts for the future. *J Surg Oncol* 4:482–510, 1972.

4. Dahlin DC: *Bone Tumors: General Aspects and Data on 6,221 Cases.* Springfield, Thomas, 1978.

5. Dahlin DC, Unni KK: Osteosarcoma of bone and its important recognizable variants. *Am J Surg* 1:61–72, 1977.

6. Cortes EP, Holland JF, Wang JJ, et al: Amputation and adriamycin in primary osteosarcoma. *N Engl J Med* 291:998, 1974.

7. Jaffe N, Frei E, Traggis D, et al: Adjuvant methotrexate and citrovorum factor treatment of osteogenic sarcoma. *N Engl J Med* 291:994, 1974.

8. Muhm JR, Pritchard DJ: Computed tomography for the detection of pulmonary metastasis in patients with osteogenic sarcoma. *Proc Am Assoc Cancer Res* 21:148, 1980.

9. Rab GT, Ivins JC, Childs DS, et al: Elective whole lung irradiation in the treatment of osteogenic sarcoma. *Cancer* 38:939, 1976.

10. Ritts RE, Pritchard DJ, Gilchrist GS, et al: Transfer factor versus combination chemotherapy: An interim report of a randomized post-surgical adjuvant study in osteogenic sarcoma, in Terry WD, Windhorst D (eds): *Immunotherapy of Cancer: Present Status of Trials in Man.* New York, Raven Press, 1978.

11. Carter SK: The dilemma of adjuvant chemotherapy for osteogenic sarcoma. *Cancer Clin Trials* 3:29–36, 1980.

12. Strander H: The interferon system and its possible use in the treatment of neoplastic disease. *Cancer Immunol Immunother* 3:35, 1977.

13. Spanos PK, Payne WS, Ivins JC, et al: Pulmonary resection for metastatic osteogenic sarcoma. *JBJS* 58A:624–628, 1976.

14. Rosen G, Huvos AG, Mosende C, et al: Chemotherapy and thoracotomy for metastatic osteogenic sarcoma: A model for adjuvant chemotherapy and the rationale for the timing of thoracic surgery. *Cancer* 41:841, 1978.

15. Telander RL, Pairolero PC, Pritchard DJ, et al: Resection of pulmonary metastatic osteogenic sarcoma in children. *Surgery* 84:335, 1978.

16. Taylor WF, Ivins JC, Dahlin DC, et al: Osteogenic sarcoma experience at the Mayo Clinic, 1963–1974. *Prog Cancer Res Ther* 6:251–268, 1978.

17. Taylor WF, Ivins JC, Dahlin DC, et al: Trends and variability in survival from osteosarcoma. *Mayo Clinic Proc* 53:695–700, 1978.

18. Taylor WF, et al: Personal communication, unpublished data.

19. Edmonson JH, Green SJ, Ivins JC, et al: Post-surgical treatment of primary osteosarcoma of bone: Comparison of high dose methotrexate versus observation: Preliminary Report (abstract). *Proc Am Assoc Cancer Res* 21:476, 1980.

15

Adjuvant Chemotherapy of Brain Tumors

Shiao Y. Woo

Lucius F. Sinks

Primary brain tumors are the second most common malignancy and the most common solid tumor in children and adolescents. In adults, although the relative incidence of brain tumors is much lower and brain tumors account for only about 2% of deaths due to cancer, malignant brain tumors still present major therapeutic problems.

The most common varieties of primary malignant brain tumors encountered are astrocytomas of various grades of malignancy, including glioblastoma multiforme, occurring both supratentorially and infratentorially (brain stem glioma), medulloblastoma, and ependymoma, which are more frequently seen in children and adolescents. These malignant tumors of the CNS will be the primary focus of the discussion of the role of chemotherapy and its present and future value in the overall management of patients suffering with these malignancies.

SURGERY

Although surgery is historically the first modality of therapy for primary malignant brain tumors, it is now well recognized that a primary surgical attack has been either ineffective or fraught with excessive morbidity or mortality. In fact, less than 20% of patients with glioblastoma are likely to be suitable for radical resection because of the extent or location of the tumor (1). Currently, the role of surgery is in biopsy of the tumor for histologic diagnosis, resection (partial or total) of the tumor bulk where feasible, and decompression of the ventricles to reduce intracranial pressure. In a small series, a second surgical look after initial surgery, radiotherapy, and chemotherapy of glioblastoma was found to be beneficial in providing better diagnostic and therapeutic information and led to greater survival for patients with glioblastoma (2). Nevertheless, for almost all patients with malignant brain tumors, surgery alone cannot be expected to produce cure.

RADIOTHERAPY

Astrocytomas, medulloblastomas, and ependymomas are all radiosensitive. Radiotherapy, given postoperatively, has improved survival rates to various degrees in patients with these tumors. Radiation alone cures about one-third of patients with medulloblastoma. Postoperative irradiation of the entire craniospinal axis in patients with medulloblastoma can now achieve a five-year survival rate of about 50%. Similar results can be achieved with ependymomas (3). Radiation produces five-year survival rates of 15% to 40% in brain stem gliomas. Stage and Stein reported five-year survival rates of 40% and 15% for grades 2 and 3 astrocytomas, respectively, after surgery and irradiation (4). Sheline (5) after reviewing data from the University of California in San Francisco and selected data from the literature concluded that the five-year survival rate for grade III astrocytomas is near zero without radiotherapy but about 20% with radiotherapy. The efficacy of radiotherapy in glioblastoma multiforme is far less impressive. Survival may be prolonged in a few patients, but the cure rate is exceedingly low. The improvement in survival also seems to be limited to the first two years following presentation. Furthermore, with tumor dose radiation up to 6,000 rad, 90% of glioblastomas recurred within a 2-cm margin of the primary site (6), suggesting that current radiation doses are inadequate to eradicate the primary tumor. However, it seems unlikely that much further improvement in survival rate can be achieved with even higher doses of radiation without concurrently producing severe side effects such as brain necrosis. More realistic areas of improvement in radiotherapy are probably in radiation volume and scheduling. Newer experimental approaches using hyperbaric oxygen or using a radiosensitizer such as 5-bromodeoxyuridine (BUDR) as reported by Japanese investigators have shown some promise but are certainly not perfected enough for wide application.

Are brain tumors, like many other solid tumors, susceptible to a chemotherapeutic attack? To answer this question, one has to examine available data concerning the blood-brain barrier in relation to pharmacokinetics of drugs, the in vitro study of brain tumor cells in culture, the kinetics of brain tumors, and the available clinical experience with chemotherapy.

BRAIN TUMORS AND THE BLOOD-BRAIN BARRIER

The concept of blood-brain barrier, a mechanism that restricts the entry of certain blood-borne materials into normal brain parenchyma, arose from Ehrlich's classic experiment in 1885 (7). Since then, significant progress has been made in understanding this barrier. It is generally accepted that the blood-brain barrier is a functional barrier, the anatomical basis of which probably lies in the cerebral capillary endothelium (8,9). Several morphologic features of the cerebral capillary endothelium distinguish it from the capillary endothelium of other organs. Tight junctions exist between adjacent cells of the cerebral capillary endothelia, whereas intercellular passages are common in other capillary endothelium. A paucity of cytoplasmic pinocytotic vesicles exists in cerebral capillary endothelia. A perivascular glial sheath and a relative lack of fenestration also characterize cerebral capillary endothelium.

Because of this functional barrier, the rapidity with which an intravascular substance enters the brain depends on its lipid-partition coefficient, its molecular size, its degree of ionization in plasma, its degree of protein binding, and the presence or absence of a specific transport system for its influx into or efflux from the brain fluid (10). Thus a drug like 1,3-bis(2-chlorethyl)-1-nitrosourea (BCNU) or one of the other nitrosureas that is nonpolar and lipid-soluble crosses the brain capillaries more readily than a polar and relatively lipid-insoluble drug such as methotrexate. Brain tumors, especially malignant ones, are known to be associated with localized alterations of the blood-brain barrier, and ultrastructural aberrations of their capillaries have been observed (11). These aberrations include hyperplastic endothelial cells with irregular patent intercellular junctions, overabundance of pinocytotic vesicles, deformed basement membranes, and disruption of the perivascular glial sheath. This regional alteration of capillary permeability has been well used in diagnostic brain scans in which the contrast media or radioactive material that is protein-bound selectively passes through the capillaries at the region of the tumor. Similar increases in capillary permeability to several chemotherapeutic agents into brain tumors as opposed to normal brain tissues have been documented (12). It therefore appears that malignant brain tumors frequently disrupt the normal gliovascular and glioneuronal relationships and alter the functional barrier of brain to blood-borne materials, including drugs, which are otherwise largely excluded from the cerebrospinal fluid.

A second route of administering drugs to the brain is by direct instillation of a drug into the subarachnoid space or into the ventricles. It has been shown in rhesus monkeys that drugs such as hydroxyurea and methotrexate that cross the brain capillary complex slowly are also cleared from the cerebrospinal fluid slowly after ventriculocisternal perfusion, thereby rendering them suitable for intrathecal administration (13). Methotrexate reaches levels of 10^{-5} M in CSF after intrathecal injection, although its distribution is variable (14). Wang et al. demonstrated that MTX levels of 10^{-7} M were obtainable with intravenous injection of MTX at 500 mg/m^2 (15). Concurrent IT Methotrexate has an additive effect and results in a better distribution throughout the entire central nervous system.

IN VITRO RESPONSE OF BRAIN TUMORS TO CHEMOTHERAPEUTIC AGENTS

There is evidence that different types of brain tumor cells in culture are responsive to several chemotherapeutic agents. Lassman et al. (16) demonstrated disintegration of medulloblastoma cells in vitro after exposure to vincristine. Kornblith et al. (17) have successfully cultured and maintained several types of brain tumors and have demonstrated in vitro response of glioblastoma cells to BCNU.

MALIGNANT GLIAL CELL CYCLE KINETICS

Malignant glial cells either in culture or in vivo show a high proportion of cells in G_1 phase and a low percentage of cells in S phase. Malignant gliomas are therefore solid tumors with a low growth fraction. In addition, within the tumor the cells, depending on the proximity to blood capillaries and the diffusion coefficient of oxygen, frequently exhibit different growth characteristics and different drug sensitivities. Cells in G_1 phase are relatively insensitive to many chemotherapeutic agents. This problem can be overcome, however, by the use of the non-cycle-specific agents such as the nitrosureas. Such drugs would be expected to be more effective than S-phase-specific agents such as cytosine arabinoside. There have also been attempts to synchronize replication of glioblastoma cells in vitro with L-warfarin (18). Synchronization renders cells more susceptible to the effect of cell cycle-specific chemotherapeutic agents. Suggestive results with warfarin as an adjuvant to chemotherapy have been observed in an uncontrolled clinical trial(18).

IN VIVO RESPONSE OF BRAIN TUMORS TO CHEMOTHERAPY

Treatment of Recurrent Brain Tumors

Medulloblastoma and Ependymoma

Lassman, Pearce, and Garg in 1966 (16) reported a group of patients with recurrent brain tumors treated with vincristine. Among these were two patients with medulloblastoma treated initially with surgery and radiotherapy. The recurrent tumors were not responsive to further radiotherapy, and the patients received vincristine and both improved clinically. At the time of the report, the two patients had survived 22 months and 8 months, respectively, from the onset of vincristine therapy. Lassman et al. (19) also reported two cases of skeletal metastases from cerebellar medulloblastoma responding to vincristine. Smart et al. (20) reported one patient with recurrent medulloblastoma who had a 50% to 100% decrease in measureable tumor after vincristine that lasted three months.

Newton et al. (21) administered intrathecal methotrexate to 30 children with brain tumors that recurred after conventional therapy. These were 11 patients with medulloblastoma and 4 with ependymoma. In 18 of the 30 patients, the effect of methotrexate alone could be evaluated. Fifteen of these patients manifested subjective and objective improvement after intrathecal methotrexate therapy. Among these were 9 patients with recurrent medulloblastoma. One patient with ependymoma also responded to methotrexate.

Rosen et al. (22) using high-dose intravenous methotrexate (300 to 500 mg/kg) with citovorum factor rescue demonstrated objective response, as judged by CT scan, in 5 of 7 patients with recurrent medulloblastoma.

At Georgetown University's Vincent T. Lombardi Cancer Research Center, 2 children with recurrent medulloblastoma and 1 with recurrent ependymoma were treated with intravenous infusion of intermediate-dose methotrexate (500

mg/m^2), and all 3 patients demonstrated a >50% response (23). One patient with recurrent medulloblastoma has been in continuous remission for 17 months.

Several other agents have been reported to be effective against recurrent medulloblastoma. These include BCNU (24,25), 1,2-(chloroethyl)-3-cyclohexyl-1-nitrosourea (CCNU) (26,27), procarbazine (28), and 4-demethyl-epidodo-phyllotoxin-B-D-thenylidene-glucoside (VM-26) (29).

In addition to single-agent chemotherapy, combination chemotherapy has also been shown to be efficacious. Duffner et al. (30) reported 5 children with recurrent medulloblastoma who were treated with a combination of vincristine, BCNU, methotrexate, and dexamethasone at Roswell Park Memorial Institute. All 5 patients responded to therapy. Two patients had no recurrence 30 and 40 months later. Two others recurred but responded to further chemotherapy and are currently disease-free.

Levin and Wilson used a combination of procarbazine, CCNU, and methotrexate in 5 patients all of whom responded (31). Mealey and Hall (32) used various combinations of vincristine, methotrexate, BCNU, and CCNU in malignant cerebral astrocytoma. Response rates to the various agents were as follows: BCNU (50%) CCNU (45%), procarbazine (50%) BCNU plus vincristine (50%), and 5-(3,5-bis(2-chloroethyl)-1-triazeno) imidazole-4-carboxide (DTIC) (25%). The response rate of brain stem glioma to BCNU was 67% and to BCNU plus vincristine was 20%. The authors also stated that a limited experience with the combination of procarbazine, CCNU, and vincristine had been highly encouraging, although no response rate was quoted.

Rosen et al. (22) in a small series reported responses of recurrent pontine glioma to high-dose methotrexate in 2 of 4 patients. Sklansky et al. (29) in their phase II study of 4-demethyl-epidodophyllotoxin-β-D-thenylidene-glucoside (VM26) in brain tumors reported responses in 5 of 12 patients with progressive malignant gliomas.

A phase II study using *cis*-diammino-dichloro platinum (DDP) in recurrent brain tumors was initiated in 1976 (23). Eight patients aged 4 to 16 years received DDP, and 6 responded favorably as judged by CT scan or neurologic improvement. Among the 6 responders, 1 patient had a cerebral glioblastoma (Figs. 1 and 2), 1 had a pontine glioma, and 1 had a thalamic glioma. The response to this relatively new agent is certainly encouraging and warrants further studies.

Adjuvant Chemotherapy

Medulloblastoma

There have thus far been only a few studies conducted to explore the feasibility and possible value of adjuvant chemotherapy after surgery and postoperative irradiation in patients with medulloblastoma. In 1970, a pilot study using vincristine, oral CCNU, and intrathecal methotrexate in children with medulloblastoma was initiated at the Royal Marsden Hospital in England (37). The two-year survival rate was 60% versus 48% in a historical group of patients with recurrent medulloblastoma and produced significant extension of survival time and good palliation in most cases.

A pilot study conducted at M. D. Anderson Hospital with nitrogen mustard,

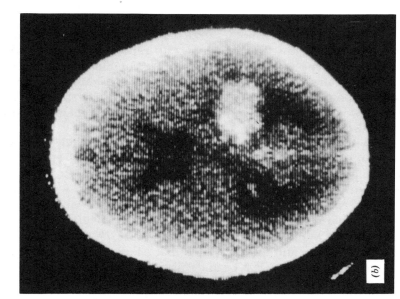

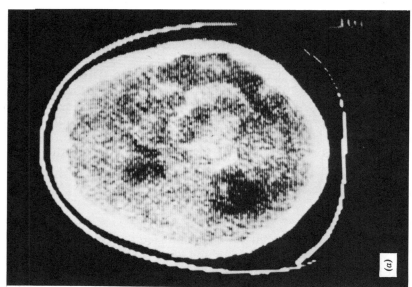

Figure 1. CT scan of an 18-year-old white man with glioblastoma multiforme in the right cerebral hemisphere. (*a*) Tumor size before treatment with *cis*-platinum; (*b*) pronounced decrease in tumor size after treatment with *cis*-platinum.

200

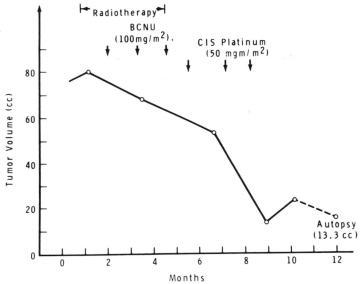

Figure 2. Volumetric estimation of tumor size (from CT scans) of above-mentioned patient with relation to treatment.

vincristine, procarbazine, and prednisone (MOPP) (33) demonstrated responses in 6 of 8 fully evaluable patients with recurrent medulloblastoma. Their survival ranged from 4 to 17 months.

Thus, there is ample evidence that medulloblastomas are sensitive to various forms of chemotherapy, and it is possible to prolong survival time and improve quality of life in patients with recurrent medulloblastoma. The experience with chemotherapy in ependymoma is much more limited, but a few patients seem to have responded favorably to various chemotherapeutic agents.

Malignant Astrocytoma, Including Glioblastoma Multiforme

Wilson et al. (34) in 1970 reported the response of recurrent brain tumors to 1,3-bis(2-chloroethyl)-1-nitrosurea (BCNU). There were 25 patients with astrocytoma or glioblastoma. The response rate of glioblastoma to BCNU was 39% and astrocytoma, 66%, with an overall response rate of 46%. No serious complications of treatment were encountered. The investigators concluded that BCNU was an effective agent against malignant glioma.

Fewer et al. (35) investigated the efficacy of 1-(-2-chloroethyl) 3-cyclohexyl-1-nitrosurea (CCNU). Five of 15 patients (33%) with recurrent glioblastoma who were not previously treated with BCNU responded to CCNU, but none of 4 patients with recurrent glioblastoma who received BCNU previously responded. The authors concluded that CCNU was as effective as BCNU against recurrent brain tumors, but cross resistance to CCNU occurred in patients previously treated with BCNU.

Wilson et al. (36), in 1976, published their review of five years of experience with single-agent chemotherapy of brain tumors. The response rates of patients treated by surgery and radiotherapy without chemotherapy were inferior to those of patients treated with all three modalities. The adjunctive chemotherapy was well tolerated without serious toxicity.

Another study was initiated in 1976 (23), in which patients with medulloblastoma were treated with surgery, cerebrospinal irradiation, and chemotherapy with intermediate-dose intravenous methotrexate (500 mg/m^2) and BCNU. There have been 12 evaluable patients aged two years who have been followed for 4 to 32 months (median 13.2 months). All the patients tolerated the chemotherapy well, and all are disease-free since treatment as evidenced by normal CT scan and stable clinical neurologic status.

The results of the Royal Marsden Hospital pilot study were sufficiently encouraging so that a randomized trial by the International Society of Pediatric Oncology (SIOP) was initiated in 1976. In this study there are two treatment groups with medulloblastoma or ependymoma: (1) those who received surgery and irradiation to the entire cerebrospinal axis and (2) those who received, in addition, adjuvant chemotherapy (vincristine and CCNU). In the last analysis, 273 patients were evaluable, and the overall three-year survival rate was about 80%. The patients receiving chemotherapy fared better than the conventionally treated group, and, in male patients and in patients under 2 years of age, the results were statistically significant.

A comparable randomized study was started in 1976, by the Children's Cancer Study Group in the United States. In this study, the chemotherapy used was vincristine, CCNU, and prednisone. In contrast to the Royal Marsden study analysis to date of the survival of 103 patients entered in the study has not yet shown a significant difference between the chemotherapy arm and the non-chemotherapy arm.

One should not come to premature conclusions from these studies because the follow-up time is inadequate. It is well known that medulloblastoma can recur up to 10 years after diagnosis. There appears, however, to be an emerging trend in favor of adjuvant chemotherapy. Even if some of these studies eventually show no demonstrable benefit of chemotherapy, one cannot conclude that adjuvant chemotherapy is of no value. Perhaps the combination of agents selected in the studies or the scheduling was not optimal. Further aggressive trials of other drug combinations based on sound knowledge of pharmacology and tumor kinetics are warranted. Such research may ultimately lead to the development of an effective adjuvant therapy for this disease.

Malignant Astrocytomas, Including Glioblastoma Multiforme
Carefully designed randomized controlled trials of adjuvant chemotherapy for malignant astrocytomas have not yet been reported.

Walker and Hurwitz (24) initially tested BCNU in 27 patients with primary or metastatic brain tumors after surgery. Sixty percent of these patients also received radiotherapy. Twenty patients had malignant or brain stem glioma, and 50% of them showed some response. The authors judged the initial experience to be sufficiently encouraging to warrant additional trials.

Subsequently, Walker and Gehan (38) reported preliminary results of the Brain Tumor Study Group in which patients were randomized to surgery alone, surgery and radiation (6,000 rad in six to seven weeks to the entire brain), surgery and BCNU, and surgery, radiation, and BCNU. The median survivals were 17, 28, 20, and 41 weeks, respectively. Postoperative irradiation as well as irradiation plus BCNU resulted in prolonged survival when compared with surgery alone. The combination of BCNU and radiation therapy appeared to yield the best results.

Shapiro and coworkers at Memorial Hospital (27) randomized patients into two groups after surgery: those who received chemotherapy alone and those who received a combination of radiotherapy and chemotherapy (vincristine and BCNU). The preliminary results showed no discernible difference between the two groups. Adjuvant chemotherapy alone appeared at least as effective as radiotherapy plus chemotherapy.

Armentrout et al. (39) in 1974 reported favorable results in their 14 patients with malignant glioma treated by a combination of surgical excision, radiotherapy (5,000 to 6,000 rad), and chemotherapy (BCNU). Nine out of the 14 patients were alive in stable or improved clinical condition with a median survival of 9.0 months.

Weir and coworkers in Canada (40) randomized patients after surgery to receive radiotherapy alone (4,000 to 4,500 rad in four to five weeks), CCNU alone, or radiation plus CCNU. The median survival time in these groups was 188, 257, and 212 days. It appears that adjuvant CCNU was as effective as radiotherapy. Although there was no statistical difference among any of these groups, the authors felt that concurrent use of CCNU may be a useful addition to radiotherapy in the treatment of astrocytoma grades III and IV, as this group had a 25% increase in mean survival time (329 days) over the other two groups (263 and 262 days).

In summary, malignant brain tumor cells are responsive to chemotherapeutic agents in vitro, and pharmacokinetic studies indicate that many of the agents can penetrate the brain and reach the tumor. There is now convincing clinical evidence that recurrent medulloblastoma is responsive to a variety of chemotherapeutic agents. The value of adjuvant chemotherapy added to surgery and radiotherapy is thus far less well established.

Malignant astrocytoma, including glioblastoma multiforme, is also responsive to chemotherapy, especially with the nitrosureas and cis-diamino-dichloro-platinum, although long-term survival is rare. Early experience with adjuvant chemotherapy suggests a beneficial role comparable in degree with that of adjuvant radiotherapy.

FUTURE DIRECTIONS

Based on the experience of treating other solid tumors, the best approach for managing patients with brain tumors is a well-coordinated multimodality one involving close cooperation among the neurosurgeon, radiotherapist, and chemotherapist. Despite ample evidence indicating effectiveness of chemotherapy in brain tumors, the state of the art is still in its infancy. A great deal of effort is needed to improve the adjuvant role of chemotherapy with the ultimate objective of producing cure in a high proportion of patients. Along this line more and larger well-planned controlled trials will be necessary in order to devise the best drug combinations with the least toxicity. Concurrently a continuous search for more effective and perhaps more specific agents with pharmacological properties ideally suited for the treatment of brain tumors needs to be carried out. In addition, a more uniform system of monitoring objective response to therapy, such as the use of CT scan, including perhaps the new technique of volumetric analysis (41), should be encouraged so that different studies can be compared more precisely.

Many chemotherapists of today are mindful of the fact that one major obstacle to the effective treatment of malignancies with drugs is a relative lack of selectivity of almost all anticancer agents. Another obstacle is resistance of the tumor to the specific agent used. For many important drugs, this resistance has been largely explained by the failure of neoplastic cells to take up the agent in a cytotoxic concentration. Any approach enabling an agent to reach its target in a selective and controlled fashion would represent a major breakthrough in cancer chemotherapy. One feasible method of achieving selective delivery of an agent to the target organ or tissue is the use of a carrier system for the agent. Recent work indicates that liposomes (phospholipids vesicle) composed of concentric lipid bilayers enclosiog aqueous spaces fulfill many requirements of a carrier system. Their synthesis from naturally occurring and thus biodegradable components, their relative lack of toxicity, their similarity to biologic membranes, and their ability to entrap a wide variety of agents have made them potentially useful carriers for targeting the delivery of antineoplastic agents.

Although the intact central nervous system does not take up liposomes avidly after systemic injection, pharmacokinetic studies on liposome-entrapped drugs in monkeys and rats (42,43) showed drug levels in brain several fold higher than after injection of the free drug. Moreover, the localized alteration of blood-brain barrier at the brain tumor potentially enables selective entry of macromolecules, such as the liposomes into the brain tumor as opposed to the normal brain. At Georgetown University's Vincent T. Lombardi Cancer Research Center, a recent study was carried out treating intracranial L1210 leukemia bearing mice with liposomal methotrexate, free MTX, and saline (44). Liposomal methotrexate was significantly superior to the free drug in prolonging survival of the mice and actually produced cure in a proportion of the mice treated. Experiments on other brain tumor systems are in progress. Thus liposomes represent a potentially useful tool for chemotherapists treating brain tumors in the future.

CONCLUSION

There is now convincing evidence of the efficacy of chemotherapy in malignant brain tumors. Clinicians caring for patients with brain tumors need to shed the prevailing cloak of pessimism and concentrate on development of better treatment regimens. Much can be learned from the experience of treating another solid tumor in children, namely, Wilms' tumor. The same pessimism existed amongst clinicians caring for patients with Wilms' tumor three decades ago. However, with a long series of studies combining surgery, radiotherapy, and chemotherapy the overall cure rate of Wilms' tumor has risen dramatically to 75% to 80%. In addition, it has been possible to refine treatment in good risk patients so that toxicity is reduced to a minimum. We are hopeful that the treatment of brain tumors will follow a similar direction to the ultimate benefit of all patients afflicted with these malignancies.

REFERENCES

1. Hitchcock E, Sato F: Treatment of malignant gliomata. *J Neurosurg* 21:497, 1964.
2. Balcueva EP, Field EM, de los Santos RS, et al: Second surgical look (SSL) following adjuvant treatment of glioblastoma. *ASCO Abstract* C-259:371, 1978.
3. Salazar OM, Rubin P, Bassano D, et al: Improved survival of patients with intracranial ependymomas by irradiation: Dose selection and field extension. *Cancer* 35:1563, 1975.
4. Stage WS, Stein JJ: Treatment of malignant astrocytoma. *Am J Roentgenol Radiat Ther Nucl Med* 120:7, 1974.
5. Sheline GE: The importance of distinguishing tumor grade in malignant gliomas: Treatment and prognosis. *Int J Radiat Oncol Biol Phys* 1:781, 1976.
6. Pruitt A, Hochberg FH: Assumptions in the radiotherapy of malignant glioblastoma, GS 29. *Neurology* 29:583, 1979.
7. Ehrlich P: Das Sauerstoffbedurfnis des Organismus, *Eine Farbenanalytische Studie.* Berlin, Hirschwald, 1885, pp 69.
8. Karnovsky MJ: The ultrastructural basis of capillary permeability studied with peroxidase as a tracer. *J Cell Biol* 35:213, 1967.
9. Reese T, Karnovsky M: Fine structural localization of a blood-brain barrier to exogenous peroxidase. *J Cell Biol* 34:207, 1967.
10. Wilbrandt W, Rosenberg T: The concept of carrier transport and its corollaries in pharmacology. *Pharmacol Rev* 13:109, 1961.
11. Long DM: Capillary ultrastructure and the blood-brain barrier in human malignant brain tumors. *J Neurosurg* 32:127, 1976.
12. Levin VA, Lindahl H, Patlak CS: Considerations in selecting effective brain tumor agents in capillary permeability and sequestered cell populations. *AACR Abstract* 806:202, 1976.
13. Blasberg RG, Patlak CS, Fenstermacher JD: Intrathecal chemotherapy: Brain tissue profiles after ventriculo-cisternal perfusion. *J Pharmacol Exp Ther* 195:73, 1975.
14. Shapiro WR, Young DF, Bipin MM: Methotrexate: Distribution in cerebrospinal fluid after intravenous, ventricular and lumbar injections. *N Engl J Med* 293:161, 1975.
15. Wang JJ, Freeman AI, Sinks LF: Treatment of acute lymphocytic leukemia using high-dose methotrexate. *Cancer Res* 36(4):1441, 1976.
16. Lassman LP, Pearce GW, Gang J: Effect of vincristine sulphate on the intracranial gliomata of childhood. *Brit J Surg* 53(9):774, 1966.
17. Walsh JM, Cassady JR, Frei E II, et al: Recent advances in the treatment of primary brain tumors. *Arch Surg* 110:696, 1975.
18. Kirsch WM, Van Buskirk JJ, Schulz DW, et al: The biologic basis of malignant brain tumor therapy. *Adv Neurol* 15:301, 1976.
19. Lassman LP, Pearce GW, Banna M, et al: Vincristine sulphate in the treatment of skeletal metastases from cerebellar medulloblastoma. *J Neurosurg* 30:42, 1969.
20. Smart CR, Ottoman RE, Rochlin DB, et al: Clinical experience with vincristine (NSC-67574) in tumors of the central nervous system and other malignant diseases. *Cancer Chemo Rep* 52(7):733, 1968.
21. Newton WA, Sayers MP, Samuels LP: Intrathecal methotrexate (NSC-740) therapy for brain tumors in children. *Cancer Chemo Rep* 52(2):257, 1968.
22. Rosen G, Chanimi F, Nirenberg A, et al: High dose methotrexate with citrovorum factor rescue for the treatment of central nervous system tumors in children. *Cancer Treat Rep* 61(4):681, 1977.

23. Sinks LF: Personal communication.

24. Walker MD, Hurwitz BS: BCNU (1,3-bis(2-chloroethyl)-1-nitrosourea; NSC-409962) in the treatment of malignant brain tumor in a preliminary report. *Cancer Chemo Rep* 54:263, 1970.

25. Fewer D, Wilson CB, Boldrey EB, et al: The chemotherapy of brain tumors: Clinical experience with carmustine (BCNU) and vincristine. *JAMA* 222:549, 1972.

26. Ward HWC: CCNU in the treatment of recurrent medulloblastoma. *Brit Med J* 1:642, 1974.

27. Shapiro WR: Malignant brain tumor chemotherapy: II. Clinical studies. *Clin Bull* 3:2, 90, 1973.

28. Kumar ARV, Renaudin J, Wilson CB, et al: Procarbazine hydrochloride in the treatment of brain tumors: Phase II study. *J Neurosurg* 40:365, 1974.

29. Sklansky BC, Mann-Kaplan RS, Reynold J, AF, et al: 4'-demethyl-epipodophyllotoxin-β-D-thenylidene-glucoside (PTG) in the treatment of malignant intracranial neoplasms. *Cancer* 33:460, 1974.

30. Duffner PK, Cohen ME, Thomas PRM, et al: Combination chemotherapy in recurrent medulloblastoma. *Cancer* 43:41, 1979.

31. Levin VA, Wilson CB: Chemotherapy: The agents in current use. *Semin Oncol* 2:63, 1975.

32. Mealey J, Hall PV: Medulloblastoma in children. *J Neurosurg* 46:56, 1977.

33. Sutow WW: Personal communication.

34. Wilson CB, Boldrey EB, Enot KJ: 1,3-bis(2-chloroethyl)-1-nitrosourea (NSC-409962) in the treatment of brain tumors. *Cancer Chemo Rep* 54(4):273, 1970.

35. Fewer D, Wilson CB, Boldrey EB, et al: Phase II Study of 1-(2-chloroethyl)-3-cyclohexyl-1-nitrosoureas (CCNU; NSC-79037) in the treatment of brain tumors. *Cancer Chemo Rep* 56(3):421, 1972.

36. Wilson CB, Gutin O, Boldrey EB, et al: Single agent chemotherapy of brain tumors in a five-year review. *Arch Neurol* 33:739, 1976.

37. Bloom HJG: Combined modality therapy for intracranial tumors. *Cancer* 35:111, 1975.

38. Walker MD, Gehan EA: An evaluation of 1,3-bis(2-chloroethyl)-1-nitrosourea (BCNU) and irradiation alone and in combination for the treatment of malignant glioma. *Proc Am Assoc Cancer Res* 13:67, 1972.

39. Armentrout SA, Foltz E, Vernund H, et al: Management of malignant glioma with surgery, irradiation and BCNU. *Proc Am Soc Clin Oncol* 15:183, 1974.

40. Weir B, Bond P, Urtasun R, et al: Radiotherapy and CCNU in the treatment of high-grade supratentorial astrocytomas. *J Neurosurg* 45:129, 1976.

41. McCullough DC, Huang HK, DeMichelle D, et al: Correlation between volumetric CT imaging and autopsy measurement of glioblastoma size. *Compu Tomog* 3:133,1979.

42. Kimelberg HK, Atchison MA: Effects of entrapment in liposomes on the distribution, degradation and effectiveness of methotrexate *in vivo*. *Ann NY Acad Sci* 308:395, 1978.

43. Kimelberg JK, Tracy TF, Watson RE, et al: Distribution of free and liposome-entrapped ^{3}(H) methotrexate in the central nervous system after intracerebroventricular injection in a primate. *Cancer Res* 38:706, 1978.

44. Dilliplane DP, Woo Sy, Rahman A, et al: Enhancement of chemotherapeutic efficacy of methotrexate entrapped in liposomes against murine intracranial L1210 leukemia. Personal communication.

16

Is Chemotherapy Useful in the Most Frequently Encountered Brain Tumors?

Philip H. Gutin

The application of empirically derived, single-drug and multidrug regimens has led to palliative control of leukemias, lymphomas, and a small group of solid tumors, including choriocarcinoma, testicular tumors, rhabdomyosarcoma, Wilms' tumor, osteogenic sarcoma, and breast carcinoma. Despite the hopeful fervor of the 1960s, however, cure by chemotherapy remains uncommon.

The chemotherapy of brain tumors has consistently been among the most disappointing failures in clinical oncology, achieving at best only short-term palliation. The results with chemotherapeutic agents against primary malignant glial tumors are a case in point (Table 1).

As a rule, it is the drugs that readily cross the blood-brain barrier and are cell-cycle phase nonspecific in their mode of action, such as the nitrosoureas (BCNU, CCNU) and procarbazine, that yield the best results as single agents against tumors of the brain (1); and it is drug combinations, rather than single agents, that have the greatest impact. But even with combinations that include potent, cell-cycle nonspecific drugs that readily cross the blood-brain barrier, the results have been poor.

THE CASE AGAINST BRAIN TUMOR CHEMOTHERAPY

For medulloblastoma, the usefulness of chemotherapeutic agents is regrettably restricted, as bone marrow reserves that have been compromised by previous craniospinal radiation do not tolerate the challenge of systemic chemotherapy. Chemotherapy of recurrent medulloblastoma at our institution (2) has achieved responses in about 60% of patients, the subsequent median time to tumor pro-

Table 1. Relative Efficacy of Chemotherapeutic Agents Against Primary Malignant Gliomas

Drug	Primary Chemotherapy	Adjuvant Chemotherapy
Single Agents		
Cell Cycle Specific Agents		
Bromodeoxyuridine (BudR)	NE	+
5-Fluorouracil (5-FU)	NE	$\emptyset$
Hydroxyurea (HU)	NE	+
Methotrexate (MTX)	+	$\emptyset$
Vinblastine	+	NE
Vincristine (VCR)	+	NE
Epipodophyllotoxin (VM-26)	+	NE
Cell Cycle Nonspecific Agents		
1,3-Bis(2-chloroethyl)-1-nitrosourea (BCNU)	+ + +	+ +
Bleomycin	NE	+
Bis(2-chloroethyl-1-triazeno)imidazole-4-carboxamide (BIC)	+	NE
1-(2-Chloroethyl)-3-cyclohexyl-1-nitrosourea (CCNU)	+ +	+
Dianhydrogalactitol (DAG)	$\emptyset$	+
Mithramycin	+	$\emptyset$
Nitrogen mustard	+	NE
Procarbazine (PCB)	+ +	$\emptyset$
Thiotepa	$\emptyset$	NE
Combination chemotherapy		
Adriamycin-VM-26-CCNU	+ +	NE
BCNU-5-FU	+ + +	NE
BCNU-MTX-VCR	NE	+
BCNU-PCB	+ + +	NE
BCNU-VCR	+	$\emptyset$
BCNU-VM-26	+	$\emptyset$
CCNU-PCB-VCR	+ + +	+ +
CCNU-VCR-MTX	+ +	$\emptyset$
BCNU-HU	NE	+ +

NE = nonevaluable because of incomplete information, less than 6 patients with similar tumors, method of evaluation not defined, or no study reported.

$\emptyset$ = no evidence of activity when evaluated as a primary form of chemotherapy, or no better than irradiation alone when evaluated in adjuvant chemotherapy studies.

+ + + = good activity defined as a median increase in survival time or time to tumor progression of 6–9 months for primary chemotherapy; an increase in survival time or time to tumor progression of 2–4 months for adjuvant chemotherapy, or doubling of long-term survivors over radiation therapy alone.

+ + = moderate activity.

+ = slight activity.

Reprinted with permission from Levin VA: Current trends in brain tumor therapy, in Paoletti P, Walker MD, Butti G, Knerich R (eds): *Multidisciplinary Aspects of Brain Tumor Therapy.* Amsterdam, Elsevier/North Holland Biomedical Press, 1979.

gression being 45 weeks. For the patients responding, deterioration usually began when bone marrow toxicity dictated a reduction in drug doses. The value of adjuvant chemotherapy for medulloblastoma is still equivocal; two large, cooperative study groups, the Children's Cancer Study Group and the Société Internationale Oncologica Pediatrica, have generated conflicting results. At best, conjoint therapy with surgery, craniospinal irradiation, and chemotherapy produces five-year survival in only 40% to 50% of patients (3).

For recurrent glioblastomas and anaplastic astrocytomas, a remission of 26 to 30 weeks can be induced by chemotherapy in 50% of patients, but a longer period of remission (52 weeks) can be expected in only 20% (4). Adjuvant chemotherapy is even less effective, adding little time, if any, to the survival of patients who undergo surgery and radiation therapy for these tumors (5).

More than 90% of anaplastic astrocytomas and glioblastomas are localized to a single area of the brain (6). Metastases from these tumors within the central nervous system are uncommon (7), and systemic metastases are rare (8,9). Almost all solid tumors that have not metastasized by the time they are detected are curable by surgery and radiation (10). Yet, despite the localized nature of almost all malignant brain tumors, the principal experimental thrust in their treatment has been the application of systemic chemotherapy—a modality for which the traditional target has been disease that spreads beyond its site of origin. The emphasis on systemic chemotherapy for malignant brain tumors seems particularly misguided when one considers the multitude of obstacles to its efficacy: (1) the difficulties in achieving adequate surgical resection, (2) the problems in delivering adequate drug to tumors, and (3) development of resistance to drugs.

Difficult Surgical Resection

Computerized tomography (CT) scanning is a major factor contributing to our ability to diagnose brain tumors earlier; but by the time clinical indications are clear and a scan is obtained, the tumor is at least 0.5 cm in diameter and contains from 10^{10} to 10^{11} cells (10 to 100 g). These tumors have a significant population of nonproliferating (G_0) cells and have approached a growth plateau consistent with Gompertzian kinetics. Large tumors, with their sizable fraction of nondividing cells, are more resistant to cytotoxic therapy than are smaller tumors of the same type (11).

In 1964, Skipper et al (12) showed that cell kill by chemotherapeutic agents follows first-order kinetics, a fraction of the cells, rather than a definite number, being inactivated by a given dose. Shackney's computer simulation studies (13) show that large tumors are more resistant to chemotherapy, not because of the inability of drugs to eradicate the larger numbers of cells present, but because a progressive reduction in fractional cell kill per course of therapy takes place in the larger, and consequently slower-growing, tumors. Steel and his coworkers (14) confirmed this dependency of efficacy on tumor size when they showed that BCNU produced greater fractional cell kill per dose in smaller Lewis lung tumors than in larger ones.

It is perhaps because of the increased fractional cell kill (per unit drug dose) possible in smaller tumors that cytoreductive surgery is so valuable to the subsequent chemotherapy of many solid tumors. When resection of at least 90% of the abdominal tumor bulk has been achieved in patients with Burkitt's lymphoma, chemotherapy-induced remissions and long-term survivals are comparable with those achieved in patients with jaw involvement only (15). Patients who do not have gross residual ovarian carcinoma after surgery respond better to chemotherapy also (16).

Widespread metastasis and local invasion are the major limitations to the surgical resection of cancer of any kind (17). Although primary brain tumors metastasize infrequently, except in the case of medulloblastoma, local invasion poses a nearly insurmountable problem in accomplishing adequate surgical resection of these tumors.

As the great majority of malignant brain tumors are surgically accessible (18), and particularly in view of the increased response to chemotherapy that can be anticipated after reducing tumor volume, the decision not to biopsy a suspected tumor, or to perform only a needle biopsy, is patently nihilistic in all but the most extreme circumstances. However, because a malignant brain tumor has never been cured by surgery, the principle of aggressiveness in good cancer surgery must be tempered with the principle of preservation of neurological function in good brain surgery. The invasiveness of brain tumors into cerebral areas that subserve important functions precludes extensive surgical resection of tumor. One does not recklessly pursue infiltrative tumors deep into the dominant hemisphere without the risk of reducing the patient to a vegetative state.

Another factor preventing more extensive surgical reduction of malignant brain tumors is the network of thin-walled blood vessels entering, exiting, and coursing within them (Fig. 1). These vessels, particularly those associated with high-flow arteriovenous shunts, bleed profusely when opened and are difficult to close using the customary hemostatic maneuvers. The surgeon must use a variety of techniques, one of the most effective being coagulation with the correct application of bipolar forceps. Hemostasis by tamponade and the application of foreign materials that promote coagulation prove relatively ineffective in brain tumor surgery because transected neoplastic arteries have little tendency to contract. When there is brisk arterial bleeding, which is often the situation near the tumor's deep surface, the surgeon may elect either to leave this portion of the tumor in situ, after achieving a dry field, or to remove the remaining tumor rapidly and control bleeding from the less fragile vessels at the tumor's surface. Few neurosurgical decisions require finer judgement because, if resection has not achieved adequate internal decompression, postoperative edema of the residual tumor and surrounding brain may cause serious complications.

The application of microsurgical techniques to the surgery of malignant brain tumors has helped the surgeon to differentiate tumor from normal tissue and to identify small points of persistent bleeding for coagulation. In addition, some surgeons have relied on the effects of adjuvant radiation and chemotherapy to reduce tumor vascularity, so that additional tumor can be removed at a "second look" operation (19).

Nonetheless, even the most aggressive resection of a malignant glioma fails to reduce the number of tumor cells by more than about 1 log. This leaves, in the best circumstances, 10^9 to 10^{10} cells to be eradicated by radiation and chemotherapy. With so great a residual burden of tumor after surgery, subsequent therapy can hardly be considered adjuvant. Before the impressive results

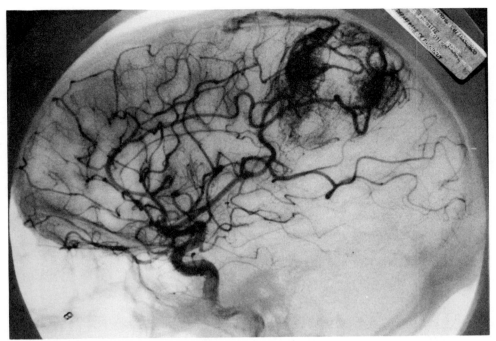

Figure 1. Lateral projection of a left internal carotid arteriogram showing hypervascularity and rapid arteriovenous shunting in a glioblastoma of the dominant parietal lobe.

achieved by the adjuvant chemotherapy of breast carcinoma and osteogenic sarcoma can be emulated in cases of brain tumor, the means for more completely reductive surgery must be perfected, so that residual tumor burden no longer exceeds the cell kill potential of available chemotherapeutic agents (20).

Delivering the Drug

Of all the barriers to any drug leaving the circulation and entering the extracellular space of any tumor, none matches the vigilance of the blood-brain barrier in excluding chemotherapeutic agents. Whereas the capillaries of almost all tissues have gaps between their capillary endothelial cells to allow relatively free exchange of substances, the brain capillary endothelium has "tight junctions" that permit the exchange of only certain molecules (21). Rall and Zubrod (22) characterized these molecules as lipid-soluble, minimally ionized, and of low molecular weight.

Vick, Khandekar, and Bigner (23) have minimized the role of the blood-brain barrier in impeding the penetration of antitumor agents into malignant brain tumors. Their argument is based on the morphology of the capillary endothelium in brain tumors, their assertion being that there are extensive defects in the tight junctions that allow penetration of even very large molecules. Nevertheless, it is drugs capable of crossing the normal blood-brain barrier that are most effective against intracerebral tumor models (1) and against malignant brain tumors in humans (24,25). An understanding of the principles of drug delivery to the brain makes this apparent paradox less mysterious.

All chemotherapeutic agents require a specific exposure to tumor in order for them to kill tumor cells effectively. On the basis that this exposure depends on the concentration of drug and the time that the drug is present in the critical area, Skipper and his coworkers (26) promulgated the concept of concentration $\times$ time (C $\times$ T) to reflect the total amount of drug reaching a tumor cell. The C $\times$ T for an individual tumor cell and an individual drug depends on the distance of the tumor cell from a capillary, the permeability of that capillary to the drug, the extracellular-intracellular partition of the drug, and the rate of breakdown of the drug (27). Since the slopes of most drug dose-response curves are quite steep, when derived from tumor cells cultured in vitro where drug

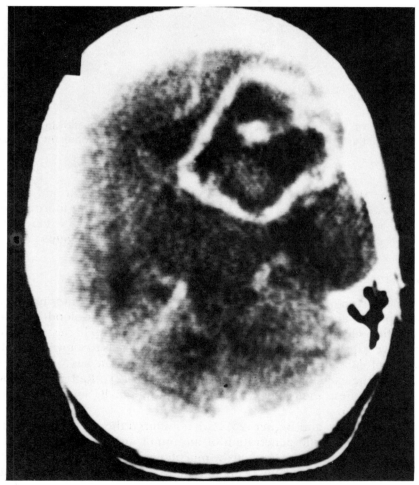

Figure 2. Axial computerized tomographic scan of a patient with a glioblastoma multiforme. The periphery shows contrast enhancement; the large central necrotic zone does not.

delivery is virtually assured, the failure of chemotherapy to cure certain solid tumors suggests that the C × T is often inadequate in the clinical situation.

Two areas of the malignant brain tumor offer the greatest challenge to the chemotherapist seeking to optimize C × T: (1) the "growing edge" of the tumor infiltrating adjacent brain and (2) the tumor's central, necrotic core, seen as a low-density region on the CT scan (Fig. 2).

The growing edge of a malignant brain tumor infiltrates the surrounding normal brain; the cells in this advancing front are among the most actively proliferative cells in the tumor. As the blood-brain barrier in the capillaries of brain adjacent to the tumor is relatively intact, a drug's ability to cross the barrier is an important prerequisite to there being an adequate C × T in this region (28,29). The strict physical requirements (lipid solubility, minimal ionization, low molecular weight) for a chemotherapeutic agent effective against brain tumors prevail, therefore, despite the defects in tumor capillary tight junctions seen by Vick, Khandekar, and Bigner (23) in the tumor itself. The superior therapeutic impact of lipid-soluble, low-molecular-weight, and relatively un-ionized drugs against malignant brain tumors can be explained, in part, by their ability to traverse the intact barrier at the growing edge.

A central necrotic core develops when a malignant brain tumor reaches a critical size. Despite the hypoxia and poor perfusion of this core, it contains viable tumor cells (many of them G_0). Experimental trials have shown that cells from this region grow into tumors when transplanted (30) or into colonies when cultured (31). To achieve a C × T adequate for cell kill in this necrotic tumor core, drugs must penetrate inward from the leaky, well-perfused tumor shell. Levin and his coworkers (27) have shown, however, that even lipid-soluble drugs with a high diffusion coefficient penetrate little more than a few millimeters from the shell, even if the concentration gradient is maintained for 24 hours.

Perhaps a prolonged intravenous infusion of any chemotherapeutic agent with its attendant prolonged concentration gradient would successfully enhance the C × T at the growing edge or in the necrotic core, but the consequent systemic toxicity would likely be profound. There is a close relationship between systemic toxicity and drug delivery. To achieve a C × T adequate for cure, while restricting toxicity to tolerable levels, is the goal for every chemotherapist; for the brain tumor chemotherapist, this goal seems remote.

Resistance to Drug

The resistance of tumor cells to oncolytic agents is a primary cause of chemotherapeutic failure. Tumor cells may be resistant to certain drugs for several reasons, including poor uptake of drug by the cell, insufficient drug activation in the cell, rapid breakdown of drug in the cell, an increase in the number of the cell's target molecules, and rapid cellular repair of drug-induced lesions. Because the problem of drug resistance is not unique to brain tumors, this factor is discussed only briefly.

Two scenarios have been proposed for drug resistance: (1) certain tumor cells are inherently resistant to certain drugs from the beginning of therapy, and (2) tumor cells acquire resistance during therapy. Most likely, both situations arise and contribute to the overall problem.

It is not difficult to conceive that there may be inherent resistance of a clone, or several clones, in a glioblastoma multiforme, given the tremendous cellular diversity present in these and other malignant brain tumors. The heterogeneity of cells with respect to morphology, chromosome numbers, biochemical markers, immunogenicity, clonogenicity, cell kinetics, and response to chemotherapy, both within and among a number of human glioblastoma and anaplastic astrocytoma cell lines, has been described in reports of tissue culture and nude mouse passage by several groups (32,33). Figure 3 shows the effect of chemotherapy on a tumor burden of 10^{10} cells when a mere 10 cells are resistant to the drug used. After initial regression and under continuing chemotherapy, proliferation of the resistant cells results in tumor regrowth.

The regression and eventual regrowth of tumor under continuing therapy can also be explained by the cells' development of resistance to drug during therapy. Some hold that it is exposure to the agent that induces the tumor cell's resistance to it. If this is true, a sublethal $C \times T$ in a brain tumor could be a major contributor to the development of resistance. Others believe, however, that spontaneous mutations occur. Spontaneous mutation to resistance has been

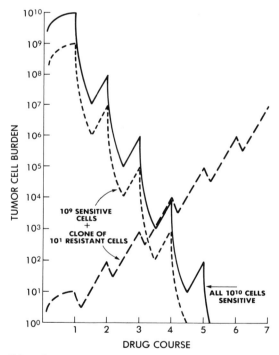

Figure 3. Tumor cell burden when all 10^{10} cells are sensitive (—) to a drug that produces a 3 log cell kill pretreatment and when a mere 10 cells are resistant to the drug (---). When a few cells are resistant, objective tumor remission occurs, but long-term survival does not because of proliferation of the resistant cells. (Reprinted with permission from Levin VA: Current trends in brain tumor therapy, in Paoletti P, Walker MD, Butti G, et al (eds): *Multidisciplinary Aspects of Brain Tumor Therapy.* Amsterdam, Elsevier/North Holland Biomedical Press, 1979.)

demonstrated in bacteria (34) and in L1210 leukemia (35). Of course, since spontaneous mutations taking place before a tumor is clinically detected could well account for the de novo resistant cell clones, there may be no distinction between inherent and acquired resistance.

ALTERNATIVES—BRAIN TUMOR AS LOCALIZED DISEASE

Since the bulk of anaplastic astrocytomas and glioblastomas are localized to one area at the time of diagnosis (6) and since systemic chemotherapy, with all its problems, may not be a rational approach to such local disease, alternatives should be explored. There are, at the moment, a number of promising innovations.

Radiation

Because ionizing radiation crosses physiological barriers with impunity, conventional whole-brain radiation has been the mainstay of adjuvant brain tumor therapy. It has been used in a standard, unvarying fractionation scheme for nearly every patient treated in almost all the chemotherapy protocols used over the years. The Brain Tumor Study Group (5) reported the first adequately controlled trial comparing adjuvant chemotherapy with radiation therapy and showed that radiation therapy after surgery contributed significantly more than chemotherapy to the patient's survival: the higher the radiation dose, the longer the survival (36).

The brain's tolerance to radiation is soon reached, however, and the cure of the malignant brain tumor, for the most part a localized disease entity, is beyond the ability of any radiation modality that affects not only the tumor but also significant areas of brain surrounding it (37). Nowhere is this principle better illustrated than in the clinical study from the University of Washington (38), where cyclotron-generated fast neutrons were used to treat patients with glioblastomas. Almost all these patients died from radiation necrosis: the radiation "cure" was achieved, but only at the cost of fatal destruction of brain.

Because radiation therapy has shown significant activity against malignant brain tumors and because high radiation doses damage normal brain, ways have been sought to increase the therapeutic ratio of brain irradiation. These efforts have focused on the development of new radiation techniques and on the identification of drugs that increase the radiosensitivity of tumor cells and so effectively reduce the dose of radiation necessary for cure.

Radiation biologists have identified cells in solid tumors that, because of their distance from adequate capillary nutrition, are depleted of oxygen (39). Because oxygen is essential in the chemical process that causes damage from radiation, these hypoxic cells are radioresistant and therefore a barrier to cure (40). A number of nitroimidazole compounds have the ability to sensitize the hypoxic cells in tumors to radiation. Metronidazole (Flagyl) has shown activity in patients with glioblastomas (41), and the testing of new nitroimidazoles (most prominently, misonidazole) against malignant brain tumors is already underway (40). As these trials have shown that a factor limiting the efficacy of these agents is their toxicity to peripheral nerves, nitroimidazole compounds are being designed that have less toxicity but the same ability to sensitize hypoxic cells (40). Another potential problem is that the delivery of radiation sensitizers to the central necrotic (hypoxic) core of a tumor is as difficult as delivery of conventional chemotherapeutic agents. The advantage of these sensitizers is that the concentration of the sensitizer in the cell must be adequate only at the instant when the cell is irradiated. The T in the C × T requirement is eliminated.

Although it is unlikely that neurosurgeons can make further significant technological innovations in the surgical resection of tumor volume in the foreseeable future, they are helping in a tangible way to develop means to increase the therapeutic ratio of radiation therapy for brain tumors. European neurosurgeons have used stereotactic techniques to implant radioisotopes directly into brain tumors for therapeutic purposes (42). These interstitial implants irradiate the tumor continuously at dose rates of 10 to 100 rad/hr. Using this technique, it is possible to deliver a therapeutic dose of radiation at these low dose rates over several days while sparing normal tissue; the same total dose given at conventional (high) dose rates must be divided into multiple fractions over several weeks to avoid necrosis of the normal tissue (43).

One reason for the increased therapeutic ratio obtained with low-dose-rate interstitial therapy is the rapid decline in radiation exposure of tissue at any increment of distance from an implanted radioactive source (inverse square law), which consequently spares surrounding normal tissues. In addition, the radiation that normal tissues do receive from implants is better tolerated, because normal cells have a better capacity for repairing sublethal low-dose-rate radiation damage than tumor cells (44) and possibly because tumor cells become increasingly radiosensitive under continuous low-dose-rate exposure as a result of tumor reoxygenation and cell-cycle redistribution (45,46).

Because of the increased therapeutic ratio that is possible with interstitial radiation therapy, surgeons at the University of California, San Francisco (UCSF) (47), have stereotactically implanted various radioisotopes (^{192}I, ^{198}Au, ^{125}I) into 27 patients who had recurrent malignant brain tumors. We have recorded a promising number of palliative responses and are now planning trials of adjuvant interstitial radiation to the tumor to provide a local boost after conventional whole-brain radiation and trials of interstitial radiation therapy administered with hypoxic cell sensitizers.

Other efforts to improve the therapeutic ratio of brain tumor radiation therapy have evolved from the development of high linear-energy transfer (LET) radiation modalities for cancer treatment. As the cytocidal effectiveness of high LET radiation is less dependent on the oxygenation of the target cells, these modalities have greater activity against hypoxic cells than conventional photon therapy (48). The efficacy and attendant difficulties with neutron therapy have been discussed elsewhere (38). However, charged particles with high LET, like pi-mesons or heavy ions (neon, carbon, helium, argon), have an advantage over neutrons, in that they are subject to the Bragg effect: enormous amounts of energy can be deposited in well-localized regions, and normal brain can be spared (49). Pi-meson irradiation of brain tumors is being investigated at Los Alamos, New Mexico, and trials with accelerated heavy ions at the BEVALAC facility at the Lawrence Berkeley Laboratory in California will soon be underway.

Chemotherapy

Recognizing that the malignant brain tumor is, for the most part, a local disease and recognizing the brain's pharmacokinetic obstacles to the penetration of many of the most potent antitumor agents, a number of investigators (50–52) have instilled drugs directly into brain tumors, hoping to drive the local concentration to cytotoxic levels. Because intratumoral concentrations must remain consistently high to create a gradient for diffusion of drugs to all parts of the tumor (3), the intermittent injection protocols used in these studies proved largely ineffective. With the recent advent of implantable pumps that continuously deliver predictable volumes of drug (53), intratumoral chemotherapy again becomes an exciting possibility. The continuous delivery of drug to the center of a brain tumor over many days could maintain the concentration gradient long enough to allow its diffusion out to the tumor's growing edge. Even a drug that has a suboptimal diffusion coefficient could, theoretically, be delivered in this fashion if it were not biotransformed too rapidly (3). At UCSF, we are planning trials of intratumoral chemotherapy with cytotoxic agents and with hypoxic cell radiosensitizers in combination with radiation.

CONCLUSION

During the decade of brain tumor chemotherapy that began with optimism and ended with frustration, time and effort have not been wasted. We have identified drugs and drug combinations that have provided useful palliation for many patients. More important, we have identified the problems involved in obtaining a better therapeutic ratio. Perhaps the inherent optimism of clinical and laboratory research oncologists will be more measured, and its direction more finely focused, as the next decade begins with fresh approaches to the treatment of brain tumors.

REFERENCES

1. Geran RI, Congleston GF, Dudeck LE: A mouse ependymoblastoma as an experimental model for screening potential antineoplastic drugs. *Cancer Chemother Rep* 4:53, 1974.
2. Crafts DC, Levin VA, Edwards MS, et al: Chemotherapy of recurrent medulloblastoma with combined procarbazine, CCNU, and vincristine. *J Neurosurg* 49:582, 1978.
3. Levin VA: Current trends in brain tumor therapy, in Paoletti P, Walker MD, Butti G, Knerich R (eds): *Multidisciplinary Aspects of Brain Tumor Therapy*. Amsterdam, Elsevier, North Holland, Biomedical Press, 1979, p 165.
4. Levin VA, Hoffman WF, Pischer TL, et al: BCNU-5-fluorouracil combination therapy for recurrent malignant brain tumors. *Cancer Treat Rep* 62:2071, 1978.
5. Walker MD, Alexander E Jr, Hunt WE, et al: Evaluation of BCNU and/or radiotherapy in the treatment of anaplastic gliomas. A cooperative clinical trial. *J Neurosurg* 49:333, 1978.
6. Pruitt A, Hochberg FH: Assumptions in the radiotherapy of malignant glioblastoma (abstract). *Neurology* 29:583, 1979.
7. Erlich SS, Davis RL: Spinal subarachnoid metastasis from primary intracranial glioblastoma multiforme. *Cancer* 42:2854, 1978.
8. Alvord EC: Why do gliomas not metastasize? *Arch Neurol* 33:73, 1976.

9. Smith DR, Hardman JM, Earle KM: Metastasizing neurectodermal tumors of the central nervous system. *J Neurosurg* 31:50, 1969.

10. Zubrod CG: Chemical control of cancer. *Proc Natl Acad Sci* (USA) 69:1042, 1972.

11. Schabel FM Jr: Concepts for systemic treatment of micrometastases. *Cancer* 35:15, 1974.

12. Skipper HE, Schabel FM Jr, Wilcox WS: Experimental evaluation of potential anticancer agents. XIII. On the criteria and kinetics associated with "curability" of experimental leukemia. *Cancer Chemother Rep* 35:1, 1964.

13. Shackney SE: A computer model for tumor growth and chemotherapy, its application to L1210 leukemia treated with cytosine arabinoside (NSC-63878). *Cancer Chemother Rep* 54:399, 1970.

14. Steel GG, Adams K, Stanley J: Size-dependence of the response of Lewis lung tumors to BCNU. *Cancer Treat Rep* 60:1743, 1976.

15. Magrath IT, Lawanga S, Carswell W, et al: Surgical reduction of tumor bulk in management of abdominal Burkitt's lymphoma. *Br Med J* 2:308, 1974.

16. Griffiths CT, Parker LM, Fuller AF: Role of cytoreductive surgical treatment in the management of advanced ovarian cancer. *Cancer Treat Rep* 63:235, 1979.

17. Skipper HE: Adjuvant chemotherapy. *Cancer* 41:936, 1978.

18. Bartal AD, Heibronn YD, Schiffer J: Extensive resection of primary malignant tumors of the left cerebral hemisphere. *Surg Neurol* 1:337, 1973.

19. Balcueva EP, Field EM, de los Santos RS, et al: Second surgical look (SSL) following adjuvant treatment of glioblastoma. *Proc Am Soc Clin Oncol* 19:371, 1978.

20. Schabel FM: Surgical adjuvant chemotherapy of metastatic murine tumors. *Cancer* 40:558, 1977.

21. Brightman MW, Reese TS: Junctions between intimately opposed cell membranes in the vertebrate brain. *J Cell Biol* 40:648, 1969.

22. Rall DP, Zubrod CG: Mechanism of drug absorption and excretion: Passage of drugs in and out of the central nervous system. *Ann Rev Pharmacol* 2:109, 1962.

23. Vick NA, Khandekar JD, Bigner DD: Chemotherapy of brain tumors: The "blood-brain barrier" is not a factor. *Arch Neurol* 34:523, 1977.

24. Levin VA, Wilson CB: Chemotherapy: Agents in current use. *Semin Oncol* 2:63, 1975.

25. Levin VA, Kabra PM: Effectiveness of the nitrosoureas as a function of their lipid solubility in the chemotherapy of experimental rat brain tumors. *Arch Neurol* 32:785, 1975.

26. Skipper HE, Schabel FM, Mellett LB, et al: Implications of biochemical, cytokinetic, pharmacologic, and toxicologic relationships in the design of optimal therapeutic schedules. *Cancer Chemother Rep* 54:431, 1970.

27. Levin VA, Patlak CS, Landahl HD: Heuristic modeling of drug delivery to brain tumors. *J Pharmacokinet Biopharm* (in press).

28. Levin VA, Freeman-Dove M, Landahl HD: Permeability characteristics of brain adjacent to tumors in rats. *Arch Neurol* 32:785, 1975.

29. Levin VA, Landahl HD, Freeman-Dove M: The application of brain capillary permeability coefficient measurements to pathological conditions and the selection of agents which cross the blood-brain barrier. *J Pharmacokinet Biopharm* 4:499, 1976.

30. Goldacre RJ: Viable tumor regions inaccessible to chemotherapeutic agents and a possible new strategy for inactivating them (abstract). *Br J Cancer* 36:406, 1977.

31. Wright DC, Levin VA: Unpublished observations, 1979.

32. Bigner DD, Bullard D, Schold C, et al: Cellular heterogeneity and diversity as a basis for therapeutic resistance of human gliomas, in Paoletti P, Walker MD, Butti G, Knerich R (eds): *Multidisciplinary Aspects of Brain Tumor Therapy*. Amsterdam, Elsevier, North Holland, Biomedical Press, 1979, p 329.

33. Shapiro WR, Basler GA, Chernik NL, et al: Human brain tumor transplantation into nude mice. *J Natl Cancer Inst* 62:447, 1979.

34. Luria SE, Delbruck M: Mutations of bacteria from virus sensitivity to virus resistance. *Genetics* 28:491, 1943.

35. Law LW: Origin of the resistance of leukemic cells to folic acid and antagonists. *Nature* 159:628, 1952.

36. Walker MD, Strike TA, Sheline GE: An analysis of dose-effect relationship in the radiotherapy of malignant gliomas. *Int J Radiat Oncol Biol Phys* (in press).

37. Sheline GE: Radiation therapy of primary tumors *Semin Oncol* 2:29, 1975.

38. Shaw CM, Sumi SM, Alvord EC, et al: Fast-neutron irradiation of glioblastoma multiforme. *J Neurosurg* 49:1, 1978.

39. Thomlinson RH, Gray LH: The histological structure of some human lung cancers and the possible implications for radiotherapy. *Br J Cancer* 9:539, 1955.

40. Gutin PH, Wara WM, Phillips TL, et al: Hypoxic cell radiosensitizers in the treatment of malignant brain tumors. *Neurosurgery* vol. 6 (567–576), 1980.

41. Urtasun RC, Band P, Chapman JD, et al: Radiation and high-dose metronidazole (Flagyl) in supratentorial glioblastomas. *N Engl J Med* 294:1364, 1976.

42. Mundinger F, Hoefer T: Protracted long-term irradiation of inoperable midbrain tumors by stereotactic curie-therapy using iridium-192. *Acta Neurochirurg* 21 (suppl):93, 1974.

43. Pierquin B: The destiny of brachytherapy in oncology. *Am J Roentgenol* 127:495, 1976.

44. Kal HB, Sissingh HA: Effectiveness of continuous low dose-rate gamma-irradiation on rat skin. *Br J Radiol* 47:673, 1974.

45. Kal HB, Barendsen GW: Effects of continuous irradiation at low dose-rates on a rat rhabdomyosarcoma. *Br J Radiol* 45:279, 1972.

46. Fu KK, Phillips TL, Kane LJ, et al: Tumor and normal tissue response to irradiation *in vivo:* Variation with decreasing dose rates. *Radiology* 114:709, 1975.

47. Gutin PH, Hosobuchi Y, Phillips TL: Stereotactic interstitial radiation for the treatment of brain tumors. *Cancer Treat Rep* (in press).

48. Broerse JJ, Barendsen GW, van Kersen GR: Survival of cultured human cells after irradiation with fast neutrons of different energies in hypoxic and oxygenated conditions. *Int J Radiat Biol Phys* 13:559, 1967.

49. Grunder HA, Hartsough WD, Lofgren EJ: Acceleration of heavy ions at the Bevatron. *Science* 174:1128, 1976.

50. Garfield J, Dayan AD: Postoperative intracavitary chemotherapy of malignant gliomas: A preliminary study using methotrexate. *J Neurosurg* 39:315, 1973.

51. Rinkjob R: Treatment of intracranial gliomas and metastatic carcinomas by local application of cytostatic agents. *Acta Neurol Scand* 44:318, 1968.

52. Weiss SR, Raskind R: Treatment of malignant brain tumors by local methotrexate: A preliminary report. *Int Surg* 51:149, 1969.

53. Blockshear PJ: Implantable drug-delivery systems. *Sci Am* 241:66, 1979.

Part 3

SUPPORTIVE CARE

17

Prophylactic Granulocyte Transfusion

Kenneth B. McCredie

The use of leukocyte replacement therapy in man was first reported in 1934, and scattered reports continued to appear in the literature until 1960 (1). In the last 25 years, the introduction of instrumentation to collect enough granulocytes from normal donors has led to a dramatic increase in the collection and transfusion of granulocytes.

Leukocytes, and particularly granulocytes, have a specific gravity close to that of red cells. A simple centrifugation of 1 unit of whole blood would yield less than 50% of the circulating white cells, the majority being lymphocytes. Buffy coats of 40 units of whole blood would be required to raise the granulocyte count in the peripheral blood by $1,000/mm^3$ in a granulocytopenic recipient (2). Another major limitation in white cell transfusion is the short half-life of circulating granulocytes after transfusion. Red cell half-life can be measured in weeks and platelets in days; the half-life of circulating granulocytes is four to six hours. Problems related to storage and short half-life pose a major challenge to the development of a successful granulocyte transfusion program.

Initially, to overcome the problem of inadequate amounts of leukocytes, patients with chronic myelogenous leukemia who had granulocyte counts 30 to 50 times normal were used as donors. The total number of granulocytes that could be collected from these patients ranged from 3×10^9 to 2×10^{11} with a median of 6×10^{10}. In these initial studies, a direct relationship was demonstrated between the dose transfused and the increase in granulocytes in the recipient. With transfused doses of fewer than 1×10^{10} granulocytes/M^2, no significant increase in granulocyte count could be detected in the recipient one hour later. However, when doses of 5×10^{10} cells from donors with chronic myelogenous leukemia were given to leukopenic recipients, increases of 1,000 granulocytes/ M^2 body surface area could be demonstrated regularly one hour after transfusion, and after doses of 1×10^{11}, granulocyte increments of 4,000 to 5,000

Supported in part by Grants CA05831 and CA19806 from NIH, Bethesda, Maryland.

granulocytes/mm^3/M^2 body surface area were observed. The importance of transfusion of large quantities of granulocytes was also demonstrated in leukopenic infected patients. Among those patients who received 1×10^{11} granulocytes, 90% showed a clinical response as measured by reduction of fever, whereas of patients who received 3×10^{10} granulocytes, only 25% responded (3).

The fraction of transfused cells that can be recovered one hour after transfusion was estimated by multiplying the posttransfusion increment per milliliter by the estimated blood volume and dividing by the number of transfused cells and multiplying this figure by 100. The percent recovery can be estimated for cells collected and transfused from donors with chronic myelogenous leukemia. The recovery at one hour has been demonstrated to be less than 5% in the ideal situation when there has been no previous donor sensitization. Such transfusions to patients with granulocytopenia have been shown to result in reduction of fever, cure of septicemia, healing of local lesions, and eradication of bacterial infections that massive antibiotics had been unable to control (4).

The small number of chronic myelogenous leukemia patients available to donate cells has led to the development of the blood cell separator and improved techniques for collection. To collect the required number of granulocytes for effective transfusion therapy, large volumes of blood must be processed. Instrumentation has been developed by which sufficient quantities of leukocytes can be obtained from whole blood and leukocyte-poor blood can be returned to the patients. The initial instrument designed specifically for the collection of leukocytes was jointly developed by the National Cancer Institute and the International Business Machines Corporation in 1963 (5).

Initial studies of the blood cell separator showed that patients with chronic lymphocytic and chronic myelogenous leukemia could donate substantial quantities of leukocytes. However, initial attempts to control these diseases with the blood cell separator alone were not successful, as sufficient leukocytes could not be collected at any one donation. Attempts have been made to improve granulocyte collection by various modifications of the blood in the in vitro circuit of the blood cell separator and by stimulation of the donor with agents known to cause leukocytosis.

Hydroxyethyl starch has been used, along with dextran and gelatin, to increase rouleaux formation of the red cells in the in vitro circuits of the blood cell separator and to improve the separation of granulocytes from the red cell layer. Hydroxyethyl starch is a highly branched polymer of glucose and an analog of glycogen. Extensive testing in dogs has shown that it is superior to dextran and that it is nontoxic and nonallogenic. In vitro studies of hydroxyethyl starch as a red cell sedimenting agent have yielded a marked increase in the number of granulocytes collected (6). A 6% solution of hydroxyethyl starch in normal saline has been used to sediment the cells in the centrifugal field of the blood cell separator. With this method, an increase in the total number of leukocytes collected from 0.5×10^{10} to 1.8×10^{10} could be achieved by performing leukapheresis in a normal donor with 1.1×10^{10} of the cells being granulocytes. There was no major change in the total number of lymphocytes collected.

In vivo granulopoiesis can regularly be demonstrated after the administration of purified bacterial endotoxin (7). Prednisone has also been used to stimulate the release of granulocytes from the bone marrow reserve and to produce maximum granulocytosis six hours after administration (8).

Etiocholanolone, a naturally occurring steroid metabolite, regularly causes granulocytosis when administered intramuscularly in man. This granulocytosis reaches its maximum 12 to 14 hours after administration. Studies have demonstrated that the increase in the circulating granulocytes is associated with expansion of the body granulocyte pool and suggest a mobilization of cells from the bone marrow granulocyte reserve in response to etiocholanolone. Repeated use of etiocholanolone has shown no diminution in the granulocytic response and has demonstrated consistent response from various individuals.

Bacterial endotoxin, prednisone, and etiocholanolone appear to cause similar mobilization of granulocytes from the bone marrow granulocyte reserve, with granulocyte increments of approximately 2,500 $\mu\ell$ regularly observed after such treatment. However, from a practical standpoint, etiocholanolone and prednisone or dexamethasone offer advantages over other agents, since they are of known chemical composition, can be standardized, and are nonantigenic.

Preliminary studies with etiocholanolone showed that the total number of granulocytes that could be collected was increased by a factor of 4. When etiocholanolone was given to the donor before leukapheresis and hydroxyethyl starch was added to the in vitro circulation through the blood cell separator, a total of 3.0×10^{10} white cells could be collected of which 2.2×10^{10}, or 73%, were granulocytes. This is a 10-fold increase over the control data (9). Similar results have been achieved with dexamethasone, gelatin, and dextran (10,11). With the increase in the number of granulocytes that can be collected from normal donors, it has been possible to study the effects of these transfusions on related leukopenic recipients. In recent studies, we have demonstrated that 14.5% of transfused granulocytes collected from normal donors can be detected in the peripheral circulation of the recipient. This is almost three times the yield after transfusion of unmatched chronic myelogenous leukemic cells. In isogeneic transfusions from identical twins, the granulocyte increment one hour after transfusion was 29%, whereas, in donors in whom HLA matching was done before transfusion and in patients who were shown to have no mismatches between donor and recipient, the percentage of transfused granulocytes present at one hour was 18%. In transfusions from parents in whom at least two antigens were mismatched at the HLA locus, the percentage was 9%. Fewer normal cells are required to achieve therapeutic results similar to those obtained with transfusion of granulocytes collected from chronic myelogenous leukemic donors. Since the number of cells from donors with chronic myelogenous leukemia required to reduce fever and control infection in leukopenic patients is approximately 1×10^{11}, one-third of this number could be adequate when the donor is an HLA-compatible sibling. This suggests that the minimum required dose for maximum effective control of infection in leukopenic patients is 3×10^{10} normal granulocytes.

Using the modifications above for collection of granulocytes from the blood cell separator, we administered 716 transfusions to 130 patients who were leukopenic, infected, and unresponsive for at least 48 hours on the current antibiotic program. One hundred twelve had an organism or organisms that could be identified in culture as causing their infection, and, in the remainder, the site of infection could be identified, but no pathogenic organism identified. The majority of these patients had pulmonary infiltrates identified clinically and on x-ray examination. A single transfusion had little or no beneficial effect on these patients, but responses were seen in patients who received multiple transfusions, particularly those who had four to eight transfusions in whom a response rate of 81% was achieved. Response was seen in 77 of 112 patients in whom the organism could be identified (69%). Sixteen of 17 (94%) patients with localized infections responded, and 60% of patients with septicemia and pneumonia responded (12).

In a further series of transfusions, response rate has been related to HLA typing and ABO compatibility and to the percentage of granulocytes recovered. It was demonstrated in that study that the degree of HLA and ABO compatibility, which appeared to affect the percentage of granulocytes circulating in the recipient one hour after the transfusion, did not markedly affect clinical response. These data made clear that further efforts would be necessary to identify the role of HLA and ABO compatibility, as well as the presence or absence of circulating leukoagglutinating and nonleukoagglutinating antibodies, to define finally the efficacy of granulocyte transfusions.

Similar results have been seen in a number of other studies, including a pediatric study in which a control group was compared with a group who received granulocyte transfusions. In that study, approximately 45% of the patients treated with granulocyte transfusions responded compared with 30% of the patients who did not receive transfusions. All 12 patients who received 4 to 14 transfusions survived more than five days compared with 5 of 19 who did not receive transfusions (13).

Cells collected by the leukoadhesive technique have been demonstrated in infected neutropenic patients to be effective in clearing clinical infections (14). Higby et al. reported that 80% of their patients receiving transfusions were alive at 30 days after the onset of treatment compared with 13% of the control group (15). Similar results have been reported by Graw et al. (16) and Vogler (17) using cells collected by the filtration method or by continuous flow centrifugation. Djerassi has reported clinical recovery in 20 of 24 infected patients, and others have reported similar findings (18).

Short-term survival of patients receiving granulocyte transfusions has been studied, but questions have frequently been raised regarding long-term survival in this group of seriously ill, infected patients. We analyzed a group of 76 patients with adult acute leukemia, one-half of whom received therapeutic granulocyte transfusions when indicated, during primary induction therapy for their disease.The patient characteristics and eventual response data for patients who received white cell transfusions and those who did not were similar. In patients, aged 50 and above, the number of patients with acute myeloblastic leukemia was slightly higher in those who did not receive white cell transfusions. Similar numbers of patients were febrile on admission. White cell counts on admission varied between the groups with a median of $29.0 \times 10^9/\mu\ell$ in the group who received transfusions and $11 \times 4 \times 10^9/\mu\ell$ in those who did not, the higher value suggesting a poorer prognosis.

The overall response rate was 76% in patients who received transfusions and

69% in those who did not. Of patients who received white cell transfusions, 75% were alive at 12.5 weeks and 25% were alive at 121 weeks with a median duration of survival of 72.6 + weeks. Patients who did not receive white cell transfusions had a 75% survival at 16 weeks, and only 25% were alive after 75 weeks. Only 5 remain alive 119 + and 171 + weeks from their diagnosis. Fifteen of 76 patients are still alive, and 13 are still in their original complete remission. Median survival for the two groups combined was 52 weeks, and the difference between the two groups was significant at the $P = .05$ level.

This study suggests that response rate is not influenced by the use of granulocyte transfusions, except to the extent that many of the transfused patients might have died of their infection before achieving a complete remission if they had not received transfusions. The difference in response rates was more marked in patients under the age of 50. Median durations of survival in this group achieving a complete remission were 70 weeks in the untransfused group and 115 weeks in the group that was transfused. Seven of 17 in the transfused group remained alive, compared with 4 of 22 in the untransfused group (19).

Because of these encouraging results in the treatment of documented infection in previously untreated, febrile patients, we embarked on a program of prophylactic granulocyte transfusion therapy. In the initial group of patients who had enough relatives with HLA identity in at least two antigens, 10 patients were studied, their ages ranging between 19 and 50; another 10 had documented infection. Prophylactic granulocyte transfusions were administered to these patients when their granulocyte counts fell below $500/\mu\ell$ after the first course of chemotherapy and were administered daily until evidence of bone marrow recovery. The minimum number of transfusions administered was 4 and the maximum 10. All 10 patients responded to chemotherapy and entered complete remission. Animal studies have demonstrated clearly that prophylactic granulocyte transfusions cause substantial reductions in morbidity and mortality (20). Studies of prophylactic granulocyte transfusions have been conducted in humans using 1.5×10^{10} granulocytes administered at approximately 48-hour intervals or a maximum of three times per week (21). Those studies clearly demonstrated that ineffective doses of granulocytes given at prolonged intervals could not prevent infection. In contrast, we used daily granulocyte transfusions in doses of $2 \times 5 \times 10^{10}$ granulocytes.

Since the prophylactic granulocyte transfusion program has been initiated, 26 patients have been entered in the program, 25 of whom are evaluable. Fourteen patients with previously untreated acute myeloblastic leukemia, 8 patients with acute lymphoblastic or acute undifferentiated leukemia, and 3 patients with chronic myelogenous leukemia (CML) in blastic transformation have been entered. These patients were compared with 258 patients who were treated with similar chemotherapy for incidence of infection, deaths with infection, and infectious deaths. Improved collection techniques have been developed using new instrumentation that should benefit both the prophylactic and therapeutic transfusion programs.

The prophylactic granulocyte transfusion program was designed to investigate the use of prophylactic granulocyte transfusions during remission induction therapy for patients with a diagnosis of acute leukemia. This group of patients had been previously demonstrated to be at major risk of fatal infection during

Table 1. Prophylactic Granulocyte Transfusions

Total entered	26
Not evaluable	1
Evaluable	25
Acute myeloblastic leukemia	14
Acute lymphoblastic leukemia/ acute undifferentiated leukemia	8
Chronic myelogenous leukemia— blastic crisis	3

the periods of severe myelosuppression associated with therapy. Because of the potential risk of sensitization to HLA antigens not present in the recipients and the possible problems this would cause, particularly for platelet replacement therapy, only patients who had two or more relatives with at least two compatible antigens were selected for prophylactic granulocyte replacement therapy during remission induction chemotherapy.

All patients were admitted to the hospital and treated with our primary chemotherapeutic protocol for adult acute leukemia (22,23). The regimen consisted of combinations of Adriamycin or rubidazone combined with cytosine arabinoside as a continuous infusion. In addition to these drugs, patients were treated with vincristine intravenously on day 1, and prednisone was administered P.O. for a maximum of five days.

In a pilot study using this combination, 50% of the patients had developed a documented infection that failed to respond to the appropriate antibiotic therapy administered for a maximum period of 96 hours and required therapeutic granulocyte transfusions. Those patients who received therapeutic granulocyte transfusions derived both short-term and long-term benefit, and the administration of transfusions allowed them to survive with infection long enough to achieve a complete remission. Those in this group who achieved complete remission survived longer than those patients who did not receive granulocyte transfusions. Whether this was because of more sensitive tumors, transfer of immunological information by the lymphocytes transfused from a normal healthy donor, or interferon or transfer factor released from the transfused cells is not known.

Table 2. Prophylactic Transfusions Clinical Response

Acute myeloblastic leukemia	12/14	85%
Acute lymphoblastic leukemia Acute undifferentiated leukemia	7/8	88%
Chronic myeloblastic leukemia— blastic crisis	2/3	66%
Total	21/25	84%

Table 3. Control Patients Treated With Adriamycin/Oncovin/Ara-C/Prednisone (Ad-OAP) and Rubidazone/Oncovin, Ara-C, and Prednisone (ROAP)

No. of patients	258
Complete remission	173 (67%)
Partial remission	10 (4%)
Total	183 (71%)

One of the 26 patients entered on the prophylactic study was not evaluable because the donor, after a few transfusions, refused to continue to support the patient during a period of myelosuppression. A breakdown of the evaluable patients by diagnosis is shown in Table 1. The majority of the patients had acute myeloblastic leukemia and the remainder acute lymphoblastic, acute undifferentiated, or CML blastic transformation. The clinical response of these patients is shown in Table 2. Twelve of 14 patients with acute myeloblastic leukemia achieved a complete remission. The overall response rate was 84%.

Two hundred fifty-eight patients being treated with the same protocols, either Adriamycin or rubidazone in combination with cytosine arabinoside, vincristine, and prednisone, were used as controls. These patients received no granulocyte transfusions or limited numbers of therapeutic transfusions from donors who were compatible at less than two antigens. Data on the control population are shown in Table 3. A complete remission was achieved in 173 of the 258 with an additional 10 patients achieving a partial remission, for an overall response rate of 71%. These 258 patients were similar in age to those in the prophylactic transfusion group, and all were between 15 and 65.

In the prophylactic transfusion group, 4 patients failed to achieve a complete remission, 2 of whom died with infection, for an overall infectious mortality rate of 8% (Table 4).

In the control group, 75 patients failed to achieve a complete remission, and 53 of 75, or 73%, died with infection. The infectious death rate for both groups was 21%, compared with 8% for the prophylactic transfusion group alone (Table 5). The survival curves for the control patients and the patients who were evaluable in the prophylactic transfusion group are shown in Figure 1. Three transfused patients with CML-blastic transformation were excluded, as there were no patients with CML-blastic transformation in the control group. The median duration of survival in patients receiving prophylactic granulocyte transfusion exceeds that of the control group, although the numbers are too small at this

Table 4. Prophylactic Granulocyte Transfusion

Failures	4
Death with infection	2 (50%)
Infectious deaths	2/25 (8%)

Table 5. Controls

Control failures	75
Deaths with infection	53 (73%)
Infectious deaths	53/258 (21%)

point to draw a meaningful conclusion about survival. However, there appears to be no disadvantage to reducing the incidence of infection in the prophylactically treated group during remission induction and intensification therapy.

The effectiveness of prophylactic granulocyte transfusions has been demonstrated in a limited number of studies in animals and humans. It appears reasonable to assume that, because of the limited number of granulocytes that can be collected and transfused into the average adult, granulocyte transfusions during a reduced bacterial burden in the period before a patient's becoming infected could be as effective as, if not more effective in reducing the incidence of infection. Problems yet to be solved include sensitization to donor antigens in red cells, lymphocytes, and granulocytes that are transfused and the timing of the dosage administered and the period over which these transfusions can be given.

The limited clinical experience is encouraging, and further well-designed studies in an appropriate setting in which adequate quantities of granulocytes can

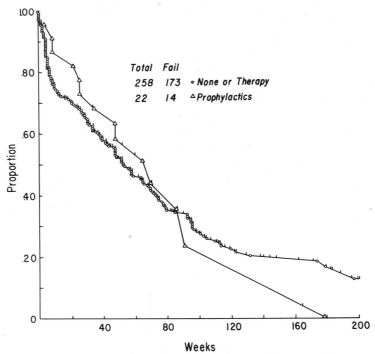

Figure 1. Survival by PMN transfusion in patients of age less than 65 years.

be collected and delivered should continue to demonstrate the beneficial effects of prophylaxis.

REFERENCES

1. Strumia MM: Effect of leukocyte cream injections in treatment of neutropenias. *Am J Med Sci* 187:527, 1934.

2. Yankee A, Freireich EJ, Carbone PP, et al: Replacement therapy using normal and chronic myelogenous leukocytes. *Blood* 24:844, 1964.

3. Freireich EJ, Levin RH, Whang J, et al: The function and fate of transfusion leukocytes from donors with chronic meylocytic leukemia in leukopenic recipients. *Ann NY Acad Sci* 113;1091, 1965.

4. Vallejos C, McCredie KB, Bodey GP, et al: White blood cell transfusions for control of infections in neutropenic patients. *Transfusion* 15:28–33, 1975.

5. Judson G, Jones A, Kellogg R, et al: Close continuous-flow centrifuge. *Nature* 217:816, 1968.

6. Thompson WL, Walton RF: Parenteral administration of hydroxyethyl starches, in *National Academy of Sciences Conference on Artificial Colloids for Intravenous Use.* 1962, pp 168–206.

7. Mechanic RC, Frei E III, Landy M, et al: Quantitative studies of human leukocytic and febrile response to single and repeated doses of purified bacterial endotoxin. *J Clin Invest* 41:162, 1962.

8. Cream JJ: Prednisone induced granulocytosis. *Br J Haematol* 15:259, 1968.

9. Kimball HR, Vogel JM, Perry S, et al: Quantitative aspects of pyrogenic and hematologic responses to etiocholanolone in man. *J Lab Clin Med* 69:415, 1967.

10. Bussel A, Benbunan M, Tanzer J, et al: Report of a simple method of collecting leucocytes from patients with chronic myeloid leukaemia, in Goldman JM, Lowenthal RM (eds): *Leucocytes: Separation, Collection and Transfusion.* London, Academic Press, 1975, pp 112–120.

11. Lowenthal RM: Chronic leukaemias: Treatment by leukapheresis. *Exp Hematol* 5(suppl):73–84, 1977.

12. McCredie KB, Freireich EJ: Increased granulocyte collection from normal donors with increased granulocyte recovery following transfusion. *Proc Am Assoc Cancer Res* 12:58, 1971.

13. Graw RB Jr, Herzig GP, Perry S, et al: Normal granulocyte transfusion therapy. *N Engl J Med* 287:367, 1972.

14. Djerassi I, Kim JS, Mitrakul C, et al: Filtration leukapheresis for separation and concentration of transfusable amounts of normal human granulocytes. *J Med (Basel)* 1:358, 1970.

15. Higby DJ, Yates J, Henderson ES: Filtration leukapheresis for granulocyte transfusion therapy. *N Engl J Med* 292:761, 1975.

16. Graw RG Jr, Stout FG, Herzig RH, et al: in Greenwalt TJ, Jamieson GA (eds): *The Granulocyte: Function and Clinical Utilization.* New York, Alan R Liss, Inc, 1977, pp 267–280.

17. Vogler WR, Winton EF: The efficacy of granulocyte transfusions in neutropenic patients (Abstract C-64). *Proc Am Soc Clin Oncol* 17:252, 1976.

18. Djerassi I, Kim JS: Problems and solutions with filtration leukapheresis, in Greenwalt TJ, Jamieson GA (eds): *The Granulocyte: Function and Clinical Utilization.* New York, Alan R Liss, Inc, 1977, pp 305–313.

19. McCredie KB, Hester JP, Freireich EJ: Leucocyte collection and transfusion physiology. *Exp Hematol* 5(suppl):33–38, 1977.

20. Epstein RB, Zander AR, in Greenwalt TJ, Jamieson GA (eds): *The Granulocyte: Function and Clinical Utilization.* New York, Alan R Liss, Inc, 1977,- pp 227–241.

21. Ford JM, Cullen MH: Prophylactic granulocyte transfusions. *Exp Hematol* 5(Suppl):65–72, 1977.

22. Benjamin RS, Keating MJ, Swenerton KD, et al: Clinical studies with rubidazone. *Cancer Treat Rep* 63:925–929, 1979.

23. McCredie KB, Bodey GP, Freireich EJ, et al: Chemoimmunotherapy of adult acute leukemia. *Cancer* 47:1256–1261, 1981.

18

Is Prophylactic Granulocyte Transfusion in the Best Interest of the Patient?

Charles A. Schiffer

In the last decade, a number of techniques have been developed and widely marketed that permit the relatively simple, safe, and efficient collection of granulocytes from normal donors for transfusion. Although the numbers of granulocytes obtainable by these techniques are marginal compared with the pyogenic response noted after infections in normals, many investigations have documented the efficacy of granulocyte transfusion in the treatment of established bacterial infection (1–7). General acceptance of the role of therapeutic granulocyte transfusion has resulted in increased interest in the next logical investigative question, that is, can the incidence and associated morbidity from infection be reduced by the prophylactic transfusion of granulocytes?

In view of the well-known relationship between the degree and duration of granulocytopenia and the incidence and severity of infection (8), one might, at first glance, consider prevention of infection by granulocyte transfusion to be a straightforward matter analogous to the successes achievable in the prevention of hemorrhage by the liberal, prophylactic use of platelet transfusion in patients with leukemia (9). Unfortunately, despite many recent advances, the same problems that confused the interpretation of earlier therapeutic granulocyte trials and in fact resulted in delay of the scientific acceptance of granulocyte transfusion have made the implementation and understanding of the results of prophylactic transfusion more difficult. These problems include donor selection, inadequate granulocyte "dose," histocompatibility factors, heterogeneity of patient population, variations in collection techniques, and quality of cells transfused. In addition, in contrast to therapeutic transfusions that are usually administered to patients refractory to conventional antibiotic therapy, alternative means of infection prophylaxis are available, varying in complexity and expense from a program of rigorous personal hygiene to the use of gastrointestinal tract microbial suppression and reverse isolation in protected environments. The controversies surrounding the latter technology are discussed in another section of this volume. In the following pages, the difficulties encountered in the use of prophylactic granulocyte transfusion are described, which, in my estimation, preclude their use in any but investigational settings.

POTENTIAL RECIPIENTS

The number of patients with cancer receiving intensive combination chemotherapy has increased substantially in the last five years, related in part to improvements in therapy as well as proliferation of the subspecialty of medical oncology. Nonetheless, few patients receiving conventional high-dose therapy for either solid tumors or almost all hematopoietic malignancies would be candidates for prophylactic granulocyte transfusion because of the relatively short periods of aplasia and the predictable return of marrow function in these patients. Indeed, despite an aggressive approach toward chemotherapy of solid tumors, only a few patients with oat cell carcinoma and bone marrow involvement have been considered candidates for therapeutic granulocytes transfusions at our center in recent years.

Changes have also occurred in the induction treatment of adult leukemia in the last five years that have resulted in a trend toward a decreased requirement for therapeutic granulocyte transfusions at the BCRP. The most important factor has been the development of more intensive regimens combining anthracyclines and cytosine arabinoside that paradoxically result in shorter overall periods of aplasia (two to four weeks on average) because of the high probability of achieving remission after single courses of therapy. Although infections of variable severity develop in almost all such patients, the incidence of Gram-negative bacteremia is low, and the response rate to antibiotic therapy alone is excellent (10). In addition, patients who are initially uninfected tend to acquire infections late in the induction course, frequently shortly before endogenous marrow recovery. It has been well demonstrated that the response rate to antibiotics alone is in excess of 90% if even minimal (100 to 200/mm^3) rises in granulocyte count occur (10–12). To some extent the same arguments pertain to recipients of bone marrow transplants, who, along with adults with leukemia, represent the other large group in whom prophylactic granulocytes have been investigated. The regeneration of myeloid elements occurs reliably within 14 to 21 days of transplantation in most patients making the time at risk from granulocytopenia comparable if not shorter than that seen in patients with leukemia (13).

In both groups, patients who are in otherwise reasonable health and uninfected at presentation tend to tolerate their initial infections well, and it therefore has been difficult, as described below, to demonstrate improved survival in recipients of prophylactic granulocyte transfusion. In this regard, one must carefully define the goals of prophylactic transfusion. Obviously, the overall goal is to achieve an increased remission rate and hence increased survival. If this cannot be demonstrated because of the good overall responses observed because of other support mechanisms, a secondary goal, and indeed the goal that corresponds to the purest "scientific" question, would be to decrease the acquisition and severity of infection and its associated morbidity and expense. In this case, one must balance the expense and side effects of transfusion, including potential side effects to donors, with the morbidity incurred by the infection that theoretically may have been prevented.

The previous discussion was not intended to suggest that all severely aplastic patients do well and would not stand to benefit from effective prophylactic transfusion if such technology were easily available. Rather, it was designed to put the potential requirement for such technology in perspective. Certainly there are large numbers of patients, and in particular elderly patients with other associated medical problems, who tolerate infection poorly and have unacceptably high mortality during induction chemotherapy. It is because of these patients and the possibility that more effective regimens may in the future incur longer periods of aplasia that studies of prophylactic granulocyte transfusion are of importance and deserve to be examined critically.

ANIMAL STUDIES

Two studies, one in dogs and the other in rats, are available that purport to demonstrate the value of prophylactic granulocyte support. Debelak et al. rendered dogs severely granulocytopenic by cyclophosphamide and administered granulocytes collected by filtration leukopheresis during the two days of maximum count suppression (14). All five nontransfused control dogs died with bacteremia, whereas bacteremia was not detected in six transfused dogs, three of whom survived and three of whom died hemorrhagic deaths. Higher doses of granulocytes than can be routinely achieved in humans were used, and some dogs were febrile at the time of administration of granulocytes, suggesting that transfusions may have been given early in the course of infection rather than strictly prophylactically. Tobias et al. rendered rats granulocytopenic by irradiation and administered a single granulocyte transfusion prepared by filtration leukopheresis two hours before an intravenous challenge with a dose of *Escherichia coli* that proved lethal to 17 out of 18 nontransfused controls (15). In contrast 10 out of 14 transfused rats survived at least four days, with 8 animals surviving the challenge completely. As in the previous study, a disproportionately higher dose of granulocytes was used than is available for humans. More important, however, was the observation that the nadir granulocyte counts produced by the irradiation was only about 1,000/mm³, a level at which spontaneous bacteremia in humans is rare. In addition, granulocyte recovery to normal levels apparently not related to the low immediate posttransfusion count increments that were noted occurred within 24 hours of transfusion and not in the control group. There is no obvious mechanism to account for this phenomenon, and the question must be raised as to whether it was the circulation of infused granulocyte that exerted the salutary effect.

Although technically prophylactic in design, both studies are perhaps more akin to the therapeutic granulocyte transfusion situation. Certainly the short-term nature of both studies provides no insight into the immense logistic problems encountered in the management of long-term aplasia in humans and cannot be used as evidence promoting the use of prophylactic granulocytes in humans.

HUMAN STUDIES

Data on six randomized studies of prophylactic granulocyte transfusion are available (13,16–21), only three of which have been published in final, detailed form (13,16,17). An additional multi-institutional study is in progress with the results still coded at this time, and observations in a group of nonrandomized patients with leukemia will be presented by Dr. McCredie in an accompanying chapter. The overall results of the randomized studies are summarized in Table 1. Although some studies also report data on patients who were infected at the time of admission, Table 1 includes only those patients who were felt to be infection-free initially. A significant number of criticisms can be made about each study:

1. Relatively small numbers of patients are available in most single institutions, and two of the studies (16,20) have less than a total of 30 patients randomized. Obviously with clinical settings as complicated as acute leukemia or marrow transplantation larger patient groups are required to demonstrate the value of a single modification of therapy definitively. Complicating the problem of patient accrual is the observation made during our study that at least 30% to 40% of newly referred patients were not eligible for randomization usually because they required antibiotic therapy at presentation for fevers caused by either severe or more commonly minor (e.g., cutaneous, gingival) infections.

2. Intermittent schedules (16,20,21) or relatively marginal doses of granulocytes were used, which, even under ideal conditions, could have produced greater than a few hundred circulating granulocytes for only short periods immediately after transfusion. Although it is possible that the transfused cells partially replenish "tissue pools" (22) that in turn may exert some protective effect, it would at least theoretically be ideal to have larger numbers of circulating granulocytes capable of migrating to and dealing with potential subclinical areas of infection. Again, technical limitations, particularly with intermittant flow centrifugation, are a major factor in that the low dose of 11.5 $\times$ 10^9 granulocytes used in our study (16) was obtained despite the fact that all donors were premedicated with corticosteroids.

3. Granulocytes prepared by filtration leukopheresis (FL) were used in the two marrow transplant studies, one of which was "successful" (13), the other of which failed to demonstrate a protective effect (17). The functional quality of granulocytes prepared by FL is notoriously variable, and quanity control of this product is difficult to achieve even in the same laboratory (23–26). There are wide differences in FL technique, and no details are provided in either paper about the technique used or the morphologic and functional integrity of the granulocytes infused. In the UCLA study 17 of 19 recipients developed clinically significant transfusion reactions (17), a well-described phenomenon usually ascribed to infusion of granulocytes damaged by the FL process (7,25). Thus, it is possible that the "negative" findings in this study are related at least in part to transfusion of imperfect granulocytes administered in much lower doses (12 $\times$ 10^9) than are usually obtained using FL. Conversely, because granulocytes obtained by any of the differential centrifugation techniques are more uniformly normal in function (26), the quality

Table 1. Prophylactic Granulocyte Transfusion

Reference	Recipients	Donors	Collection Method	Schedule	Mean Granulocyte Dose $\times 10^9$	Results (Infected/Total)	
						Control	Treatment
13	Marrow transplant	Marrow donor	FL, CFC	OD	22.3–FL 15.7–CFC	17:40	2:29
19	Adult leukemia	Nonmatched	CFC, IFC	OD	20	11:28	1:21
21	Adult leukemia	"HLA compatible"	CFC	...	25.9	19:25	1:13
20	Adult leukemia	Nonmatched	IFC	QOD	14.9	6:11	3:13
17	Marrow transplant	Nonmatched	FL	OD	12	9:19	7:19
16	Adult leukemia	Nonmatched	IFC	QOD	11.5	3:9	0:9

FL = filtration leukopheresis.

CFC = continuous flow centrifugation.

IFC = intermittent flow centrifugation.

OD = daily.

QOD = alternate days.

237

of the cells transfused is not an important factor in interpreting trials using fresh granulocytes obtained by centrifugation.

4. Available evidence indicates that poorly matched granulocytes are of no benefit and may in fact be harmful when administered to alloimmunized recipients (27–30). Clearly, therefore, the immunologic status of the recipients can have a major effect on the outcome of transfusion trials. Histocompatibility considerations were not mentioned in the UCLA study, perhaps accounting for some of the transfusion reactions, and it is not clear whether any of the patients reported by Ford et al. (20) had evidence of alloimmunization before beginning transfusion. Alloimmunized patients were excluded from randomization on the BCRP study (16), and lymphocytotoxic crossmatch was used as screening by Cooper et al. (21) and Mannoni et al. (18) with only "histocompatible" family members used as donors in the former report. Clift et al. (13) avoided the histocompatibility problem in perhaps the most ideal fashion by using the marrow donor as the sole source of granulocytes, although it is still possible that even HLA-MLC identical family members could have been histoincompatible with respect to granulocyte specific antigens (31).

5. There is some confusion in the data presented on the same group of patients by Mannoni et al. in different publications. As presented in initial abstract form (18) "documented" infections developed in 3 out of 15 patients receiving prophylactic granulocyte compared with 13/24 controls. In a subsequent "letter to the editor" (19), "major" infections occurred in 1/21 granulocyte recipients and 11 out of 28 controls. Both differences are highly statistically significant, the study appears to be thoughtfully planned and implemented, and it is hoped that these apparent discrepancies will be clarified in the final publication.

Despite these criticisms, important information and some conclusions can be drawn from these studies. The last three studies cited in Table 1 do not demonstrate statistically significant differences in infection acquisition between transfused and control groups. In each report, however, the rate of infection was lower in the transfused patients, and although it is certainly not scientifically accurate to "pool" the data, it is interesting that the rate of infection was 24% (10 out of 41) in granulocyte recipients compared with 46% (18 out of 39) in controls. A similar trend was noted by Cooper et al. (21), but, because this study was not strictly randomized in that patients were allocated according to the availability of a compatible donor, the results must be regarded as tentative. The low frequency (twice weekly) of granulocyte transfusion and the unusually high incidence of severe, sometimes fatal hemorrhage in the control group suggest that other factors may account in part for the observed results. In addition, the very high rate of severe infection (19 out of 25 patients) in the controls is of concern when interpreting the results of this study.

The studies by Clift et al. (13) and Mannoni et al. (19) are the most rigorous in terms of frequency of transfusion and numbers of patients evaluable and have few if any critical faults in terms of study design. Both demonstrate statistically, and clinically, significant declines in infection acquisition that are particularly notable in the French study (19) because the control group received oral nonabsorbable antibiotics as "baseline" infection prevention. These two studies demonstrate convincingly that prophylactic granulocyte transfusion can prevent the development of infection in certain patient populations. The three available "negative" studies (16,17,20) do not detract from this conclusion, particularly in view of the criticisms of these investigations discussed above.

Of note is that the overall survival from infection was not altered by the prophylactic transfusions in either "positive" study (13,19), attesting to the value of antibiotics and therapeutic granulocyte transfusions. None of 21 granulocyte recipients versus 3 out of 28 controls died of infection in the French study (19), with figures of 0 out of 9 versus 4 out of 40 respectively in the Seattle report (13). Thus, although the important scientific point about prevention of infection seems to have been adequately demonstrated, it is unclear whether this translates into increased patient survival because of the excellent "salvage"!rate with conventional infection treatment.

SIDE EFFECT OF TRANSFUSION

Whether the reduction in infection acquisition and presumed morbidity is "worth" the multiple side effects that accompany prophylactic granulocyte transfusion can never be answered quantitatively. Nonetheless, this is the critical remaining issue that must be considered before recommending prophylactic granulocytes for use on a wider scale. The problems that have been identified are discussed in detail in this section.

Expense

Although the cost is rarely the determining factor in making therapeutic decisions in individual patients, the overall expense is an important consideration when attempting to decide about the large-scale implementation of new technology, particularly when the impact on total patient survival may be marginal. Presently the average charge for a granulocyte transfusion is approximately $250 to $300, such that a series of 10 to 15 prophylactic transfusions would increase the charge per patient by $3,000 to $5,000 per induction course. Each granulocyte transfusion also consumes three to six hours of "donor time," including "travel time," which represents a considerable potential loss of donor income and productivity. This donor time is usually not considered in the "cost equation" but certainly does represent a hidden and difficult to quantitate cost to society, particularly if prophylactic transfusion were to become standard practice.

Rosenshein et al. (32) have attempted to determine the cost effectiveness of prophylactic transfusion compared with therapeutic granulocyte transfusion once infection is acquired. The authors necessarily depend on broad estimates of the effectiveness of transfusion, leukemia incidence in the population, and remission and infection rates, all of which can be quibbled with because of the imprecision of the available data. Given these imperfections, it was estimated that the cost of prophylactic transfusion was $36,000 to $54,000 per expected life year, would add 35% to the average patient's hospital bill, and cost $50 to

$60 million if applied widely to all adults with newly diagnosed leukemia. Corresponding figures for therapeutic transfusions were $16,000, 17%, and $18 million, considered by the authors to be expensive, but more cost effective. Although these figures are certainly exaggerated in that they unrealistically assume that all patients would receive either prophylactic or therapeutic transfusions during all granulocytopenic stages of their illness, they are an example of the type of thinking that should, but usually does not, take place prior to advocating expensive new technology.

Donor Factors

In contrast to other methods of infection prevention, prophylactic granulocyte transfusion demands the active participation and cooperation of nonmedical personnel, that is, the family member or volunteer donor. Although granulocyte donation is a safe procedure in terms of serious morbidity, minor side effects inevitably occur, ranging from the inconvenience of missing work to the anxiety associated with needle sticks and citrate reactions. In addition more serious reactions can occur rarely, particularly with filtration leukopheresis, a procedure that is declining in usage as a consequence (25,33). With respect to centrifugation techniques it is necessary to use corticosteroid stimulation and rouleauxing agents, most commonly hydroxyethyl starch (HES), in order to achieve effective yields (34). Corticosteroids are probably innocuous when administered in occasional single doses, and significant short-term side effects are infrequent with HES administration, although fluid retention and rare atopic reactions have been described (35). There is evidence however that HES is retained in normals for periods of weeks to months, and any possible longer-term effects are unknown (36). These factors are of particular importance when it is necessary to use small numbers of donors repeatedly because of histocompatibility considerations. In the Seattle study the marrow donors served as granulocyte donors, and many had arteriovenous fistulae constructed to permit donation for as many as 14 to 21 consecutive days (13). Iron supplementation was used in all donors, and ten donors required transfusion because of anemia. Obviously this approach is extreme and impossible outside of highly specialized centers but serves as a reminder of the burden and risks faced by donors. Physicians using granulocyte transfusions, and indeed even single donor platelet preparations, should be mindful of the donor risks and consider the indications for transfusion carefully. This is particularly true in the prophylactic setting.

Availability of Facilities

The initiation of a course of prophylactic granulocyte transfusion implies a daily commitment for a two- to three-week period to a particular patient. Few hospital-based or regional centers presently have the capacity to support large numbers of such patients concurrently. It would be inappropriate to compromise support of other patients with single donor platelets or therapeutic granulocytes, both of which require the use of the same machines, given the marginal benefit of prophylactic transfusions.

RECIPIENT SIDE EFFECTS

Alloimmunization

Despite the high doses of immunosuppressive and cytotoxic drugs administered to patients with leukemia, the majority of such patients become alloimmunized after multiple transfusions from random donors (37–39). Clinically, alloimmunization is associated with transfusion reactions and associated refractoriness to random donor platelets with a consequent increased risk of hemorrhage. There is suggestive evidence that leukocytes are more "immunogenic" than platelets (40), and therefore the development of alloimmunization has always been of concern in recipients of granulocyte transfusion. Surprisingly, there is little literature on the subject before recent publications dealing with prophylactic transfusion. In recipients of therapeutic granulocyte transfusions, Thompson et al. noted the development of a variety of granulocyte specific antibodies in 74% of patients over a period of days to weeks (41). In addition, it is well recognized clinically that transfusion reactions often occur toward the end of a series of therapeutic transfusions, suggesting the development of immunization.

In our study at the BCRP, alloimmunization characterized by moderately severe transfusion reactions, the presence of lymphocytotoxic antibody, and refractoriness to random donor platelets developed in 7 of 10 patients, in some as early as a week after beginning transfusions (16). The fever and chill reactions caused significant anxiety and increased antibiotic usage in transfused patients and in at least one, and possibly two patients, were associated with transient presumably immunologically mediated pulmonary infiltrates. Because of this high rate of immunization it was elected to terminate our study prematurely, before accruing a sufficient number of patients to answer the question of infection prevention. Mannoni et al., who also used nonmatched donors, noted a high rate (approximately 70%) of immunization to HLA antigens, necessitating a switch to HLA matched donors in many recipients (18). Lastly, Zaroulis et al. have also recently described apparent accelerated rates of immunization, particularly to granulocyte-specific antigens after granulocyte transfusion (42).

In addition to the immediate side effects, and the difficulties encountered in subsequent platelet support, the development of alloimmunization makes future granulocyte donor selection difficult, given the present confused state of the art of granulocyte crossmatching (43). Although it is theoretically attractive to use "matched" donors from the onset of transfusion, it is presently possible to type reliably only for HLA antigens and not other, clinically important granulocyte-specific antigens. Because few centers have large numbers of HLA-typed donors available, it would seem to be most appropriate to reserve HLA matched family and nonrelated donors for use in the therapeutic setting rather than risking sensitization to difficult to detect antigens by prophylactic transfusion.

Graft versus host disease (GVHD)

Fatal GVHD has been described following transfusion of nonirradiated prophylactic granulocytes to a recipient with leukemia (44), and one patient in our study developed a syndrome highly suggestive of acute GVHD, although this could not be documented by skin biopsy. This complication can be avoided by irradiation of the bag before transfusion, but this would be cumbersome for many institutions and could conceivably delay transfusions to the point where functional lesions produced by storage (45) could significantly affect the quality of the granulocyte product. Because GVHD is so unusual in nontransplant recipients, it would be premature to recommend irradiation of granulocyte preparations routinely. Furthermore, there is no reason to assume that the incidence of GVHD would be greater after granulocyte transfusion than after administration of other blood products (e.g., single-donor platelets) that also contain large numbers of viable lymphocytes. Thus, although GVHD can occur after granulocyte transfusion, it is such a rare occurrence that it should not be a major consideration on the "balance sheet" in the debate about prophylactic granulocytes.

Cytomegalovirus (CMV) Infections

An increased incidence of CMV infection was noted in the UCLA study in both bone marrow transplant and leukemic recipients of granulocyte transfusions (17). This was most prominent in patients with negative CMV titers before transfusion, suggesting transmission of the virus by the transfused cells rather than reactivation of latent infection. Although CMV also was detected in six controls, two of these patients had received therapeutic granulocyte transfusions. Six of the nine previously seronegative prophylactic granulocyte recipients developed CMV pneumonia, attesting to the clinical importance of this observation. The incidence of CMV infection was not described by Clift et al. (13), although interstitial pneumonia was seen in transfused and control patients in equal rates. If the observations about CMV infections are confirmed in other studies, this would represent another important deterrant to the indiscriminate use of prophylactic granulocyte transfusion.

SUMMARY AND CONCLUSIONS

Based on the reports of Clift et al. and Mannoni et al. it would appear that the pure "scientific" question about prevention of infection by prophylactic granulocyte transfusion has been answered in the affirmative. However, in view of the expense, the substantial problems created by alloimmunization, the potential strain on existing transfusion services and donors, the possible increased transmission of CMV, and particularly because of the absence of a demonstrable effect on patient survival, it would be totally inappropriate even to consider providing prophylactic granulocytes for all patients with leukemia. Furthermore, because of the complexities involved with histocompatibility issues, prophylactic transfusion should not be used outside of investigative centers. Relatively simple, inexpensive, and nontoxic means of infection prevention with trimethoprim-sulfamethoxazole or nalidixic acid have shown initial promise (46) and, if proved effective, would provide an alternative to more cumbersome technology (protected environments, gut sterilization, prophylactic granulocytes) for use in the community at large. The conclusions above do not indicate that research dealing with prophylactic granulocytes from normal donors represents "irrelevant" technology. Future successes in leukemia treatment may depend on longer periods of aplasia, a circumstance in which prophylactic granulocyte transfusion may have a greater import, particularly if improvements in our understanding of granulocyte immunology occur.

It is also possible that for selected patients at high risk a different approach to prophylactic transfusion may be appropriate therapy at this time. The patient described in Figure 1 illustrates this point. The patient was an elderly man with acute nonlymphocytic leukemia with poor dentition, gingival hypertrophy, and a tooth abscess. Therapeutic leukocyte transfusions from a donor with chronic myelogenous leukemia (CML) were administered, resulting in prompt healing of the abscess and marked improvement in the gingiva. The patient had not been previously transfused, and temporary engraftment documented by the presence of Ph[1] chromosome took place, resulting in a sustained production of granulocytes for about two weeks. The patient remained afebrile, off antibiotics, for almost all this time, and achieved remission without further signs of infection. We have seen similar clinical courses in two other high risk patients with extensive rectal and cutaneous lesions in whom temporary CML grafts served as effective infection prophylaxis as well as initial therapy for infection. As previously described (47), leucocyte alkaline phosphatase levels were increased in the engrafted cells, suggesting an "environmental" influence on the elaboration of this enzyme by the CML clone. GVHD has been described in recipients of CML

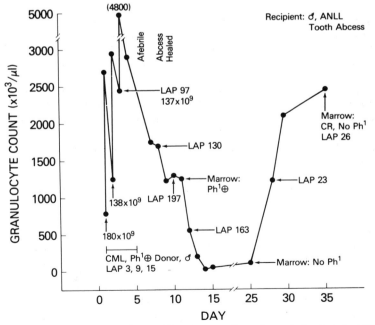

Figure 1. Clinical course of a patient with acute nonlymphocytic leukemia (ANLL) who received three transfusions from a donor with chronic myelogenous leukemia (CML). See text for details. LAP = leukocyte alkaline phosphatase; CR = complete remission.

transfusions (48) but was not seen in these three patients all of whom achieved complete remission. Although this approach is experimental and cannot be recommended except for certain high risk nonimmunized patients, it serves as a reminder of what may be achievable if doses of granulocytes sufficient to produce a sustained rise in granulocyte count could be collected.

ADDENDUM

The results of the collaborative study mentioned in the text have recently become available (Strauss et al., *Proc. Amer. Soc. Clin. Oncol.* 22:495, 1981). A total of 102 patients receiving initial induction therapy for acute nonlymphocytic leukemia (ANLL) were randomized to receive daily prophylactic granulocyte transfusions or standard supportive care. Although there was a reduction in the number of bacteremias in the transfused group (5 bacteremias/54 transfused patients vs. 13/48 controls, $P < .05$), there were no significant differences in the overall rates of infection or in the survival or remission rates. There was a high incidence (78% of patients) of reactions to the granulocyte transfusions and the incidence of possibly immunologically induced pulmonary infiltrates was much increased in granulocyte transfussion recipients. Similar to the present commentary, the authors conclude that: "prophylactic granulocyte transfusions cannot be recommended as standard therapy during remission induction for ANLL."

REFERENCES

1. Higby DJ, Yates JW, Henderson ES, et al: Filtration leukapheresis for granulocyte transfusion therapy: Clinical and laboratory studies. *N Engl J Med* 292:761, 1975.

2. Herzig RH, Herzig GP, Graw RG Jr, et al: Successful granulocyte transfusion therapy for gram-negative septicemia: A prospectively randomized controlled study. *N Engl J Med* 296:701, 1977.

3. Alavi JB, Root RK, Djerassi I, et al: A randomized clinical trial of granulocyte transfusions for infection in acute leukemia. *N Engl J Med* 296:706, 1977.

4. Schiffer CA, Buchholz DH, Aisner J, et al: Clinical experience with transfusion of granulocytes obtained by continuous flow filtration leukopheresis. *Am J Med* 58:373, 1974.

5. Vogler WR, Winton EF: A controlled study of the efficacy of granulocyte transfusions in patients with neutropenia. *Am J Med* 63:548, 1976.

6. McCredie KB, Freireich EJ, Hester JP, et al: Leukocyte transfusion therapy for patients with host-defense failure. *Transplant Proc* 3:1285, 1973.

7. Aisner J, Schiffer CA, Wiernik PH: Granulocyte transfusions: Evaluation of factors influencing results and a comparison of filtration and intermittent centrifugation leukapheresis. *Br J Haematol* 38:121, 1978.

8. Bodey GP, Buckley M, Sathe YS, et al: Quantitative relationships between circulating leukocytes and infection in patients with acute leukemia. *Ann Intern Med* 64:328, 1966.

9. Schiffer CA, Aisner J, Wiernik PH: Platelet transfusion therapy for patients with leukemia, in Greenwalt TJ, Jamieson GA (eds): *The Blood Platelet in Transfusion Therapy*. New York, Alan R Liss, Inc, 1978, p 267.

10. Love LJ, Schimpff SC, Schiffer CA, et al: Improved prognosis for granulocytopenic patients with gram-negative bacteremia. *Am J Med* 68:643, 1980.

11. EORTC Antimicrobial Therapy Project Group: Three antibiotic regimens in the treatment of infection in febrile granulocytopenic patients with cancer. *J Infect Dis* 137:14, 1978.

12. Keating MJ, Bodey GP, Valdivieso M, et al: A randomized comparative trial of three amino-

glycosides: Comparison of continuous infusions of gentamicin, amikacin and sisomicin combined with carbenicillin in the treatment of infections in neutropenic patients with malignancies. *Medicine* 58:159, 1979.

13. Clift RA, Sanders JE, Thomas ED, et al: Granulocyte transfusions for the prevention of infection in patients receiving bone-marrow transplants. *N Engl J Med* 298:1052, 1978.

14. Debelak KM, Epstein RB, Andersen BR: Granulocyte transfusions in leukopenic dogs: *In vivo* and *in vitro* function of granulocytes obtained by continuous-flow filtration leukopheresis. *Blood* 43:757, 1974.

15. Tobias JS, Brown BL, Brivkalns A, et al: Prophylactic granulocyte support in experimental septicemia. *Blood* 47:473, 1976.

16. Schiffer CA, Aisner J, Daly PA, et al: Alloimmunization following prophylactic granulocyte transfusion. *Blood* 54:766, 1979.

17. Winston DJ, Ho WG, Young LS, et al: Prophylactic granulocyte transfusions during human bone marrow transplantation. *Am J Med* 68:893, 1980.

18. Mannoni P, Rodet M, Radeau E, et al: Granulocyte transfusion: Efficiency of prophylactic granulocyte transfusions in care of patients with acute leukemia, in Hogman CS, Lindahl-Kiessling K, Wigzell H (eds): *Blood Leucocytes: Function and Use in Therapy*. Stockhold, Almquist and Wiksell Int'l, 1977.

19. Mannoni P, Brun B, Rodet M, et al: Correspondence. *N Engl J Med* 299:489, 1978.

20. Ford JM, Cullen MH: Prophylactic granulocyte transfusions. *Exp Hematol* 5:65–72, 1977.

21. Cooper MR, Heise E, Richards F, et al: A prospective study of histocompatible leucocyte and platelet transfusions during chemotherapeutic induction of acute myeloblastic leukemia, in Goldman JM, Lowenthal RM (eds): *Leucocytes: Separation, Collection and Transfusion*. New York, Academic Press, 1979, p 436.

22. Rosenshein M, Price T, Dale D: Neutropenia, inflammation and the kinetics of transfused neutrophils. *Clin Res* 26:507A, 1978.

23. Wright DG, Kauffmann JC, Chusid MJ, et al: Functional abnormalities of human neutrophils collected by continuous flow filtration leukopheresis. *Blood* 46:901, 1975.

24. Klock JC, Boyles J, Bainton DF, et al: Nylon-fiber-induced neutrophil fragmentation. *Blood* 54:1216, 1979.

25. Schiffer CA: Filtration leukapheresis: Summary and perspectives. *Exp Hematol* 7(suppl 4):42, 1979.

26. McCullough J, Weiblen BJ, Deinard AR, et al: In vitro function and post-transfusion survival of granulocytes collected by continuous-flow centrifugation and filtration leukapheresis. *Blood* 48:315, 1976.

27. Goldstein IM, Eyre HJ, Terasaki PI, et al: Leukocyte transfusions: Role of leukocyte alloantibodies in determining transfusion response. *Transfusion* 2:19, 1971.

28. Graw RG Jr, Goldstein Im, Eyre JH, et al: Histocompatibility testing for leucocyte transfusion. *Lancet* 2:77, 1970.

29. Appelbaum FR, Trapani RJ, Graw RG Jr: Consequences of prior alloimmunization during granulocyte transfusion. *Transfusion* 17:460, 1977.

30. Westrick MA, Debelak-Fehir KM, Epstein RB: The effect of prior whole blood transfusion on subsequent granulocyte support in leukopenic dogs. *Transfusion* 17:611, 1976.

31. Lalezari P: Neutrophil antigens: Immunology and clinical implications, in Greenwalt TJ, Jamieson GA (eds) *The Granulocyte: Function and Clinical Utilization*. New York, Alan R Liss, Inc, 1977, p 209.

32. Rosenshein MS, Farewell VT, Price TH, et al: Cost effectiveness analysis of therapeutic and prophylactic leukocyte transfusion *New Engl J Med* 302:1058, 1980.

33. Dahlke MB, Shaf SL, Sherwood WC, et al: Priapism during filtration leukapheresis. *Transfusion* 19:482, 1979.

34. Mishler JM, Higby DJ, Rhomberg W, et al: Hydroxyethyl starch and dexamethasone as an adjunct to leukocyte separation with the IBM Blood Cell Separator. *Transfusion* 14:352, 1974.

35. Rock G, Wise P: Plasma expansion during granulocyte procurement: Cumulative effects of hydroxyethyl starch. *Blood* 53:1156, 1979.

36. Maguire LC, Strauss RG, Koepke JA: Elimination of hydroxyethyl starch from donor blood after single and multiple leukapheresis. *Transfusioo* 19:650, 1979.

37. Schiffer CA, Lichtenfeld JL, Wiernik PH, et al: Antibody response in patients with acute non-lymphocytic leukemia. *Cancer* 37:2177, 1976.

38. Howard JE, Perkins HA: The natural history of alloimmunization to platelets. *Transfusion* 18:496, 1977.

39. Green D, Tiro A, Basiliero J, et al.: Cytotoxic antibody complicating platelet support in acute leukemia: Response to chemotherapy. *JAMA* 236:1044, 1976.

40. Brand A, Van Leuwen A, Eernisse JG, et al: Platelet immunology with special regard to platelet transfusion therapy, in *Platelet Immunology*, Proceedings of the 16th International Congress of Hematology, Kyoto, 1976.

41. Thompson JS, Burns CP, Herbick JM: Stimulation of granulocyte antibodies by granulocyte transfusion. *Blood* 50(suppl):303, 1977.

42. Zaroulis CG, Weiser B, Jaramillo S: Granulocyte-specific antibodies in leukocyte transfusion therapy. *Blood* 54(suppl):131a, 1979.

43. Ungerleider RS, Appelbaum FR, Trapani RJ, et al: Lack of predictive value of antileukocyte antibody screening in granulocyte transfusion therapy. *Transfusion* 19:90, 1978.

44. Ford JM, Lacey JJ, Cullen MH, et al: Fatal graft-versus-host disease following transfusion of granulocytes from normal donors. *Lancet* 2:1167, 1976.

45. Price TH, Dale DC: Neutrophil transfusion: Effect of storage and of collection method on neutrophil blood kinetics. *Blood* 51:789, 1978.

46. Gurwith MJ, Brunton JL, Lank BA, et al: A prospective controlled investigation of prophylactic trimethoprim/sulfamethoxazole in hospitalized granulocytopenic patients. *Am J Med* 66:248, 1979.

47. Schiffer CA, Aisner J, Daly PA, et al: Increased leukocyte alkaline phosphatase activity following transfusion of leukocytes from a patient with chronic myelogenous leukemia. *Am J Med* 66:519, 1978.

48. Schwarzenberg L, Mathe G, Amiel JL, et al: Study of factors determining the usefulness and complications of leukocyte transfusions. *Am J Med* 43:206, 1967.

19

Protected Environments for the Treatment of High Risk Cancer Patients

Stephen C. Schimpff

INTRODUCTION

Infections in the granulocytopenic cancer patient are often life-threatening. The use of protective isolation, prophylactic antibiotics, or both has lessened the risks of infection, but there remains much room for improvement in both the concepts and applications of infection prevention techniques. New approaches to infection prevention are needed because, as therapy has improved for diseases such as acute nonlymphocytic leukemia (ANLL), the number of patients experiencing prolonged (>14 days), profound (<100 granulocytes/$\mu\ell$) granulocytopenia with attendant high risk of infection also has increased.

The incidence of infection is directly related to the absolute level of circulating granulocytes (1,2). As the granulocyte count drops, the incidence of infection increases with a marked rise as the count drops below 500/$\mu\ell$. Severe infections tend to occur at granulocyte levels below 500/$\mu\ell$; nearly all Gram-negative bacteremias occur when the granulocyte count is below 100/$\mu\ell$ (Fig. 1). Stable granulocytopenia, at any level, is less likely to be associated with infection than is rapidly developing granulocytopenia. For example, patients with either aplastic anemia or slowly developing cyclic neutropenia have few infections compared with patients with acute leukemia who have a rapidly dropping granulocyte count after remission induction chemotherapy. A single peripheral granulocyte count does not take into account the total bone marrow reserve, the marginated pool of granulocytes, or granulocyte function. Nevertheless, the granulocyte count is an excellent indicator of patients who require intensive attention to infection prevention.

Current therapy of ANLL with agents such as daunorubicin and cytosine arabinoside generally induces about 20 to 30 days of granulocytopenia with levels below 100/$\mu\ell$ for 10 to 20 days—longer if more than one course of therapy is required. Patients with acute leukemia undergoing bone marrow transplantation experience about three weeks of nearly absolute granulocytopenia pending mar-

GRANULOCYTOPENIA

(e.g., Acute Nonlymphocytic Leukemia)

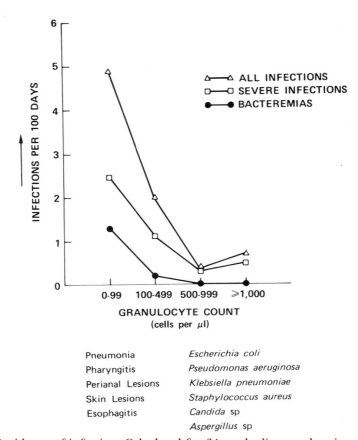

Pneumonia	Escherichia coli
Pharyngitis	Pseudomonas aeruginosa
Perianal Lesions	Klebsiella pneumoniae
Skin Lesions	Staphylococcus aureus
Esophagitis	Candida sp
	Aspergillus sp

Figure 1. Incidence of infection. Calculated for 64 newly diagnosed patients with acute nonlymphocytic leukemia treated with daunorubicin and cytosine arabinoside for remission induction. From Schimpff et al, *Leuk Res* 2:231–240, 1978, with permission of publisher.

row engraftment. An additional consequence of intensive chemotherapy is damage to the alimentary mucosa that establishes multiple potential foci for infection development that, in the presence of granulocytopenia, often progresses rapidly to bacteremia.

ORIGIN OF INFECTION

Almost all infections in granulocytopenic patients, in the absence of other factors predisposing to infection such as tumor obstruction or iatrogenic procedures, occur along the alimentary tract or in the lungs. Thus, the most common infections are pharyngitis, esophagitis, colitis, perianal lesions, and pneumonitis (3). Urinary infections are uncommon except in patients with anatomical abnormalities; skin infections are principally associated with damage to the integument, for example, venipuncture or bone marrow aspiration. The organisms that cause infection at each of these sites are those expected by an understanding of the dynamics of the microbial flora that colonize in the local area. Almost all cases of pharyngitis, esophagitis, colitis, perirectal lesions, and pneumonitis are caused by Gram-negative bacilli, or, in those who have received broad spectrum antibiotic therapy in the recent past, infections may be caused by yeasts *(Candida, Torulopsis)* or, in some settings, *Aspergillus* species. In addition, patients colonized in the anterior nares with *Staphylococcus aureus* have a propensity to develop staphylococcal infection (2).

Sites of Infection and Pathogenic Organisms

Not only is pneumonia common, but it has the highest associated mortality. The presumed pathogenesis is that cytotoxic therapy damages the tracheobronchial mucosa and its ciliary function so that organisms that reach this area either through inspired air or through minor aspiration of oral content are not cleared upward but reach the alveoli, where parenchymal infection can be instituted. In the absence of adequate numbers of granulocytes or functional alveolar macrophages, the infection can rapidly progress to involve large areas, frequently with hematogenous dissemination. Shifts in the pharynx and gingiva toward a Gram-negative flora during the first few days of hospitalization are consistent with the observation that pharyngitis also is caused by Gram-negative bacilli. Studies of Johanson and colleagues have indicated that an individual not receiving antimicrobial therapy who has an acute severe illness has a very high likelihood of shifting his microbial flora of the pharynx to include and perhaps be predominated by Gram-negative bacilli (4). Additional studies by Johanson indicated that this is related to change in binding sites on the squamous epithelial cells of the oral mucosa such that these cells bind Gram-negative bacilli to the exclusion of the usual normal oral flora. If a patient also receives broad spectrum antimicrobial therapy, the colonizing flora will be shifted further either toward more resistant bacteria or toward yeasts such as *Candida* species and *Torulopsis glabrata*. The shift of pharyngeal flora toward Gram-negative bacilli occurs even in complete reverse isolation such as a laminar air flow room, suggesting that colonization of the upper alimentary and respiratory tracts arises from the patient's endogenous intestinal flora. Routine surveillance cultures of the oral cavity of ANLL patients reveal Gram-negative bacilli and frequently *S. aureus* from nearly all patients within one to two weeks after admission to the hospital. The majority of pneumonias, therefore, especially those which occur within the first few weeks of induction chemotherapy, are caused by Gram-negative bacilli such as *Escherichia coli, Klebsiella pneumoniae,* and *Pseudomonas aeruginosa* as well as *S. aureus*. Pneumonias occurring later in the patient's hospitalization may also be caused by these organisms, but if the patient has received prolonged courses of broad spectrum antimicrobials, the risk of fungal pneumonia increases. Antibacterial therapy helps the yeast *T. glabrata* to colonize the oropharynx with resultant invasion of the lung. *Aspergillus fumigatus* or *flavus* and the agents of mucormycosis reach the patient via the air, colonize in the nose and sinus area, invade, and may progress to pulmonary infection. Alternatively, the fungal spores in the air may reach the trachea and bronchi directly and, in the appropriate setting of ciliary dysfunction and mucosal damage, locally colonize and lead to pneumonia (5).

Pharyngitis is a frequent complication following chemotherapy and may be related to the mucosal alterations caused by cytotoxic therapy. Almost all cases are probably due to local invasion of a mixed flora, but, as from other sites, *P. aeruginosa*, *Klebsiella* spp., and occasionally *S. aureus* are responsible for almost all bacteremias arising from the infected pharynx. *Candida albicans* and other *Candida* species are frequent causes of a disabling pharyngitis that may seriously limit swallowing, but almost all candidemias probably arise from the esophagus or intestinal tract.

Esophagitis is much more common than generally appreciated and is the major process from which *Candida* disseminates. Inflammation usually begins in the lower third of the esophagus, where a combination of cytotoxic related, mucosal alterations and gastric acid reflux predisposes to microbial invasion. The initial invaders may be viruses such as cytomegalovirus or herpes simplex or bacteria such as *P. aeruginosa; Candida* spp. may invade either initially or later.

Perianal and perirectal lesions frequently develop in patients with acute monocytic or myelomonocytic leukemia (30% to 60% incidence) but seldom in acute myelocytic leukemia and acute lymphocytic leukemia (10%). Even a very minor appearing lesion can be the source of a bacteremia, more often caused by *P. aeruginosa* than by *E. coli* or *K. pneumoniae*.

Many skin lesions are related to trauma, such as venipuncture, bone marrow aspiration, axillary shaving, ecchymosis, or bleeding. Many are caused by *S. aureus*, especially in nasal carriers. Gram-negative bacilli as a group, however, are the most frequent invaders of the skin. Normal skin bacteria such as *S. epidermidis* and diphtheroids less frequently invade.

Urinary infections are uncommon in the absence of specific predisposing factors, for example, catheter, leukemic infiltration of the prostate with obstruction, or recurrent urinary tract infections. In the granulocytopenic as in the normal individual, the etiologic agent correlates with the stool flora and hence is usually a Gram-negative bacillus. *Candida* spp. or *T. glabrata* urinary infections tend to occur only in patients with marked alterations in their microbial flora and, unless secondary to septicemia, are usually catheter-related.

The many blood product transfusions required during remission induction therapy of acute leukemia predispose to hepatitis. Because of improved screening, hepatitis B is now uncommon but non-A, non-B hepatitis persists as a major problem; more than 50% of patients develop this infection within a few months of leukemia diagnosis.

Epidemiology

Our first study of the origin of infection, conducted in 1969 to 1971 before specific infection control measures were instituted, evaluated 48 patients with ANLL who were hospitalized for one or more courses of induction therapy (3). There were 84 microbiologically documented infections of which about one-half (40) had an associated bacteremia. The most common origins for the development of bacteremia were pneumonias and anorectal lesions. Gram-negative bacilli overall caused approximately two-thirds of the infections, with *P. aeruginosa* being preeminent (23 of the 87 isolated organisms).

The great majority of infections were caused by organisms already colonizing the patient. Of the 87 organisms isolated from 84 separate infections, 75 were preceded by isolation of the same organism from surveillance cultures. Furthermore, there was a close correlation between the site of infection and the surveillance culture site from which the same organism was isolated. Organisms causing pharyngitis, pneumonitis, and esophagitis had usually been isolated from oral cavity cultures before infection, and organisms causing perirectal lesions or urinary tract infections had been isolated from previous rectal cultures. Most *S. aureus* infections, which usually occurred in the lungs or skin, were preceded by nasal carriage of *S. aureus*.

Table 1 lists the potential pathogens isolated from surveillance cultures at the time of admission and during hospitalization and indicates the number that were associated with subsequent infections. Overall, among 265 organisms present at the time of admission among these 48 patients, 40 were associated with subsequent infections. Similarly, among 285 organisms that were acquired during hospitalization, 35 were associated with a subsequent infection; that is, 47% of these infections were caused by organisms that were nosocomially acquired.

Considering the frequency of acquisition of new organisms, one would predict that methods that would interrupt the sequence of acquisition-colonization should reduce the incidence of bacteremia in these patients. That such is the case can be deduced by comparing the data in Table 1 (1969 to 1971) with those in Table 2 (1971 to 1976) (6). Since completion of the earlier study, the BCRC instituted stricter environmental controls, more intensive staff and patient hygiene, a cooked food (low microbial content) diet, increased patient and staff education, and use of oral nonabsorbable antibiotics. Substantially fewer potential pathogens were acquired in the second period, and, for those organisms that did colonize the patient, fewer progressed to bacteremia. With *P. aeruginosa* as an example, in 1969 to 1971, 22 (46%) of the 48 patients acquired *P. aeruginosa*, and 13 (59%) of the 22 developed a subsequent bacteremia. During 1971 to 1976, only 19 (24%) of 80 acquired *P. aeruginosa*, and, of these, only 3 (16%) of 19 had a subsequent bacteremia. Thus, infection was very substantially reduced, presumably as a result of improved environmental controls that reduced acquisition and reduced colonization of *P. aeruginosa* along the alimentary canal through the use of oral nonabsorbable antibiotics. Further analyses of Tables 1 and 2 will show that, for Gram-negative bacilli overall, a substantial reduction in acquisition of these organisms resulted in reduced chance for infection and, additionally, for those Gram-negative bacilli which did colonize the patient, there was a marked decline in their ability to induce bacteremia.

GENERAL CONCEPTS OF INFECTION PREVENTION

To recapitulate, damage to mucosa and other body barriers affords entry by organisms, frequently hospital-acquired, that usually are not considered to be highly virulent. The absence of adequate numbers of circulating, functional

Table 1. Colonization and Subsequent Bacteremia in 48 Patients with Acute Nonlymphocytic Leukemia Baltimore Cancer Research Center, 1969–1971

Organism	Baseline Flora			Acquired Flora		
	Colonized	Bacteremia	Percent	Colonized	Bacteremia	Percent
Gram-positive cocci						
Staphylococcus aureus	14	1	7	12	1	8
Group D Streptococcus sp.	30	1	3	14	1	7
Streptococcus pneumoniae	1	0	0	1	2	100
Gram-negative bacilli						
Pseudomonas aeruginosa	9	3	33	22	13	59
Pseudomonas spp.	4	0	0	25	0	0
Escherichia coli	34	3	9	8	0	0
Klebsiella spp.	25	4	16	17	2	12
Serratia spp.	5	2	4	4	1	25
Enterobacter cloacae	11	0	0	22	0	0
Proteus spp.	29	0	0	12	0	0
Citrobacter sp.	7	0	0	16	0	0
Mima polymorpha	2	0	0	6	1	17
Other	—	2	—	—	0	—
Yeasts						
Candida albicans	21	1	5	18	1	6
Candida spp.	3	0	0	13	0	0
Total[a]	265	17	—	285	22	—

[a]Includes some less frequent organisms not listed above.

An additional 23 baseline organisms caused nonbacteremic infections of a total of 40 infections secondary to baseline organisms.

An additional 13 acquired organisms caused nonbacteremic infections for a total of 35 infections secondary to acquired organisms.

Modified from Schimpff et al., Origin of infection in acute nonlymphocytic leukemia. *Ann Intern Med 77*:707, 1972.

Table 2. Colonization and Subsequent Bacteremia in 80 Patients with Acute Nonlymphocyic Leukemia Baltimore Cancer Research Center, 1971–1976

Organism	Baseline Flora			Acquired Flora			Bacteremia Without Colonization
	Colonized	Bacteremia	Percent	Colonized	Bacteremia	Percent	
Gram-positive cocci							
Staphylococcus aureus	36	5	14	17	1	6	2
Streptococcus faecalis	21	0	0	21	4	19	0
Streptococcus pneumoniae	0	0	—	1	1	100	0
Gram-negative bacilli							
Pseudomonas aeruginosa	16	4	25	19	3	16	3
Pseudomonas spp.	4	0	0	3	0	0	1
Escherichia coli	80	12	15	25	3	12	2
Klebsiella pneumoniae	27	3	11	34	4	12	0
Klebsiella spp.	8	0	0	13	1	8	1
Serratia marcescens	0	0	—	9	1	11	2
Enterobacter cloacae	19	0	0	16	0	0	0
Proteus mirabilis	24	2	8	28	1	4	1
Proteus spp.	9	1	11	24	1	4	0
Citobacter sp.	11	0	0	18	0	0	0
Mima polymorpha	0	0	—	3	0	—	1
Flavobacterium	1	0	—	3	0	—	1
Yeasts							
Candida albicans	38	1	3	24	1	4	0
Candida spp.	12	0	0	16	3	19	1
Torulopsis glabrata	3	2	67	10	1	10	0

Modified from Remington J et al, Life-threatening infections in the compromised host, in *Current Chemotherapy*. Washington, DC, American Society for Microbiology, 1978, pp 37–42.

granulocytes allows rapid progression of infection, often with bacteremia. These severe infections may be difficult to diagnose promptly, and, despite improvement in antimicrobial and granulocyte transfusion therapy, mortality rates remain high. Prevention of infection is therefore critical and a major responsibility of all who care for these patients. Techniques of infection prevention can be logically inferred from the foregoing concepts of infection development and can be categorized under the broad headings of (1) bolstering host defense mechanisms, (2) avoiding invasive or traumatic procedures, (3) suppressing organisms that colonize at or near common sites of infection, and (4) reducing acquisition of hospital-associated organisms (7).

Bolstering Host Defense Mechanisms

At the present time, there is not a lot that can be done in a practical way to bolster the patient's host defenses. Most important, of course, is reversal of the patient's underlying condition so that the granulocytopenic state resolves as promptly as possible. Influenza vaccine is safe and probably effective if given as time-distant as possible either before or after chemotherapy or immunosuppressive therapy. Currently none of the following are standard prophylactic measures: pseudomonas vaccine, enterobacteriaceae core antigen vaccines, pneumococcal vaccine, hepatitis vaccines, or prophylactically administered granulocyte transfusions.

Avoidance of Invasive and Traumatic Procedures

As in any patient population, the avoidance of intravenous catheters and urinary catheters substantially prevents intravenous-associated and urinary tract infections. All intravenous medications should be given by a butterfly type of needle that should be changed at least every 48 hours. The dressing should be changed each day. All tubing and bottles should be changed at least every 24 hours, and all tubing should be changed after any blood product administration. Careful attention should be given to applying firm pressure after venipuncture, fingerstick, or bone marrow aspiration to reduce the opportunity for an infection nidus from blood extravasation. All shaving should be done with an electric razor to reduce the chance for integumentary damage. Axillae should not be shaved, and occlusive antiperspirants should not be used.

Microbial Suppression

Good patient hygiene, including a daily bath and shampoo with an antiseptic compound such as chlorhexidine or povidone-iodine, maintains reasonably clean skin. Dental care, including daily brushing and flossing, reduces dental plaque and may prevent the development of acute periodontal infection. Dental consultation and a thorough prophylaxis should be performed before the initiation of myelosuppressive therapy. Povidone-iodine swabsticks rubbed on the axillae three times a day substantially decrease the frequency of axillary infections. Similar swabsticks can be used to clean the perianal and vulvar regions. Oral nonabsorbable antibiotics suppress the organisms colonizing the alimentary canal. Multiple regimens have been evaluated (e.g., gentamicin, vancomycin, nystatin [GVN]; framycetin, colymicin, nystatin [Fracon]) and generally have been found effective in substantially suppressing the flora. Problems include high cost, disagreeable taste (and hence soon compliance), and the acquisition of antibiotic-resistant organisms. The last problem especially has prompted consideration of the concept of colonization resistance, which suggests that the normal anaerobic flora, if preserved, largely prevent colonization by new organisms that might reach the patient from his environment. Agents that suppress the aerobic but not the anaerobic flora include trimethoprim/sulfamethoxazole, nalidixic acid, and pipemidic acid. Their possible use is reviewed elsewhere (8).

Reduction of the Acquisition of New Organisms

Since hospitalized patients are likely to acquire many new organisms and since approximately 50% of infections during periods of granulocytopenia are caused by these acquired organisms, logic suggests that reduction of acquisition should reduce infection incidence. Recognition of the organisms which are acquired and which tend to cause infection coupled with knowledge of their environmental sources can go far in planning an appropriate infection routine. Such a program can include complex techniques such as total patient isolation in a laminar air flow room but must include the simple techniques practical for any hospital. A relatively simple program of good housekeeping, a single room, careful staff and patient hygiene (especially handwashing), a low microbial diet, and a reasonably clean water supply goes a long way toward reducing the acquisition of potential pathogens by the high risk patient. Patients should not be placed in large open wards but preferably should be housed in single bedrooms with private bathrooms to reduce patient-to-patient cross contamination. All personnel who may come in contact with the patient should be trained in a program of personal hygiene that includes careful handwashing. An effective approach is to instruct the patient to refuse contact with anyone who has not washed. The patient should be indoctrinated with a regard for personal hygiene, including daily bathing and shampooing with an antimicrobial compound such as chlorhexidine. Food is a common source of acquired potential pathogens, but a sterile diet is difficult to prepare and is usually poorly accepted by patients. A diet of low microbial content ("cooked-food diet") can be conveniently prepared by eliminating all uncooked items such as salads. Commercially canned and bottled foods and beverages generally are sterile or nearly so, as are pasteurized products. Meats, vegetables, and desserts prepared by cooking are acceptable. Products such as ground pepper and other spices usually are highly contaminated by Gram-negative bacilli. The water supply that the patient uses for drinking and bathing should be evaluated from time to time. Often, removal of a faucet aerator ensures reasonably acceptable water supplies. Sterile bottled water may be necessary if the water is found to be contaminated. The patient's room and the hospital area in general should have a satisfactory housekeeping routine that includes the use of a phenolic disinfectant in the mop water, a clean mop head, and the double-bucket system. All horizontal surfaces and bathroom fixtures in the patient's room should be wiped daily with a phenolic disinfectant.

It is useful to consider the routes of acquisition of the more commonly acquired potential pathogens, as a recognition of these routes will explain the preceding suggestions.

Gram-Negative Bacilli

The microbial flora found on green leafy vegetables generally includes Gram-negative bacilli such as *E. coli* and *P. aeruginosa* plus not infrequent colonization with *S. aureus* or *C. albicans*. The cooked-food diet substantially reduces this problem. Eliminated from the diet are all raw fruits, vegetables, salads, foods that have been prepared with uncooked ingredients such as tuna salad sandwich, and comestibles that have been properly prepared but stored in a manner that recontamination is possible, for example, iced tea where nonsterile ice has been added. It is to be emphasized that this cooked-food diet is not sterile but it is practical and acceptable in most hospitals. To place a patient in protective reverse isolation and at the same time use a diet teeming with potential pathogens makes little sense; yet such is the common approach to reverse isolation.

A sterile or nearly sterile water supply is essential. Almost all city water supplies are low in microbes, but organisms are often introduced near the point of use, for example, through the faucet aerator. The screening in the aerator collects organic material that serves as growth media for potential pathogens such as *P. aeruginosa* and *Serratia marcescens*. Removal of the faucet aerator altogether, or at least frequent removal, cleaning, and autoclaving, eliminates much of this problem. Where water supplies are unsatisfactory, it may be necessary to use sterile bottled water for patient use in bathing, dental care, drinking, and food preparation. If the water supply is reasonably free of particulate matter, final filters on each sink outlet ensure an adequate water supply. These filters tend to become clogged after a few days to a few weeks but may often preclude the need for sterile bottled water.

Common sources in hospitals of Gram-negative bacilli include ice machines, where contamination with *P. aeruginosa* is a particularly frequent problem and is extremely difficult to eliminate. Ice machines from which ice is to be used for patients with granulocytopenia should be of the type where the ice falls out of the machine into a cup and where no scoop or hand can get into the inner apparatus. Even in this situation, the ice should be checked approximately once a month to ensure that it has not become contaminated. Another source is the bedpan washer, which generally does not close tightly. The spray of water particles emitted from such equipment contaminates the area about it and may well settle on items that were believed to have been clean. Esophagoscopes and bronchoscopes are usually not sterilized between uses because of damage to the instrument by steam or gas sterilization; nevertheless, host contamination by Gram-negative bacilli is not uncommon, leading to the potential for introduction of the organisms directly into a site in the compromised patient where infection is frequent, that is, esophagus and lung. Certain antiseptic solutions, particularly the quarternary ammonium compounds (e.g., benzalkonium), are capable of supporting growth of *P. aeruginosa* and other Gram-negative bacilli. These solutions are used in many hospitals to soak esophagoscopes, thermometers, sigmoidoscopes, and so on. Most important is careful cleaning to remove residual organic matter and, then, disinfection with an effective agent such as 8% aqueous formaldehyde or 2% alkalinized gluteraldehyde. Other potential hazards are humidifiers for oxygen delivery, respiratory assist equipment, or any other area or apparatus that tends to stay moist for prolonged periods.

Gram-negative organisms also are capable of remaining viable on the hands of staff members as they go from patient to patient or from patient to bedpan to patient. Simple but thorough handwashing rapidly eliminates Gram-negative organisms from the hands because they are not part of the normal flora of the hands. At our center, pressurized cans of antiseptic hand cleansers are placed at each bedside. Application of a small amount before and after patient contact takes only a few seconds and overcomes the frequent reluctance to seek out a sink.

Staphylococci

At any given time *S. aureus* colonizes the anterior nares of 15% to 30% of the normal population, with an even larger segment of the population being colonized on an intermittent basis. From the nose, *S. aureus* can easily be picked up by the hands and carried to any body area. *S. aureus* can be shed into the air on droplets during sneezing by a normal individual who is not aware of his carrier status. Staff members may have *S. aureus* on their hands secondary to nasal carriage and may spread it to patients under their care. Patients with mycosis fungoides generally are heavily colonized with *S. aureus* and tend to contaminate the environment with desquamated scales. Likewise, patients with staphylococcal postoperative wound infections or staphylococcal pneumonia tend to shed staphylococci into their immediate environment, and these organisms may be readily carried to other patients by staff members who carry the staphylococci on their hands or clothing. The best approach to reduction of staphylococcal acquisition is to enforce a policy of personnel hygiene emphasizing handwashing along with appropriate wound and respiratory isolation for those with staphylococcal infections.

Fungi

Yeasts tend to be acquired from food products; acquisition can therefore be reduced by the use of the low-microbial diet. Filamentous fungi are acquired through the air. Relatively little can be done other than perhaps removal of live flowers and plants and routine cleaning of air-conditioning and refrigerator filters and condensors. Some hospitals now are being constructed with air handling systems for both heating and cooling that use high-efficiency particulate air (HEPA) filters with no air recirculation. Such systems, although of high initial cost, do maintain a much greater control of air. For example, many studies have shown that the average number of organisms per 1,000 cu ft of air in a standard hospital room is approximately 3,000, whereas, in a hospital room using HEPA filtration for the main air intake system with no air recirculation, viable organisms are reduced to about 300 per 1,000 cu ft of air, that is, a 10-fold reduction.

Viruses

Granulocytopenia does not, per se, predispose to viral infection. Hepatitis, however, is a frequent problem because of the intensive use of blood product transfusions. Use of multiple-unit plateletpheresis from as few donors as possible for each patient and screening of donors for disqualification of those with minor elevations in SGOT levels should reduce acquisition of these infections.

All these techniques require constant attention but, if followed carefully, substantially if not dramatically lower the rate of new organism acquisition. Greater reduction requires the use of sophisticated reverse isolation equipment such as the laminar air flow (LAF) room.

LAMINAR AIR FLOW ROOMS

Reverse isolation can take many forms, but the most efficient system devised has been the laminar air flow room. Laminar air flow rooms were first developed to provide clean rooms for the space industry (Fig. 2). The essential elements are a bank of high-efficiency particulate air (HEPA) filters along one entire wall of the room through which air, pumped by blowers, enters the room at a uniform velocity (30 to 90 ft/min) moving in a laminar pattern. The air usually exhausts at the opposite end of the room. The net effects are essentially sterile air in the room, minimal air turbulence, minimal opportunity for microorganism buildup, and a consistently clean environment. As noted previously, the standard hospital room may have approximately 3,000 potential pathogens per 1,000 cu ft of air and a regular room supplied with filtered air about 300 organisms per 1,000 cu ft. A laminar air flow room generally has nearly sterile air with ranges of zero

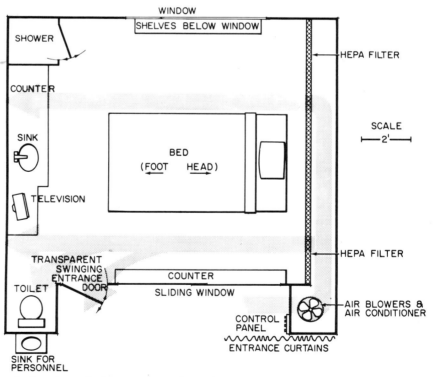

Figure 2. Laminar air flow room at the Baltimore Cancer Research Center, Baltimore, Maryland. From Schimpff et al, *Ann Intern Med* 82:351–358, 1975, with permission of publisher.

to 15 organisms per 1,000 cu ft of air during patient occupancy (9). Not only is the air itself sterile on entry, but the constant movement of air in a laminar pattern removes those organisms shed from the patient so that the room remains clean. In addition, a visitor to the room, provided he remains downstream from the patient, cannot shed organisms directly on the patient. Generally, reverse isolation in regular hospital rooms without such air exchange mechanisms may be cleaner than a conventional hospital room but does not approach the efficacy of laminar air flow. Air testing of new LAF units at the BCRC revealed a remarkably low frequency of all airborne particles and of viable airborne particles. Photooptical counts of particles >0.5 μm diameter averaged <10 per cu ft of air. Viable particles (bacteria, yeasts, fungi) detected with a large volume electrostatic precipitating air sampler (1,000 liters of air per minute operated over 10 minutes, i.e., 353 cu ft per sample) using appropriate isokinetic probes indicated <0.0005 organisms per cubic foot of air.

Before patient use, the entire room is cleaned with disinfectant and stocked with sterile supplies. All items that enter the room, including linens, examining equipment, blood drawing tubes, and personal items, must be sterile or thoroughly cleaned. Water is sterile, and food is either sterile (autoclaved) or of low microbial content (cooked food). The patient may be examined through glove ports, but everyone, staff and visitors, must wear sterile garments when inside and must remain downstream from the patient.

LAF Isolation without Microbial Flora Suppression

The use of laminar air flow units or their equivalent without oral nonabsorbable antibiotics has been evaluated in only a limited number of studies. One would predict, however, that a substantial decrease in the acquisition of new organisms, particularly those most likely to cause infection in the granulocytopenic patient, should lead to a decrease in the overall incidence of infection. Yates and Holland (10) placed leukemia patients in a laminar air flow room or similar facility, and when compared with controls, there was a decrease in pneumonias, in severe infections overall, and especially in *Pseudomonas* infections. The EORTC Gnotobiotic Group evaluation also found a decrease in infections and, in addition, noted a decrease in organism acquisition when isolation alone was compared with concurrent controls (11). Control patients had a contamination index (new bacteria isolated per patient per week) substantially higher (2.35) than that of the isolated patients (1.59), with the latter acquisitions apparently due to technique lapses. The colonization index of newly isolated bacteria per patient per week that persisted in subsequent cultures for more than one week was likewise higher for control (0.60) than for isolated (0.41) patients. Additionally, the rate of pneumonias developing during the study period was less in the isolated patients. Therefore complete reverse isolation decreases the acquisition of potential pathogens and the development of severe infection.

LAF Isolation with Microbial Suppression

In most evaluations, oral nonabsorbable antibiotics often with added topical and orificial antibiotics and antiseptics have been used in conjunction with LAF reverse isolation. Oral nonabsorbable antibiotics are usually begun one to two days before entry into the room. Among the combinations evaluated, gentamicin, 200 mg; vancomycin, 500 mg; and nystatin, 5 million units (GVN) has been most commonly used. These may be given in liquid form every four to six hours around the clock. In addition, antibiotic mouthwashes, nasal sprays, vaginal douches, and topical ointments to ears, anterior nares, and perianum have been used in some centers along with antimicrobial soap preparations.

Induction Therapy of Acute Leukemia

Bodey and colleagues (12) treated 33 patients with acute leukemia in a protected environment with prophylactic antibiotics and compared these with 66 concurrently treated leukemia patients selected retrospectively as controls based on multiple prognostic factors. The isolated patients had a greater percentage of days granulocytopenic than did the controls, and yet there was still a substantial reduction in the incidence of severe infections both at granulocyte counts $<100/\mu\ell$ and at 101 to $999/\mu\ell$. Although complete remission rates were similar, the isolated patients had an increased duration of remission apparently related to their more intensive chemotherapeutic regimen.

Yates and Holland (10) evaluated adult acute leukemia patients in (1) regular rooms, (2) reverse isolation in regular rooms with the use of prophylactic nonabsorbable antibiotics, (3) reverse isolation in laminar air flow rooms, or (4) LAF isolation with oral nonabsorbable antibiotics. When compared with controls, the LAF isolation with oral nonabsorbable antibiotic group had fewer infections, including fewer severe infections, fewer pneumonias, and fewer P. aeruginosa infections. There was no significant improvement in complete remission rates.

Levine et al. (13) distributed adult patients with acute leukemia to (1) a control group treated in regular rooms or (2) a group similarly housed but given oral nonabsorbable antibiotics or (3) a group treated in Life Islands or laminar air flow rooms along with oral nonabsorbable antibiotics. The isolated patients had substantially greater amounts of time with granulocyte counts $<100/\mu\ell$; nevertheless there were marked reductions both in septicemias, especially those caused by Gram-negative organisms, and in pneumonias. The 22 patients treated in protected environments with oral nonabsorbable antibiotics had 8 infections, whereas the 28 control patients had 22 infections. When the granulocyte count was $<100/\mu\ell$, the percentage of days spent infected was 12% for the isolated versus 40% for the control patients, and the episodes of infections per 100 days was 1.5 versus 5.5, respectively. Despite this marked reduction in infection incidence, there was no difference in the complete remission rate.

The EORTC Gnotobiotic Group (11) evaluated leukemia patients treated in (1) a ward setting, (2) isolators without use of oral nonabsorbable antibiotics, or (3) isolators with oral nonabsorbable antibiotics. The patients in the last group had a greater reduction in the rate (index) of new organism contamination/colonization (0.83/0.10) than did those in isolation alone (1.59/0.41) or those in the control group (2.35/0.60). Infections overall were not significantly reduced in the isolated groups without or with oral nonabsorbable antibiotics (35% and 45%, respectively) compared with controls (54%), but the pneumonia frequency was reduced significantly (6% and 7% compared with 24%). Remission rates were higher and survival longer for the isolated patients.

Schimpff et al. (14) evaluated adult patients with acute nonlymphocytic leukemia who were admitted for remission induction therapy. Patients were infection-free at the time of admission and were prospectively allocated to treatment in (1) an open ward or in two to three-bedded rooms (control group), (2) a ward setting with use of oral nonabsorbable antibiotics, or (3) a laminar air flow room isolator with use of oral nonabsorbable antibiotics (LAF + A). GVN was the oral antibiotic combination; other specific topical or orificial antiseptics or antibiotics were not used. The same physicians and nurses cared for patients in all three groups in the same area of one floor of the hospital. The LAF + A and the control group spend 47% and 48%, respectively, at a granulocyte count of <100/ $\mu\ell$. Compared with controls, the LAF + A group had a significantly decreased acquisition of new organisms (average of 0.45/patient/week compared with 1.24/patient/week for controls), incidence of total infections, microbiologically documented infections, severe infections, or infections with an associated bactere-

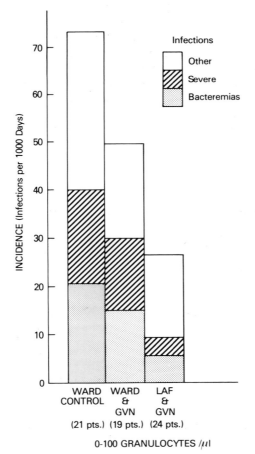

Figure 3. Incidence of infection during profound granulocytopenia for patients with ANLL enrolled in BCRC controlled trial comparing routine ward care (WARD CONTROL) to ward care plus oral nonabsorbable antibiotics (WARD + GVN) to laminar air flow room reverse isolation plus oral nonabsorbable antibiotics (LAF + GVN).

mia. Eighty-three percent of the isolated patients experienced no severe infections during remission induction therapy compared with 38% of the control group. Pneumonias were markedly reduced (3 versus 13), as were anorectal lesions (2 versus 10), pharyngitis (6 versus 11), and urinary tract infections (0 versus 6). Infections caused by Gram-negative bacilli were reduced, as were fatal infections (17% versus 52%) and infectious death occurring before the patient had had an adequate trial of remission induction chemotherapy (8% versus 30%). Most notable was the dramatic reduction in bacteremias and other severe infections during periods of profound ($<100/\mu\ell$) granulocytopenia (Fig. 3), periods that averaged 47% to 48% of the on-study time. The complete remission rate was higher in the LAF + A than in the control group (54% versus 24%) with a resultant improved survival (Fig. 4). Some patients in each group received a particularly myelosuppressive and mucosal damaging form of remission induction chemotherapy (daunorubicin, 180 mg/m² in one dose) resulting in a very high risk of infection. This risk was admirably controlled by the isolation plus oral nonabsorbable antibiotics (Fig. 3), which allowed more patients to survive long enough for induction therapy to be effective (Fig. 4).

In a study from the Institut Jules Bordet by Lohner et al. (15), 21 patients, mostly with ANLL who were receiving induction chemotherapy were randomized in a control group in which they received their chemotherapy in a single room along with sterile food and water plus oral nonabsorbable antibiotics (vancomycin, polymixin, kanamycin, and nystatin). Twenty-four additional patients were randomized to complete reverse isolation in a plastic tent type of vertical laminar air flow isolator using high efficiency particulate air filters along with sterile food and water and oral nonabsorbable antibiotics. In this evaluation, the

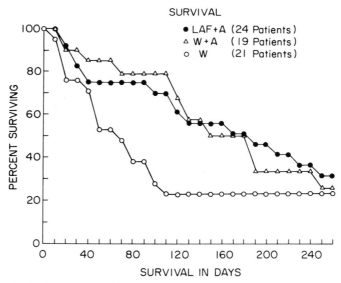

Figure 4. Survival of patients with ANLL allocated to Ward, Ward + GVN, or LAF + GVN. From Schimpff et al, *Ann Intern Med* 82:351–358, 1975, with permission of publisher.

patients in the LAF room were given more intensive chemotherapy, resulting in twice as many days of granulocytopenia below $100/\mu\ell$ than the control group. At this level of granulocyte count, the isolated group had an incidence of infection that was approximately 50% that of the control group. The incidence of bacterial septicemia was 6 per 1,000 days in the isolated group compared with 12 per 1,000 days in the control group, and the incidence of all other infections was 24 per 1,000 days in the isolated group compared with 39 per 1,000 days among the controls. Surprisingly, the frequency of *Aspergillus* infections was greater in the isolated group, but this is perhaps explained by the fact that many of these patients had been hospitalized for some period before isolation, thus allowing acquisition via the airborne route before residence in the LAF room.

Rodriguez et al. (16) randomly allocated 145 adult leukemia patients to receive remission induction therapy in or out of laminar air flow rooms with either oral (PA) or systemic (SA) prophylactic antibiotics. Infection incidence was lower in than out of the laminar air flow rooms at granulocyte counts $<500/\mu\ell$, and the occurrence of fatal infections was reduced (13% versus 28%). There was no difference between those receiving oral as opposed to systemic prophylactic antibiotics. Patients treated in the isolators had a higher complete remission rate (61% versus 45%) and longer median survival time (72 weeks versus 42 weeks).

Bone Marrow Transplantation

Buckner et al. (17) in Seattle studied the use of laminar air flow rooms for isolation of patients receiving bone marrow transplants. Patients admitted for transplantation were randomly allocated to a control group that was treated in regular patient rooms or to the laminar air flow rooms. The control group patients, placed in regular patient rooms, were given routine diets and were not isolated. The isolated patients were given a sterile diet and oral nonabsorbable antibiotics. There were 45 LAF patients and 44 control patients; about two-thirds had acute leukemia and one-third had aplastic anemia. There was a reduction in bacteremias (10 versus 23) and other severe infections (3 versus 22) among the LAF patients compared with controls. Graft versus host disease and interstitial pneumonitis frequencies were not affected.

Therapy of Lymphomas, Carcinomas, and Sarcomas

Finally, a number of studies are in progress evaluating LAF room techniques for therapy of solid tumors such as sarcomas, non-Hodgkin's lymphoma, breast carcinoma, and small cell carcinoma of the lung (18). In almost all these trials, the LAF isolated patients are being treated with increased doses of chemotherapeutic agents in an attempt to improve tumor shrinkage. Despite increased dosage, with consequent increased days of marked granulocytopenia, the incidence of infection has been reduced. In addition, for patients with non-Hodgkin's lymphoma and perhaps those with soft-tissue sarcoma, the duration of complete remission has been prolonged. This is presumably a result of the opportunity to increase drug dosage while decreasing infection morbidity and mortality (18).

Overall, it can be concluded that reverse isolation in a laminar air flow room or similar facility using careful aseptic techniques very substantially reduces organism acquisition and the incidence of infection. The additional use of oral nonabsorbable antibiotics to suppress colonizing organisms further substantially reduces the development of severe infections. There is at this time no longer any question that the LAF concept is effective for the purpose for which it was designed, namely, to prevent infection. Given that conclusion, it must be determined whether such an approach is beneficial in a practical sense.

The complete remission rate for patients with acute leukemia treated under these intensive conditions compared with controls has, in many trials, not been significantly improved. Although psychological deprivation has not been a problem, the patient is denied close contact with loved ones. The cost of isolation is high, in both equipment and supplies plus added time commitments of personnel (19).

Considered in these terms, the value of the laminar air flow room—prophylactic antibiotic regimen may be questioned when used for patients with poor long-term survival potential. Other factors should be considered, however. Not only have the combined effects of laminar air flow room reverse isolation plus oral nonabsorbable antibiotics reduced infections, but infections have been most significantly reduced in those patients with the most profound levels of granulocytopenia, that is, those patients given the most intensive bone-marrow-suppressing, mucosal-damaging chemotherapy had the most significant reduction in infections. It follows that when used for patients at less risk of infection, less protection has been recognized, and negative attitudes have been inappropriately developed. Although increased remission rates have not been uniformly observed, this represents the current status of antileukemia therapy rather than the negation of the infection prevention potential of LAF reverse isolation. In addition, it is difficult if not almost unethical to subject patients in remission to intensive remission maintenance programs (e.g., late intensification with chemotherapy continued to bone marrow aplasia or intensive ablation followed by bone marrow transplantation). In this setting of a patient at risk of infection entirely as a result of maintenance therapy, it is mandatory that every possible effort be expended to prevent infectious morbidity and mortality. To do otherwise is to subject the patient to unacceptable risk.

My own opinion is that research in these areas should continue because it is likely that more effective forms of leukemia induction or leukemia maintenance chemotherapy will be developed shortly, as will better therapy for solid tumors and improved techniques for bone marrow transplantation. This will result in the potential for prolonged survival or cure of many malignancies. In all likelihood, such new approaches will be both bone-marrow and mucosa-damaging. The availability of proved techniques to reduce infection will allow optimal use of new, effective, albeit toxic, compounds with the potential for long-term patient benefit and survival.

REFERENCES

1. Bodey GP, Buckley M, Sathe YS, et al: Quantitative relationships between circulating leukocytes and infection in patients with acute leukemia. *Ann Intern Med* 64:328, 1966.
2. Schimpff SC: Infections in patients with acute leukemia with emphasis on infections associated with granulocytopenia, in Bennett JE (ed): *Principles and Practices of Infectious Diseases.* New York, John Wiley & Sons, Inc, 1979, p 2263.

3. Schimpff SC, Young VM, Greene WH, et al: Origin of infection in acute nonlymphocytic leukemia. Significance of hospital acquisition of potential pathogens. *Ann Intern Med* 77:707, 1972.

4. Johanson WG, Pierce AK, Sanford JP: Changing pharyngeal bacterial flora of hospitalized patients. Emergence of gram-negative bacilli. *N Engl J Med* 281:1137, 1969.

5. Aisner J, Murillo J, Schimpff SC, et al: Invasive aspergillosis in acute leukemia: Correlation with nose cultures and antibiotic usage. *Ann Intern Med* 90:4, 1979.

6. Schimpff SC: Infection in adults with acute leukemia, in Williams JD, Geddes AM (eds): *Chemotherapy*. New York, Plenum Publishing Corp, 1976, p 81.

7. Schimpff SC: Infection prevention in patients with cancer and granulocytopenia, in Greico MH (ed): *Infections Complicating the Abnormal Host*. New York, Yorke Medical Books (in press).

8. Schimpff SC: Infection prevention during granulocytopenia, in Remington JS, Swartz MN (eds): *Current Clinical Topics in Infectious Diseases*. New York, McGraw-Hill Book Co, 1980, p 85.

9. Bodey GP, Johnston D: Microbiological evaluation of protected environments during patient occupancy. *Appl Microbiol* 22:828, 1971.

10. Yates JW, Holland JF: A controlled study of isolation and endogenous microbial suppression in acute myelocytic leukemia patients. *Cancer* 32:1490, 1973.

11. Dietrich M, Gaus W, Vossen J, et al: Protective isolation and antimicrobial decontamination in patients with high susceptibility to infection. A prospective cooperative study of gnotobiotic care in acute leukemia patients. I. Clinical results. *Infection* 5:3, 1977.

12. Bodey GP, Gehan EA, Freireich EJ, et al: Protected environment-prophylactic antibiotic program in the chemotherapy of acute leukemia. *Am J Med Sci* 262:138, 1971.

13. Levine AS, Siegel SE, Schreiber AD, et al: Protected environments and prophylactic antibiotics. A prospective controlled study of their utility in the therapy of acute leukemia. *N Engl J Med* 288:477, 1973.

14. Schimpff SC, Greene WH, Young VM, et al: Infection prevention in acute nonlymphocytic leukemia. Laminar air flow room reverse isolation with oral, nonabsorbable antiobiotic prophylaxis. *Ann Intern Med* 82:351, 1975.

15. Lohner D, Debusscher L, Prevost JM, et al: Comparative randomized study of protected environment plus oral antibiotics versus oral antibiotics alone in neutropenic patients. *Cancer Treat Rep* 63:363, 1979.

16. Rodriguez V, Bodey GP, Freireich EJ, et al: Randomized trials of protected environment-prophylactic antibiotics in 145 adults with acute leukemia. *Medicine* 57:253, 1978.

17. Buckner CD, Clift RA, Sanders JE, et al: Protective environment for marrow transplant recipients. A prospective study. *Ann Intern Med* 89:893, 1978.

18. Bodey GP, Rodriguez V, Cabanillas F, et al: Protected environment-prophylactic antibiotic program for malignant lymphoma. *Am J Med* 66:49, 1979.

19. Drazen EC, Levine AS: Laminar air flow rooms. *Hospitals, JAHA* 48:88, 1974.

20

Do Results Justify the Expense of Protected Environments?

Philip A. Pizzo

Since infection is the major cause of death in the patient with cancer and can serve as a deterrent to the delivery of potentially beneficial cancer therapy, considerable attention has been focused on developing methods for infection prevention. This objective requires a thorough understanding of the factors that heighten the risk of serious infection in the cancer patient, including disease- and treatment-related defects in the integumentary and mucosal physical barriers, diminished phagocytic defenses, decreased cellular and humoral immunity, and nutritional deficiency (1). In addition, careful microbial surveillance studies have shown that approximately 86% of the infections that occur in the patient with cancer arise from the patient's endogenous microbial flora and that 47% of these infecting organisms have been acquired by the patient during hospitalization (the most frequent nosocomial isolates being *Pseudomonas aeruginosa, Escherichia coli, Klebsiella pneumoniae,* and *Candida albicans*) (2–5). Numerous hospital sources also contribute to the colonization of the cancer patient, including staff-patient and patient-patient transmission, food, air, water, hospital equipment (e.g., respirators, vaporizers), and both medical and surgical manipulations and procedures. In addition, the endogenous or acquired microbial flora of the patient can also be perturbed by the antibiotics or chemotherapeutic agents frequently used in cancer treatment (6,7).

Consequently, the primary objective during the past 15 years has been directed at developing methods for suppressing or eliminating the host's endogenous microbial burden, as well as in decreasing the acquisition of new (i.e., hospital-acquired) organisms by the cancer patient. Theoretically, the reduction of the patient's microbial burden while severely immunocompromised should reduce the risk of developing a serious infection and thus permit the cancer patient to receive optimal, or even very intensive, chemotherapy that might result in longer disease-free survival. The prevention techniques that have been used have varied in complexity from simple single-room isolation to more elaborate systems using air filtration and decontamination. The most sophisticated of these regimens is

267

the total protected environment (PE) consisting of a laminar air flow room (LAFR) in which high-efficiency particulate air (HEPA) filters are used to remove all particles greater than 0.3 μm in size. When all the surfaces of the LAFR are carefully disinfected, and if all objects that then enter the facility are also steam- or gas-sterilized, a relatively sterile environment is achieved. In order to avoid contamination, patients entering the LAFR must also be fully decontaminated, usually with oral nonabsorbable antibiotics, cutaneous antisepsis, orificial antibiotics, and a semisterile diet. The cumulative data to date have shown that this total protected environment is capable of a significant, albeit incomplete, reduction in the incidence of serious infections in severely compromised cancer patients (8). In spite of this relative success, the PE regimen is elaborate, cumbersome, and expensive, and its use has not clearly permitted a consistent benefit from the cancer treatment regimens used in it. It is appropriate, therefore, to reassess critically the use of the PE as a component of current cancer therapy.

MICROBIOLOGICAL STUDIES

Evaluation of the individual components of the protected environment regimen (i.e., isolation, air filtration, prophylactic antibiotics, and antisepsis) has been clouded by inconsistent results. This is largely a consequence of noncomparable study designs, many of which have not been controlled and which have evaluated small numbers of patients who were treated in different types of isolation facilities, receiving different antibiotic decontamination regimens, and with variations in the patients' underlying malignancies, chemotherapy, and duration of granulocytopenia. It is nonetheless appropriate to summarize the results of these investigations.

Standard single-room reverse isolation has been frequently used in an attempt to reduce the nosocomial acquisition of potential pathogens by leukopenic cancer patients. Since an abundance of anecdotal data has suggested that this precaution alone is unlikely to alter significantly the airborne transmission of microorganisms or the incidence of infection arising from the patient's endogenous microbial flora, it is not surprising that a recent prospectively randomized trial of strict reverse isolation versus routine ward care has failed to demonstrate a beneficial effect in the prevention of infection in leukopenic patients (9).

However, when HEPA filtration is used in conjunction with room isolation, either in a Life Island or in a unidirectional LAFR, there is a significant reduction in the influx of exogenous microorganisms into the isolation room (10–18). Furthermore, if the surfaces of the air-filtered room are also disinfected, more than 70% of the environmental cultures obtained in the room will be sterile compared with those in a regular hospital room (19,20). However, if the patient housed in such an air-filtered isolation room does not also undergo rigorous gastrointestinal and cutaneous decontamination, the environment quickly becomes autocontaminated with the patient's endogenous microbial flora (21,22). Consequently, although the acquisition of new organisms may be reduced by the addition of air filtration to room isolation, it would be surprising if this regimen alone had a major impact on infection prevention, since the majority of infections are caused by the patient's endogenous microbial flora. This has been substantiated by a recent clinical trial in which isolation plus air filtration alone failed to demonstrate a significant reduction in the incidence of infections when compared with patients treated with routine ward care (13).

The benefit of prophylactic antibiotics designed to suppress or eliminate the host's endogenous microbial flora has also been evaluated without concomitant physical isolation. Most commonly, a combination of nonabsorbable antibiotics (e.g., gentamicin, vancomycin, nystatin, polymixin B) are used to achieve gastrointestinal decontamination. Although the microbial burden can be reduced with these agents, this is hampered in the nonisolated patient by the continued exposure to exogenous organisms from the air, water, food, and physical contacts. Moreover, the nonabsorbable antibiotics generally only suppress rather than truly eliminate the host's microbial flora. Therefore, the antibiotics must be taken daily during the period of risk, or the suppressed flora reappear within days after their discontinuation. The continued administration of the antibiotics is poorly tolerated by some patients and may result in nausea, vomiting, and diarrhea. Accordingly, patient compliance is imperfect and potentially deleterious, since the sudden discontinuation of antibiotics by the patient who is still granulocytopenic may permit certain organisms (e.g., *P. aeruginosa*) to repopulate the gastrointestinal tract rapidly and potentially lead to serious infection (23–25). The increased incidence of aminoglycoside-resistant microbial isolates from institutions where nonabsorbable antibiotics are frequently used is also of concern (26,27). Finally, there are certain body sites (e.g., oropharynx) that are very difficult to decontaminate effectively and certain organisms (e.g., *C. albicans*) that are very difficult to eliminate with currently available antimicrobial agents, irrespective of the body site. As a consequence of these problems, it is not surprising that a consistant benefit of gastrointestinal decontamination without concurrent physical isolation has not been observed in the more than dozen clinical trials that have addressed this question (13,19,24,25,27–33).

Although the individual components of the total protected environment are only inconsistently successful in reducing the rate of infectious complications in high risk patients, the combined regimen appears beneficial. However, PE patients still have 5% to 25% the number of serious infections found in comparably treated control patients (8,19). The majority of these infections occur during the first four weeks of isolation, presumably before the time that maximum microbial suppression has been achieved. Moreover, the inability of the PE regimen to eliminate the resident microbial flora from all body sites in a serious limitation, since more than three-quarters of the infections that occur in PE patients are due to these persistant organisms. Accordingly, the improved control of infection observed when PE patients were treated with trimethoprin-sulfamethoxazole in addition to nonabsorbable antibiotics is encouraging and may indicate a role for systemic antibiotic prophylaxis in conjunction with the PE regimen (34). The only other clinical trial in which systemic antibiotics were used in conjunction with the PE was the rotating systemic antibiotic schedule used by Rodriquez et al. (33). This latter schedule did not prove useful, although this is most likely a consequence of the suboptimal and inconsistant antibiotic coverage provided by this antibiotic regimen, rather than the lack of a potential benefit from systemic antibiotics.

Although the PE regimen reduces the incidence of bacterial and fungal infections, no protection is afforded against the clinically important latent herpesviruses (i.e., *Herpes simplex, Herpes zoster,* cytomegalovirus [CMV]) or protozoa (i.e., *Pneumocystis carinii*). This is particularly relevant for patients who are undergoing allogeneic bone marrow transplantation for the treatment of aplastic anemia or leukemia and who are at risk for both acute bacterial and fungal infections after transplantation, as well as severe interstitial pneumonia with CMV. Although the PE is effective in reducing the incidence of the bacterial and fungal infections during the posttransplant period of severe granulocytopenia, the incidence of interstitial pneumonitis, presumably secondary to the reactivation of latent CMV, is unaffected by protected isolation (35,36). Although this is not strictly a failure of the PE regimen per se, the onset of CMV pneumonitis nonetheless serves to limit the successful outcome from allogenic bone marrow transplantation. Clearly, a more successful decontamination program, as well as effective antiviral therapy, is necessary to improve the usefulness of the PE regimen in preventing the wide range of serious infections that occur in these high risk patients. However, even if this is successfully accomplished, the PE still has several other formidable limitations worthy of consideration.

First, the costs of establishing an isolation unit are significant: Currently, commercially available semiportable LAFRs that can be installed in a standard hospital room average approximately $28,000 per unit. Room preparation for LAFR installation, exclusive of major reconstructive requirements, adds another $5,000 to 8,000 to the initial cost. In addition, financial provision must be made for a sterile supply service, sterile kitchen, microbiology laboratory, as well as a highly skilled nursing staff and trained dietary, housekeeping, and maintenance services (37). Furthermore, a large number of consumable supplies (e.g., sterile gowns, masks, linens, disinfectants, and antibiotics) add to the daily cost of patient care, which generally ranges from $500 to $750 per day.

The psychological impact of continued isolation on the patient must also be considered in evaluating the PE regimen. Although almost all studies have described only minimal psychological complications, this is most probably related to the increased availability of occupational, psychological, and physical therapists who contribute to the supportive care of the PE patient (38–41). Our experience with children, even when younger than 5 years of age, confirms the psychological acceptability of the PE regimen (42). However, since these patients clearly require continued support by both family and professional staff, this must also be included in the cost accounting of the PE program.

In addition potential adverse effects related to the suppression of the patient's endogenous microbial flora must also be considered. For example, a decrease in the peripheral leukocyte count, diminished colony-stimulating factor, and altered humoral and cellular immunity have been described in axenic animals (43–50). The antibiotic decontamination schedule may have an adverse effect on the patient's nutrient absorption, and the suppressed microbial flora may also affect the metabolism of certain chemotherapeutic agents (e.g., methotrexate) (51–53). Clearly, the potential, and perhaps unanticipated, deleterious consequences of the protected environment regimen also deserve consideration.

APPLICATION OF THE PROTECTED ENVIRONMENT IN CANCER TREATMENT

Since the PE regimen reduces the incidence of serious infection in patients with prolonged granulocytopenia, its usefulness in cancer treatment rests on making possible the successful completion of chemotherapeutic schedules that might have been impeded by infectious complications or mortality. Therefore, in evaluating the usefulness of the PE, it is important to establish first whether the reduced rate of infection does indeed permit the successful delivery of chemotherapy to more patients. Second, it is important to determine whether this therapy then increases the rate and duration of remission of treated patients. Furthermore, since both the log-kill kinetic model and the Norton-Simon hypothesis suggest that escalation to very intensive levels of chemotherapy may enhance therapeutic efficacy, it is meaningful to also assess whether such high-dose drug regimens further improve the outcome for cancer patients. Since the application of intensive drug therapy has been limited by its resultant hematologic toxicity and the risk of infection, the beneficial effects of the PE make it feasible to assess the efficacy of such treatment strategies.

Clinical trials using the PE have been conducted, or are in progress, for the treatment of adults with leukemia, lymphoma, and solid tumors as well as for several pediatric malignancies. Unfortunately, the evaluation of many of these trials is limited by the small number of patient entries, variation of the age and sex of the patient, differences in the therapeutic regimens, and a lack of appropriate control patients. Nonetheless, several conclusions can be inferred.

At least nine clinical trials have used the PE regimen for the treatment of adults with leukemia (10,12,13,19,24,33,54–56). A significant decrease in the incidence of serious infection has been observed in all but one of these trials. Hence, infection did not serve as a deterrent to the successful administration of chemotherapy to these patients. Nonetheless, in only two of these trials was an improvement in the induction of complete remission noted, and even this benefit may have been spurious. In one of these studies, 43% of the control patients were more than 60 years of age compared with 17% of the PE patients (24). Since other studies have suggested that patients who are older than 60 years have a poorer response to therapy, this unbalanced prognostic variable could have biased the apparently better observed response to chemotherapy in the PE patients. More recently, Rodriquez et al. reported a significant difference in the complete response rate between PE and non-PE patients (61% versus 45%) as well as an improved duration of survival for PE patients (72 weeks versus 42 weeks) (33). The authors attributed these results to the administration of more intensive chemotherapy to the PE patient. Although PE patients did receive more chemotherapy than control patients, the dosage escalations were not significantly different. Moreover, the duration of complete remission did not differ between the PE and control patients, making the association of the initial chemotherapy with the duration of survival exceedingly tenuous. In addition, the response rate for the control patients (45%) was lower than that observed in other concurrent trials, and the fact that there were a large number of early deaths in the control group further compromises a valid interpretation of these data. Hence, although the hypothesis that early more intensive chemotherapy may increase the rate and duration of disease-free remission is attractive, it is not yet supported by the existing clinical trials for the acute leukemia of adults.

Perhaps a better test for this hypothesis will result from current studies using very intensive chemotherapy in conjunction with autologous or allogeneic bone marrow transplantation for patients with acute myelogenous leukemia who have achieved initial remission. The objective of this treatment strategy is to prolong remission duration and survival by eradication of residual leukemia cells with very intensive chemoradiotherapy conditioning followed by bone marrow transplantation (57). The poor long-term survival for patients with AML justifies this very intensive treatment schedule. Should this approach be successful, and if the problem of CMV reactivation pneumonia that has been associated with allogeneic bone marrow transplantation can be controlled with either new antiviral agents or interferon, the PE regimen will be useful in the treatment of acute myelogenous leukemia.

The role of intensive chemotherapy for patients whose leukemia has become refractory to standard dosages of chemotherapy has been more disappointing. In spite of the success of the PE in permitting the delivery of these chemotherapy schedules, because of the decreased incidence of infection, the remission rate has been brief in these patients (58). Clearly, the real limitation for these patients remains the lack of chemotherapy that is successful in producing durable remission. Moreover, the possibility of further intensifying the chemotherapy with the hope of attaining greater cytoreduction is ultimately limited by life-threatening extramedullary toxicity (e.g., cardiac, hepatic, gastrointestinal) that occurs at these higher dosages.

A stimulus for the potential value of intensive chemotherapy stems from the observation that the majority of patients with Burkitt's lymphoma who no longer responded to conventional dosages of chemotherapy had demonstrable responses when given very intensive chemotherapy (BACT: BCNU, cytosine arabinoside, 6-thioguoinine and high-dose cyclophosphamide). Although long-term unmaintained remissions (>3 years) have been achieved in only 10% of these patients, the value of very aggressive chemotherapy in these relapsed poor risk patients was clearly substantiated (59,60). The possibility that intensive chemotherapy might be more beneficial if administered to patients early in their treatment course (i.e., before the onset of drug resistance) is currently being tested. Bodey et al. studied this hypothesis in adults with lymphoma, the majority of patients being stage IV with either DHL, NPDL, mixed, or DPPL (61). Patients were treated with combination chemotherapy (CHOP-Bleo) with the dosages of cyclophosphamide and adriamycin being increased by 50% over three consecutive cycles. Patients in this trial received therapy in either a PE or normal ward setting, and the occurrence of severe infection precluded subsequent dosage escalation. The patients treated in a PE had a significantly decreased incidence of infection during the period of postchemotherapy granulocytopenia and hence were more able to receive full dosage escalation compared with control patients (96 versus 77%). Although there was no difference in the complete remission rate for patients in either the PE or control group, the duration of remission was longer for patients who received full dosage escalation compared with patients who did not. Although these observations are preliminary, they do suggest a potential benefit from early intensive chemotherapy and hold forth the possibility that better results may be attained with even more intensive drug schedules. If this proves true, the protected environment may be an important component of such treatment programs.

The value of early intensive chemotherapy is also being investigated in other adult tumors (e.g., sarcomas, breast cancer, and small cell carcinoma of the lung). Since these tumors are characterized by initial chemotherapeutic responsiveness but early relapse, the possibility of achieving greater cytoreduction with early dosage escalation is worth exploring. As with the lymphomas, should these therapeutic schedules prove to be beneficial, the supportive role of the PE will be an important adjunct to therapy.

The rationale for the use of intensive chemotherapy in various childhood malignancies is also based on the established initial chemotherapeutic responsiveness but early relapse rate when patients have metastatic disease. In the Pediatric Oncology Branch of the NCI we initially evaluated the role of such intensive (i.e., marrow ablative) schedules of chemotherapy for patients whose tumors had become refractory to standard dosages of therapy. Patients with non-Hodgkin's lymphoma, Ewing's sarcoma, rhabdomyosarcoma, osteosarcoma, or neuroblastoma received various three- to four-drug combinations that included vincristine, methotrexate, adriamycin, actinomycin-D, cytosine arabinoside, 6-thioguanine, mCCNU, BCNU, DTIC, or L-PAM. In addition, each regimen included high-dose cyclophosphamide in dosages ranging from 135 to 200 mg/kg over three to four days. These regimens resulted in periods of absolute granulocytopenia (PMN $<500/mm^3$) that ranged from 15 to 66 days. Seventy-two such patients have received intensive chemotherapy when their tumors had become refractory to standard dosages of chemotherapy. Fifty of these patients were treated in a PE. There was a significant decrease in the incidence of infections for PE patients whose duration of granulocytopenia was prolonged beyond 28 days compared with patients receiving comparable chemotherapy in a regular ward setting. Although more than half of these patients, both PE and non-PE, attained a complete or partial remission with the intensive chemotherapy, even though they had been unresponsive to standard dosages of chemotherapy, the mean duration of response was brief (~2 months) and was prolonged in only 10% (62). Although disappointing, the results of this trial also suggest that intensive chemotherapy may serve a role if administered early in the patient's treatment course and before the development of overt drug resistance. We are currently testing this hypothesis in patients who have metastatic rhabdomyosarcoma or in patients with central axis or metastatic Ewing's sarcoma. Eighteen patients have been treated to date with a combination of intensive chemoradiotherapy. With the PE, the therapy has been tolerated, and preliminary observations regarding its efficacy are encouraging (63).

In summary, although the initial trials evaluating the PE for adults with acute leukemia showed a significant reduction in the incidence of serious infections during periods of profound granulocytopenia, no consistent benefit could be demonstrated in the response or duration of remission for patients who received standard dosages of chemotherapy. Current experience with very intensive chemotherapy regimens, however, suggests a potential therapeutic benefit. This includes patients with acute myelogenous leukemia who are treated with ablative chemotherapy plus allogeneic or autologous bone marrow transplantation, as well as adults and children undergoing intensive chemoradiotherapy for the initial treatment of lymphomas and solid tumors. Should these studies confirm a benefit from early intensive therapy, as measured by significantly prolonged disease-free remission, the infection control benefits of the PE will be well used.

FUTURE ALTERNATIVES AND OBJECTIVES

The infection-prevention benefits attributed to the PE must also be balanced against other recent improvements in supportive management. Among these is the observation that certain systemically absorbed antibiotics, most notably trimethoprim-sulfamethoxazole:TMP/SMX, may provide prophylaxis against bacterial infections during chemotherapy-induced periods of granulocytopenia (64). This has been successfully used in hospitalized adults undergoing treatment for acute leukemia (65) and has also been used in conjunction with nonabsorbable antibiotics (34). At the NCI we are investigating the role of TMP/SMX plus erythromycin in preventing fever or infection in children with malignancy who have received bone-marrow-suppressive chemotherapy. This regimen is directed at both Gram-positive and Gram-negative organisms. Should this approach be successful and without significant toxicity (i.e., development of resistant organism or superinfections), it may serve to amplify and extend the benefits of the PE or may even provide a simple alternative to PE for some patients.

Another strategy that is aimed at controlling the patient's microbial flora is the use of *partial decontamination,* in which the aerobic flora of the patient is eliminated but the anaerobic flora is preserved. This can be accomplished with a number of oral antibiotics, including naladixic acid, TMP/SMX, polymixin B, and amphotericin. The residual anaerobic flora appears capable of protecting the host from colonization by potential pathogenic aerobic organisms and hence may be capable of diminishing the incidence of infection during high risk periods (66).

Coupled with strategies aimed at altering, suppressing, or prophylaxing the host's microbial flora are newer methods for shortening the period of risk from granulocytopenia. The first of these is the infusion of cryopreserved autologous bone marrow after the administration of intensive chemotherapy (67). Preliminary results suggest that autologous bone marrow rescue can shorten the period of granulocytopenia to 25 days or less. This maneuver, therefore, may lessen the need for patients undergoing intensive chemotherapy to be treated in a PE when autologous bone marrow is available. We are currently testing this hypothesis by randomizing patients who will receive cryopreserved bone marrow to undergo intensive chemotherapy in either a PE or routine ward setting.

In addition to the hematologic benefits of autologous bone marrow rescue, enhanced granulocyte recovery can be observed after chemotherapy when patients are treated with a number of chemical or immune adjuvants. For example, a recent trial used lithium carbonate for patients undergoing chemotherapy and demonstrated a significant acceleration in granulocyte recovery for treated patients compared with controls (68). Should this benefit be substantiated, the possibility for bolstering host defenses after chemotherapy may be achievable.

In future studies, techniques for shortening the period of chemotherapy-induced granulocytopenia (e.g., autologous bone marrow infusion or immunoregulatory agents) may be combined with systemic antibiotic prophylaxis (e.g., TMP/SMX) to provide an effective method for infection prevention. These modalites may also provide a more simple and broadly applicable alternative to the protected environment for patients undergoing chemotherapy.

REFERENCES

1. Pizzo PA: Infectious complications in the child with cancer: I. Pathophysiology of the compromised host and the initial evaluation and management of the febrile cancer patient. *J Pediatr* 98:341–354, 1981.

2. Bodey GP: Epidemiological studies of *Pseudomonas* species in patients with leukemia. *Am J Med Sci* 260:82–86, 1970.

3. Schimpff SC, Young VM, Green WH, et al: Origin of infection in acute nonlymphocytic leukemia: Significance of hospital acquisition of potential pathogens. *Ann Intern Med* 77:707–714, 1972.

4. Schimpff SC, Greene WH, Young VM, et al: Significance of *Pseudomonas aeruginosa* in the patient with leukemia or lymphoma. *J Infect Dis* 130:(suppl)S24-σ31, 1974.

5. Von der Waaij D, Tielemons-Speltie TM, de Houban-Roech AMJ: Infection by and distribution of biotypes of enterobacteriaceae species in leukaemic patients treated under ward conditions and in units for protective isolation in seven hospitals in Europe. *Infection* 5:188–194, 1977.

6. Greene WH, Schimpff SC, Young VM, et al: Empiric carbenicillin, gentamicin and cephalothin for presumed infection. *Ann Intern Med* 78:825, 1973.

7. Mackowiak PA: Microbial synergism in human infections. *N Engl J Med* 298:21–26, 83–87, 1978.

8. Pizzo PA, Levine AS: The utility of protected environment regimens for the compromised host: A critical assessment, in Brown E (ed): *Progress in Hematology,* Grune & Stratton, Inc, X, pp 311–332, 1977.

9. Maki DG, Nauseef WA: A study of simple protective isolation in patients with granulocytopenia. *19th Interscience Conf Antimicrob Ag Chemother,* 212, 1979.

10. Dietrich M, Rasche H, Rommel K: Antimicrobial therapy as a part of the decontamination procedure for patients with acute leukemia. *Eur J Cancer* 9:443–444, 1973.

11. Mathé G, Schneider M, Schwarzenberg L, et al: Five years experience in the clinical use of a pathogen-free isolation unit, in Mathé G (ed): *Recent Results in Cancer Research,* 29. New York, Springer-Verlag, 1970, pp 3–13.

12. Yates JW, Holland JF: A controlled study of isolation and endogenous microbial suppression in acute myelocytic leukemia patients. *Cancer* 32:1490–1498, 1973.

13. Dietrich M, Gaus W, Vossen J, et al: Protective isolation and antimicrobial decontamination in patients with high susceptibility to infection: A prospective cooperative study of gnotobiotic care in acute leukemia patient: I. Clinical results. *Infection* 5:3–10, 1977.

14. Shadomy S, Ginsberg MK, LaConte M, et al: Evaluation of a patient isolator system: I. Evaluation of subsystems and procedures for sterilization and concurrent sanitation. *Arch Environ Health* 11:183–190, 1965.

15. Bodey GP, Loftis J, Bowen E: Protected environment for cancer patients: Effect of a prophylactic antibiotic regimen on the microbial flora of patients undergoing cancer chemotherapy. *Arch Intern Med* 122:23–30, 1968.

16. Bodey GP, Freireich EJ, Frei E III: Studies of patients in a laminar air flow unit. *Cancer* 24:972–980, 1969.

17. Buchberg H, Lilly GP: Model studies of directed sterile air flow for hospital isolation. *Ann Biomed Eng* 2:106–122, 1974.

18. Trexler PC: Microbial isolators for use in the hospital. *Biomed Eng* 10:63–67, 1975.

19. Levine AS, Siegel SE, Schreiber AD, et al: Protected environments and prophylactic antibiotics: A prospective controlled study of their utility in the therapy of acute leukemia. *N Engl J Med* 288:477–483, 1973.

20. Bodey GP, Kim Z, Bowen E: A semiquantitative total body skin culture technique for patients in a protected environment. *Am J Med Sci* 257:100–115, 1969.

21. Shadomy S, Ginsberg MK, Zeiger E: Evaluation of a patient isolator system: II. Distribution profiles of patient microflora during prolonged isolator confinement. *Arch Environ Health* 11:191–200, 1965.

22. Shadomy S, Ginsberg MK, Zeiger E: Evaluation of a patient isolator system: III. Microbial contamination of the isolator interior. *Arch Environ Health* 11:652–661, 1965.

23. Bodey GP, Rosenbaum B: Effect of prophylactic measures on the microbial flora of patients in protected environment units. *Medicine* 53:209–228, 1974.

24. Schimpff SC, Greene WH, Young VM, et al: Infection prevention in acute nonlymphocytic leukemia: Laminar air flow room reverse isolation with oral, nonabsorbable antibiotic prophylaxis. *Ann Intern Med* 82:351–358, 1975.

25. Bodey GP, Rodriguez V: Protected environment–prophylactic antibiotic programmes: Microbiological studies. *Clin Haematol* 5:395–408, 1976.

26. Hahn DM, Schimpff SC, Fortner CL: Infection in acute leukemia patients receiving nonabsorbable antibiotics. *Antimicrob Agents Chemother* 13:958–964, 1978.

27. Klastersky J, Debusscher L, Weerts D, et al: Use of oral antibiotics in protected environment unit: Clinical effectiveness and role in the emergence of antibiotic-resistant strains. *Pathol Biol* 22:5–12, 1974.

28. Preisler HD, Goldstein IM, Henderson ES: Gastrointestinal "sterilization" in the treatment of patients with acute leukemia. *Cancer* 26:1076–1081, 1970.

29. Henderson ES, Preisler HD, Goldstein IM: Studies of components of patient protection programs: Nonabsorbable antibiotics and low bacterial diet, in Mathé G (ed): *Recent Results in Cancer Research,* 29. New York, Springer-Verlag, 1970, pp 24–30.

30. Keating MJ, Penington DG: Prophylaxis against septicemia in acute leukaemia: The use of oral framycetin. *Med. J. Aust.* 2:213–217, 1973.

31. Levi JA, Vincent PC, Jennis F, et al: Prophylactic oral antibiotics in the management of acute leukaemia. *Med J Aust* 1:1025–1029, 1973.

32. Reiter B, Gee T, Young L, et al: Use of oral antimicrobials during remission induction in adult patients with acute nonlymphoblastic leukemias. *Clin Res* 21:652, 1973.

33. Rodriguez V, Bodey GP, Freireich EJ, et al: Randomized trial of protected-environment prophylactic-antibiotics in 145 adults with acute leukemia. *Medicine* 57:253–266, 1978.

34. Enno A, Catovsky D, Darrell J, et al: Co-trimoxazole for the prevention of infection in leukemia. *Lancet* ii:395–397, 1978.

35. Buckner CD, Cliff RA, Sanders JE: Protective Environment for marrow transplant recipients: A prospective study. *Ann Intern Med* 89:893–901, 1978.

36. Winston DJ, Gale RP, Meyer DV, et al: Infectious complications of human bone marrow transplantation. *Medicine* 58:1–31, 1979.

37. Drazen EC, Levine AS: Laminar air-flow rooms. *Hospitals* 48:88–93, 1974.

38. Haenel T, Nagel GA: Das pschologische verhalten von tumorkranken mit agranulozytose under isolierbedingungen. *Schweiz Med Wochenschr* 105:839–843, 1975.

39. Holland J: Acute leukemia: Psychological aspects of treatment, in Elkerbout F, Thomas P, Zwaveling A (eds): *Cancer Chemotherapy.* Leiden, Leiden University Press, 1971, pp 292–300.

40. Kohle K, Simons C, Weidlich S, et al: Psychological aspects in the treatment of leukemia patients in the isolated-bed system, "Life Island." *Psychother Psychosom* 19:85–91, 1971.

41. Dietrich M: Reverse isolation and gut decontamination in the management of cancer patients. *Eur J Cancer* 15:45–49, 1979.

42. Sussman EJ, Hollenbeck AP, Hersh SP, et al: Separation-deprivation and childhood cancer: A conceptual re-evaluation, in Kellerman J (ed): *Psychosocial Aspects of Childhood Cancer* (in press).

43. Gordon H, Pesti L: The gnotobiologic animal as a tool in the study of host microbial relationships. *Bacteriol Rev* 35:390–429, 1971.

44. Reyniers JA, Wayner M, Luckey TD, et al: Survey of germ-free animals: The white wyandotte and white leghorn chicken, in Reyniers JA (ed): *Lobund Reports No. 3.* Notre Dame, Indiana, University of Notre Dame Press, 1946.

45. Metcalf D, Foster R, Pollard M: Colony stimulating activity of serum from germ-free normal and leukemic mice. *J Cell Physiol* 70:131–132, 1967.

46. Crabbé PA, Bazin H, Eyssen H, et al: The normal microbial flora as a major stimulus for proliferation of plasma cells synthesizing IgA in the gut: The germ-free intestinal tract. *Int Arch Allergy Appl Immunol* 34:362–375, 1968.

47. Horowitz RE, Bauer H, Paronetto F, et al: The response of the lymphatic tissue to bacterial antigen. *Am J Pathol* 44:747–761, 1964.

48. Nash DR, Crabbé PA, Bazin H, et al: Specific and nonspecific immunoglobulin synthesis in germfree mice immunized with ferritin by different routes. *Experientia* 25:1094–1097, 1969.

49. Sell S: Immunoglobulins of the germfree guinea pig. *J Immunol* 93:122–131, 1964.

50. Sell S: γ-Globulin metabolism in germfree guinea pigs. *J Immunol* 92:559–564, 1964.

51. Cohen MH, Creaven PJ, Fossieck BE Jr, et al: Effect of oral prophylactic broad spectrum

nonabsorbable antibiotics on the gastrointestinal absorption of nutrients and methotrexate in small cell bronchogenic carcinoma patients. *Cancer* 38:1556–1559, 1976.

52. Dietrich M, Rasche H, Rommel K: Antimicrobial therapy as a part of the decontamination procedure for patients with acute leukemia. *Eur J Cancer* 9:443–444, 1973.

53. Zaharko DS, Bruckner H, Oliverio VT: Antibiotics alter methotrexate metabolism and excretion. *Science* 166:887–888, 1969.

54. Lohner D, Debusscher L, Prévost JM, et al: Comparative randomized study of protected environment plus oral antibiotics versus oral antibiotics alone in neutropenic patients. *Cancer Treat Rep* 63:363–368, 1979.

55. Bodey GP, Gehan EA, Freireich EJ: Protected environment–prophylactic antibiotic program in the chemotherapy of acute leukemia. *Am J Med Sci* 262:138–151, 1971.

56. Bodey GP, Rodriguez V, McCredie KB: Early consolidation chemotherapy for adults with acute leukemia in remission. *Med Pediatr Oncol* 2:299–308, 1976.

57. Gale RP: Advances in the treatment of acute myelogenous leukemia. *N Engl J Med* 300:1189–1199, 1979.

58. Kramer B, Appelbaum RR, Herzig G, et al: Treatment of refractory acute leukemia with high dose chemotherapy. *Cancer Treat Rep* 61:1397–1398, 1977.

59. Ziegler JL, Magrath IT, Deisseroth AB, et al: Combined modality treatment of Burkitt's lymphoma. *Cancer Treat Rep* 62:2031–2034, 1978.

60. Appelbaum FR, Deisseroth AB, Graw RG, et al: Prolonged complete remission following high-dose chemotherapy of Burkitt's Lymphoma in relapse. *Cancer* 41:1059–1063, 1978.

61. Bodey GP, Rodriguiz V, Carbonillas F, et al: Protected-environment prophylactic antibiotic program for malignant lymphoma: Randomized trial during chemotherapy to induce remission. *Am J Med* 66:74–81, 1979.

62. Pizzo PA, Levine AS, Simon R: Utility of laminar air-flow rooms in the delivery of intensive chemotherapy for children with refractory malignancies. *Am Assoc Cancer Res* 19:82, 1978.

63. Glaubiger D, Makuch R, Wachenhut J, et al: Early results of current combined modality therapy trials in Ewing's sarcoma at NCI, in Jones SE, Salmon SE (eds): *Adjuvant Therapy of Cancer*, II. New York, Grune & Stratton, 1979, pp 409–418.

64. Hughes WT, Kuhn S, Chaudary S, et al: Successful chemoprophylaxis for *Pneumocystis Carinii* pneumonitis. *N Engl J Med* 297:1419–1426, 1977.

65. Gurwith MJ, Brunton JL, Lank BA: A prospective controlled investigation of prophylactic trimethoprim/sulfamethoxazole in hospitalized granulocytopenic patients. *Am J Med* 66:248–256, 1979.

66. Guiot HFL, van der Meer JWM, von Furth R: Infection prevention by partial antibiotic decontamination. *19th Interscience Conf Antimicrob Ag Chemother* 61, 1979.

67. Deisseroth A, Abrams RA: The role of autologous stem cell reconstitution in intensive therapy for resistant neoplasms. *Cancer Treat Rep* 63:461–471, 1979.

68. Lyman GH, Williams CC, Preston D: The use of lithium carbonate to reduce infection and leukopenia during systemic chemotherapy. *N Engl J Med* 302:257–260, 1980.

21

The Age-Old Question of Euthanasia

Nathan Schnaper

INTRODUCTION

Euthanasia: The word itself screams out a clarion call to controversy. Any person or group defending its position in the debate stands on belief rather than knowledge. Neither side can rationally persuade the other of its validity. No scientific support can, nor perhaps ever will, be introduced on either side of the question. There are more questions than answers. Religious, bioethical, and philosophical issues and concepts can be argued, but, again, the framework is belief rather than fact. Conceptually, death introduces a void to be filled by fantasies (1) that are colored by cultural values of emotion. The opponents to any serious consideration of application of euthanasia confuse its therapeutic possibilities for terminal cancer patients with the Hitlerian "final solution."

The term "euthanasia" has come to mean induced death ("mercy killing"), but inappropriately so. Literally it means "good death." Joseph Fletcher has offered a useful categorization of euthanasia (Table 1) (2). It dispenses with obfuscating language. "Voluntary" implies a personal wish as opposed to "involuntary." "Direct" and "indirect" relate to the manner by which one dies. Voluntary direct is suicide (a form of "active" euthanasia). Voluntary indirect is the individual's expressed wish that no extraordinary means be used to keep him alive, for example, refusal of treatment for a life-threatening complication, or the "living will" ("passive" euthanasia). Involuntary direct is termination of a person's life by a relative, a physician, or friend without the person's consent—mercy killing (active). Involuntary indirect is—again, without the person's consent—the removal of all life support systems by the physicians or other helpers (passive).

The opponents to euthanasia include abortion in their anathematic persuasion. They have little concern or compassion for those who are slowly dying, be it from starvation, criminality, or unrelenting disease. Overpopulation as well as terminal illness is granted pious mutterings and little else. The American birth rate has plummeted, but the rest of the world continues to proliferate. Modern medical technology is extending longevity. It is anticipated that in the year 2000 the world population will be 7 billion. In the United States, 40% of its citizens will be over age 65. Land for living area and food the world over will diminish.

Table 1. Euthanasia Defined

		Term Now Implies Causality (Mercy Killing)	
		VOLUNTARY (Personal Wish)	
HOW	Direct	Suicide	(Active)
	Indirect	Refusal of Treatment for Complications	(Passive)
		Living Will	
		INVOLUNTARY (No Personal Wish)	
HOW	Direct	Mercy Killing	(Active)
	Indirect	Removal of Life Support	(Passive)

After Fletcher, J., *Am. J. Nurs*, 73–760, 1973

At this writing, 800 million people now live on the verge of starvation or malnutrition (3). And the situation can only get worse.

CONSIDERATION OF THE LEGAL ISSUES

Homicide, or first-degree murder, the most judicially reprehensible of the criminal offenses causally relating one person to the death of another, is distinguished in our system of criminal law from all lesser offenses (e.g., manslaughter) and noncrimes (e.g., self-defense killing) by one crucial element—premeditation. There are at least two exceptions. An execution (the carrying out of the death penalty) by agents of the state, although all too premeditated, is not a criminal homicide. Another exception is the militarily authorized premeditated killing of other persons—hopefully, the enemy—during war.

No concession is made for the laudable motives of the doctor or relative who is trying to put an end to suffering, passively or actively. However, court decisions concerning mercy killing display an unusually great disparity between the theory and the delivery of the law.

There have been at least nine reported mercy killing court decisions involving doctors: two convicted (in Holland, suspended sentences), five acquitted, one acquitted as an abettor, and one not indicted. Sixteen other reported decisions involved nonphysicians: first-degree murder, two (one life sentence, the other paroled for life); lesser homicide, two (one suspended sentence, the other three to six years); acquitted, four; acquitted on the grounds of temporary insanity, six; refusal to indict, two (4).

What follows is a personal anecdote that affirms the reality of disapproval by certain elements of our society. Not too long ago, this author was called before the local medical society's grievance committee. The charge of murder was initiated by an antieuthanasia group. According to them, the evidence was a misquotation in a newspaper article on passive euthanasia and this author's work with the dying. The matter was clarified and dismissed, but the burden of defense was this author's responsibility.

The rights of society, vis-à-vis the rights of the individual, are defined by judicial interpretations of our Constitution, particularly the First, Fourth, and

Fourteenth Amendments of the Bill of Rights. The First Amendment guarantees each person the right to control his life through individual expressions of religious freedom. The First, Fourth, Fifth, Ninth, and Fourteenth Amendments allow the right of privacy, and the Fourteenth Amendment guards individual freedom from arbitrary interference by government, except where overriding governmental or societal interests are at stake.

The statutory criminal law of each state defines euthanasia as a crime against society. First-degree murder, implying deliberation, was a common-law offense (there are no longer common-law crimes). Suicide is a felony, but is obviously not punishable if successful, and never prosecuted in American courts if unsuccessful. However, aiders and abettors and conspirators are liable to prosecution.

In order to amend the homicide laws to make euthanasia a separate entity, several medicolegal aspects must be considered. The most important legal consideration is intent. In first-degree murder the act must not only be intentional, but it must be committed with malicious intent. Even when considered a crime, euthanasia should be far less reprehensible, because of its compassionate nature. Although it is always deliberate, it is also an act intended to relieve suffering. Grand juries commonly make this distinction between motives when they fail to indict perpetrators. However, our Judeo-Christian democratic heritage makes it difficult for us to justify homicide, even if it is done at the request of the victim. (The community takes precedence over the individual.)

Consent is the other complex issue. It involves the voluntary stipulation of the patient that his life be ended. The complexity arises through the circumstances surrounding consent. The most clear-cut form of consent would be a declaration by a person, healthy in mind and body, fully informed as to all the medical and legal implications, dictating the type of medical treatment to be used in the event of terminal illness. This declaration could be modified or revoked at any time before his death. This would relieve family and physician of personal responsibility and legal liability.

Bedside consent is less clear-cut. How does a law take into account the desperate pleas of a questionably competent, terminally ill patient who cries out between periods of unconsciousness for a peaceful end? Should he be permitted to demand death, or should that decision be left to a legal guardian? The precise distinction between rational, willful consent and unwitting emotional outbursts cannot be codified by legislators. The question of whose judgment to rely on with respect to consent cannot be strictly delineated.

Consent procured under coercion is not only illegal, should death result, but unethical (5). A patient suffering a prolonged illness with intense pain cannot consent willfully if that consent is a consequence of either blatant or subtle coercion. He or she should not be made to feel guilty for causing financial or emotional expense to family or friends. Irreversible illness, constant pain, his or her own emotional needs, and personal philosophy should be the only dictates of willful consent. The issue of patient consent is discussed later in the section "Medical Considerations."

Other legal questions involving euthanasia legislation are justiciability and standing (5). The important justiciability question here is whether compulsory medical treatment is a legal issue at all. Does euthanasia have any business being in a court of law, or should it be solely up to the individual to decide how long he or she wants to be kept alive and by what means? After this decision is made by the individual, the standing issue is who has a right to challenge that decision in court? If the physician and the hospital are relieved of liability or if they concur with the individual's request to die, does the family have the right to request a court to reverse the decision legally and, if so, under what circumstances?

These issues were paramount in the well-publicized case of Karen Ann Quinlan. Judge Robert Muir of the Superior Court of Morris County, N.J., on November 10, 1975, denied standing to Karen's father, who had requested the power to authorize discontinuance of all extraordinary means necessary to keep Karen alive. The father should have asked for guardianship, for which he did have standing. The court was then put in the position of upholding "its constitutional obligation—equal protection of life that is the right of all citizens." With respect to justiciability, Judge Muir also stated that "It is a medical decision, not a judicial one!"

On March 31, 1976, the New Jersey Supreme Court, in a 7 to 0 decision, corrected Judge Muir's ruling and allowed Karen's father, as guardian, to assert her constitutional right of privacy. (Precedent: U.S. Supreme Court decision in *Griswold v. Connecticut* 381 U.S. 479, 1965, and the Ninth Amendment.)

The controversy of omission of treatment versus commission of an act of murder has been exhaustively debated. Omission is the failure to act positively to prolong life. It is loosely defined because the relationship between a physician and patient is essentially not one of duty and therefore not liable. The patient hires the physician in good faith that he will do everything in his power to keep his patient healthy. At any time during their relationship, the patient is free to discharge the doctor, or the latter is, in turn, free to ask to be relieved. However, abandonment of a patient is considered a tort, a legally culpable act that, according to law, merits compensation. The compensatory purpose of tort law is certainly applicable in the case of accident or acute illness but loses relevance when dealing with terminal illness or euthanasia. There is no compensation necessary for consentient death, and, on these grounds alone, omission and commission are indistinguishable. If commission is to be considered homicide, the act of omission must be given the same punitive consideration.

The now well-known Massachusetts Supreme Court decision in the Saikewicz case bears witness to the judicial preempting of the medical profession (6,7). The court decided that termination of life support systems in cases of minors, mental incompetents, and unconscious persons should be a court responsibility and not left to families, committees, or physicians.

This lengthy consideration of the relevant legalistics was undertaken as an attempt at clarification and also to emphasize the confusion associated with past attempts to usurp the basic medical responsibility for the patient.

EMOTIONAL CONSIDERATIONS

Regardless of arguments to the contrary, some religious convictions are emotionally based, just as political convictions and personal likes and dislikes are. Paul appreciated pain and suffering as testimony. Jesus, in His Sermon on the

Mount felt that, "Blessed are the merciful, for they shall obtain mercy." Religionists objected to anesthesia years ago following the tenets of Paul.

Cicely Saunders, well known for her compassionate and creative concern for the terminally ill and her hospice concept, decries euthanasia in any form on religious grounds (8). Patients who are dying must find "reconciliation and peace" with God. In other words, it is "God's will." However, she does advocate sedation and relief of suffering. In my view this is passive euthanasia.

Thoughtful, concerned people are made uncomfortably guilty by the understandable association of ending a life with "murder." There are those who have lived through Hitler's holocaust who fear the inevitability of a final solution. There are those who feel that if they approve, legally, of active intervention that they will have no safeguards against premature endings for themselves. Who will decide for them whether or not there is a reasonable hope that they can be cured? Moreover, once the door is opened, what about some other (emotional) illness? Unusual political belief? Then there are those who agree enthusiastically with the concept, but "I don't want to be involved" or "Let George do it," they say (9).

ETHICAL CONSIDERATIONS

Theological arguments against euthanasia are used to counter legal abortions and vice versa. Thus, theology is equated with ethics. John Fletcher assumes a posture in opposition to Joseph Fletcher, who views abortion and selective euthanasia of defective infants as morally sound. John Fletcher states, "If we chose to be shaped by Judeo-Christian visions of the 'createdness' of God, we ought to care for the defective newborn as if our relation with the Creator depended on the outcome. If we chose to be shaped by visions of the inherent dignity of each member of the human family, no matter what his or her predicament, we ought to care for this defenseless person as if the basis of our own dignity depended on the outcome" (10).

Inherent in the controversy is denial. The heat on both sides is expressed in intellectual abstractions akin to how many angels can stand on the head of a pin. The fruit of this thinking is no resolution, no real action, and thus death is denied.

This preoccupation leads to a digression from the dying patient to a lofty consideration of intellectualized abstract concepts (11). Morality can be viewed as duty versus consequential. In other words, right versus wrong at one end or beneficial result at the other. Of course, the question arises, Is what is right always what is good? For example, duty dictates that the dying patient be told the truth. But is the consequence always good? Will the truth help him through his remaining days or shatter him? Is it the doctor's duty to treat despite the patient's request to end the suffering and indignity? Could the physician be practicing immoral deception by continuing to treat, offering the patient false hope? On the other hand, is the doctor deceiving himself when he is "too busy" to respond to a call from the patient's family because he knows that, by not going, the patient will die? Or somehow or other he unconsciously "forgets" to see the patient with the same fatal results?

Simplified, the core issue for the physician is concern for the quality of life as compared to the sanctity of biological life. When one is brain dead, the brain is destroyed and life ceases. When the cortex alone is damaged or a vital organ no longer functions adequately and cannot be repaired, mechanical means can sustain life. Here, the question of quality of life arises. Precluded from this discussion are the life-threatening or the potentially fatal illnesses such as leukemia, cancer, kidney failure, and unconsciousness. Also omitted are the emotional accusations and defenses against "scavengers" seeking organ transplants.

The problem here is how to determine what the quality of life is, and who makes the decisions concerning it. A leukemia patient allowed to bleed to death because, "life has become too unbearable for this patient and there's no point in prolonging it," might have made a "miraculous" recovery and gone into remission—sitting up and smiling, to have another six months to a year of enjoyable life. Or a patient with high spinal cord transsection, which some might feel incompatible with worthwhile living, might be felt by one who experienced it as a stumbling block, rather than an end.

On the other hand, there are patients with high spinal cord lesions who survive by the grace of life-support systems. As time goes on, they develop muscular contractures, bladder and bowel dysfunction, infections, decubiti, and other complications. They become training experiences for the residents in many of the medical disciplines. Unfortunately, the association that quickly comes to mind is that the high cord lesion patient is to the doctor in training what the cadaver is to the medical student.

Engelhardt, discussing bioethics and the process of embodiment, comments ". . . in the case of brain death, when personal life has ceased and vegetative life ensues, there are again no human rights involved, only human values. The body may be valued because it is the body of a loved person, or for the use value of its organs, but there is no longer a person present to be respected" (12).

MEDICAL CONSIDERATIONS

A view from the doctor's frame of reference is a plea for protection from publicity and criminal accusations. In other words, he wants his hands to be guided. The bioethicists approve permitting death, not causing it, and feel the patient should decide; there is the inference on their part that the doctors won't let the patient decide. The doctors argue that the patient frequently is not in a position to decide, and, therefore, legal safeguards are necessary. Yet, there are physicians who admit to practicing passive euthanasia by withdrawing life-support systems. This is not passive. Legally, this is a studied act of commission on the part of the doctor.

Jackson and Younger remind the physician of the need for some clinical caveats regarding patient consent and autonomy (13). The patients may be ambivalent, depressed, displaced from another hidden problem, fear treatment will be stopped, or have wishes that are misperceived by the family or staff. Their word of caution is useful, but implicit in their presentation is that decisions to terminate by physicians are made in a perfunctory manner. Such decisions are usually made with considerable debate and some anguish.

Oncologists can easily recall the many times their patients early in treatment have made unilateral bargains with them. "When that time comes, can I have the medicine, the fifty reds (Seconal)?" or some such statement. Even when that time arrives, it is the rare patient who asks for active intervention. Rather the request is for cessation of treatment. What many oncologists hear is stop the chemotherapy or radiotherapy. The physician unconsciously chooses to forget that blood, blood products, and antibiotics are also treatment. The result is that the patient's life is prolonged by transfusion and ancillary medicines, such as antibiotics, needlessly and against the patient's wishes.

In December, 1973, the House of Delegates of the American Medical Association adopted a resolution condemning mercy killing but condoning passive euthanasia. Rachels takes issue with this doctrine (14). Where a patient is dying a slow and painful death, a lethal injection could be quick and painless, that is, more merciful. Passive euthanasia could be interpreted as a decision to prolong agony. Rachels concludes, "So, whereas doctors may have to discriminate between active and passive euthanasia to satisfy the law, they should not do any more than that. In particular, they should not give the distinction any added authority and weight by writing it into official statements of medical ethics."

Statistically, the chances are excellent that a youngster killed in an accident will be replaced in society by an aging, possibly senile and incontinent old man. This same old man who might have died of pneumonia were it not for the old man's friend, penicillin, may be bedridden and disruptive to the entire family. The family may not be able to place him in a nursing home because of guilt.

Death is also of concern for the young who are victims of fatal illnesses and trauma. The end for them can be nearly obscene. Shoemaker, writing about the problems of trauma, portrays a graphic picture that is also applicable to the terminally ill: "All too frequently, the conduct of a relatively dignified demise gives way to a horror show, which may culminate in a rapid administration of many drugs, some of which may counteract each other. Heroic efforts . . . may suggest the appearance of pharmacologic last rites, rather than that of a well thought-out plan" (15).

Pollster Mervin Field is reported in *Time* magazine to have interviewed a cross section of 504 Californians. He found that 87% agreed that the incurably ill have a right to refuse medication to prolong life and 63% (41% of those over 70) felt they had a right to ask for and receive medication to end life if incurably ill (16).

There is the assumption that religionists are unanimous in their negative view of any sort of euthanasia. This is not true. Pope Pius XII on November 24, 1957, speaking to a Congress of Anesthesiology in Rome, sanctioned the cessation of extraordinary means of prolonging life when sound medical judgment or extensive or irreversible brain damage indicates a negative prognosis. He went on to say that the previously expressed wishes of the patient or those presumed by the next of kin should be taken into account. When this is not known, or the family defers to the doctor, the latter should not take into consideration his own feelings or scientific orientation but base his decision on the burdens his continued efforts might place on the family and the patient. In the case of Catholic patients, Extreme Unction (now Sacrament of the Sick) should be administered before resuscitation is stopped.

The Church Assembly Board for Social Responsibility, in its *Decisions about*

Life and Death, agrees with Pius: "Society cannot take the duty of decision away from the physician. It should not, without creating insurmountable practical difficulties, put it into commission by creating tribunals of some sort to decide the difficult cases—the doctor must be left with his decisions, but he must remain answerable for them to society and, the religious man would add, to God."

Physicians are dedicated to saving and prolonging life. Technological and scientific advances are greeted by them with pride, despite the fact that these signs of progress are besmudged with dire portent for the future: new medical discoveries, the use of pesticides, and amazing machines—all leading to the mixed blessing of longevity and "vegetables."

How difficult it must be for the doctor who is devoted to cure to stand there and do nothing! Radical therapy, indeed! How much easier it is to medicate or operate when one's omnipotence is threatened by the patient's irreversible disease (17).

DISCUSSION

The ethics problem is less tangibly assessed. Legalization of euthanasia could diminish society by reducing the sanctity of life. The obvious response to this statement is that the sanctity of life is reduced even more by the prolonged suffering that accompanies lengthening of the dying process. Certainly the intrinsic values of personal liberty and prevention of cruelty exalt the quality of life rather than degrade it (18).

Ethics is defined as that branch of philosophy dealing with values relating to human conduct, with respect to the rightness and wrongness of certain actions and to the goodness and badness of the motives and ends of such actions (19).

Hence, from a philosophical rather than a theological vantage point: It should be noted that being good could still have meaning, in that it implies a proper mode of conduct; that is, when we breathe, this is a proper mode of conduct in that it is an action that enables us to move toward the good, which could be extended into a discussion of the Kantian emphasis on the means as opposed to the Aristotelian stress on the ends as the right way to morality. Thus, being good has meaning, but the good would be indeterminate, as there would be nothing with which it could be compared. Many philosophers note this and say we have no real knowledge to use in our comparison (how does one know what is bad?) and therefore refrain from setting up any code of ethics (ethical nihilism). At any rate, if there is no alternative to the good, we would have to say that all being is good (20).

As alluded to earlier, theology is equated with ethics. As long as God is involved in a discussion of this topic, morality becomes the province of the servants of God. This conveys an aura of superiority, if not omnipotence, to the ethicists even above that of physicians, who are usually sarcastically viewed as all-powerful. Their arguments always beg their correctness by inferred authority vested by God on the bioethicists.

A case in point: Dr. John Fletcher in his statement quoted earlier refers to "... our relation with the Creator ..." as a basis for an antiabortion and euthanasia stand (10). Are we to assume that Buddhists, Taoists, and atheists do not care for the defective newborn or the defenseless person? Why should we who believe in the Judeo-Christian visions of the "creativeness" of God flout our provincialism by demanding of others allegiance to our political views cloaked in moral-ethical-religious bunting? If one disagrees with the bioethicists, he is ipso facto either hostile, anti-God, a nonbeliever, a nonhuman, or, at best, a pagan from some far-away aboriginal culture.

A view of death from the Judeo-Christian mountain top is reflected in the frequent request, actually a plea, from terminally ill Christians is, "I'm tired, I want to go home again, can I?" Home, of course, equating with the arms of Jesus.

There is also a Jewish approach to the naturalness of the death process. "Death is very good because it takes man to a sinless world, where the battle with impulses is ended" (21). We might add, ended also is the battle with illness and medical helpers.

Another Talmud vignette: "Better the day of death than the day of one's birth. When a person is born, all rejoice; when he dies, all weep. But it should not be so" (22). The Talmudic commentary explains that no one can comfortably foresee one's life events, but better is the man who "left the world peacefully." A parable is added concerning two ships, one departing, the other returning. The harbor crowd rejoiced over the departing ship, not over the arriving one. This should not be so, as the ship that has set out, no one knows what is in store for it, rough seas, storms, etc. The ship that has reached safely into the harbor commands our rejoicing (23).

The White House Conference on Aging (1971) makes reference to the proper concern of religious bodies and private agencies and says, "Any discussion of the spiritual well-being of man must include all aspects of life, even that of death. Although there are strong arguments in any such discussion they are best resolved in open discussion. "Religious bodies and government should affirm the right to, and reverence for life and recognize the individual's right to die with dignity" (24).

Legal considerations are punctuated by the recent explosion in the number of medicolegal suits in this country. The ensuing litigations have led to heightened awareness of the doctor's responsibility to society in a legal sense. Law is absolute, making few distinctions among the various motives for an act. The medical profession is in a unique position. It is granted the power of affecting life and death. Perhaps because of this, there is much suspicion in today's consumer-oriented society of a person who requires deep faith on the part of the recipient of healing, or even death. A physician who assumes the role of decision maker on life in a nontraditional way risks the wrath of the community through lawsuits and even legal and professional sanctions.

It is unquestionable that legal sanctions are necessary to protect unwilling victims of euthanasia. It is unconscionable to put to death a severely ill person whose religious beliefs, fear of death, or hope for restored health dictates otherwise. Even under these conditions, however, there are circumstances such as prolonged coma, continued deterioration, and irreversible damage that argue strongly in favor of leaving the decision to sustain life with the physician. In such instances, how should state law be applied to the "perpetrator?" Since there is no precedent of harsh penalties, fulfillment of the maximum sentence as prescribed by law might constitutionally be considered cruel and unusual (inhumane) punishment (25).

The pervasive legal question is, should the state regulate an individual's right to control his own body when the end result is death? What should the interest of the state be? Can the law justify societal motives in such a personal decision? The answers to these questions lie in two areas: criminal jurisprudence and ethics (culture). With regard to the first question, the abuses of euthanasia both by the medical community and by lay people are prosecutable offenses and rightly so.

Howard Rome, asks succinctly, ". . . How many Karen Ann Quinlans can be cared for? Does not her case, as it has been legally determined, set a precedent? Can we devise a system that can furnish a decent minimum health care to all, with no illusion that medical services will be equally distributed without discrimination?" (26).

The opposition to legalization of euthanasia takes both a religious and nonreligious form. In 1958, Yale Kamisar offered several arguments that remain very forceful today (27). The first is that when a physician pronounces a patient incurable, he is not only taking a great responsibility on himself for correct and final diagnosis but is also judging medical science to be nonadvancing or technologically static. There has been constant change in the scientific approach to disease and in cure rates, and the physician is disregarding this fact by making the pejorative statement that the patient's condition is irreversible. Of course the validity of this point of view varies with each case and can hardly be considered an argument for a person who is brain dead or debilitated by widely metastatic carcinoma.

Another argument involves the difficulty of getting consent from a patient who is comatose, incoherent, brain-damaged, and so on. This is also a valid point that is variable among individuals. The third argument, which has the most global ramifications and generates the most fear, is known as the *wedge theory*. Cornford describes the wedge objection as . . . "You should not act justly today, for fear that you may be asked to act still more justly tomorrow" (28). The thin edge of the wedge is euthanasia, and the thick edge is genocide. Legalizing euthanasia would necessitate myriads of legal and medical safeguards to prevent abuses. The fear that fosters this argument is well taken in our society.

Congress and the President have the capability of legislating wholesale slaughter in the form of war, during which safeguards and protections for the individual are only nominally provided for by the Geneva Convention. Our society may not be ready to tolerate the paradoxes of abhorrent murder and mercy killing. The abuses are easily imaginable: from hopelessly defective newborns to retarded children; from incurably insane adults to those with borderline insanity; from terminally ill adults to the senile and quadraplegics.

These examples are greatly exaggerated, but they underline a dilemma that rests at the crux of the euthanasia controversy: the decision is really not whether to legalize mercy killing, but how to do it with wisdom as well as compassion. (The wedge theory is invoked by the antiabortion proponents to reinforce the conviction that abortion is morally unacceptable.)

Kutner (1969) proposes that the law already recognizes a patient's right to refuse treatment, providing that he or she is capable of consent. He contends that this is not voluntary euthanasia but merely compliance. This interpretation of the law paves the way for passage of a binding living will. Kutner's proposals for the will are summarized as follows:

1. The patient should not be treated without his consent.
2. When consent is not expressed, the doctor must treat the patient or be held liable.
3. At the time the patient signs the consent form for surgery to release the hospital and doctor, he or she can also sign the living will.
4. In case of possible future accident, stroke, myocardial infarction, he or she can sign the living will at any point in his or her life when he or she is fully in control of his or her faculties and thereby committing himself or herself to the extent to which he or she would be willing to submit to treatment.
5. The document is absolutely revocable.
6. It can be revoked at any time that the person is deemed to be incompetent.
7. A person may anticipate mental illness and insert a clause to that effect beforehand.
8. The document cannot be nullified by someone else, unless instructed by the patient.
9. The will cannot be used as physician initiative to terminate life (29).

In addition to Kutner's criteria, I propose two other points. The first is that the document be written in lay language, not in medical or legal terms, so that the patient understands the division of responsibility among physician, family members, and himself or herself. Another requisite for the terminology of the will is that it have implied rather than specific obligations. In this way, the physician has the freedom to use his or her own medical judgment, instead of being bound by rigid conditions and procedures, (i.e., specific amounts of medication, a stated amount of time on the respirator, etc.) This also confers a degree of universality on the will so that it can be applied to all disease states without dealing with specifics. The vagueness of the language also makes the will timeless, so that it can take into account technological advances in medical science and breakthroughs in disease control.

It must be pointed out that if one takes into consideration the assumption that doctors are already quietly and independently terminating extraordinary means of treatment of terminally ill patients, a new issue may evolve (30,31). A complex legal structure would complicate the physician's use of his or her good judgment and compassion in order to comply with the letter of the law. The living will and the patient's wishes concerning his or her treatment should be a natural part of the doctor-patient relationship. It should not be legislated but should be dealt with as fundamentally as the professional diagnosis or any other type of consultation, that is, subject to responsible medical practice.

An alternative to euthanasia: the hospice? In a word, no. As a concept, not as an institution, it is creditable, but it is not relevant as an alternative to euthanasia. In the section "Emotional Considerations" it was noted that Cicely Saunders, the guiding light of the current hospice movement, vehemently opposes any form of euthanasia on religious grounds (8). On the surface it appears that the hospice is indeed an alternative to euthanasia. But in practice it rigidly fulfills the requirements for passive euthanasia. The hospice movement has evolved from medieval times, beginning with shelters for travelers, usually sponsored by a monastery. Then came hospitals, with a church responsibility. Historically, hospitals were foreboding and considered a place to die.

Today, the hospice movement reflects the past in its orientation—church rather than medicine, comforters rather than medicine men. The literature on the hospice movement is written by nonphysicians for the most part and filled with well-intentioned catch phrases. Perhaps it is a testimonial to an assumed default on the part of the medical profession. Dying and death have come full cycle. Once upon a time people died at home. Later they died in hospitals. Today they die in intensive care units. Now there is an effort again to have people die at home, or at least in a simulated homelike atmosphere. The suggested rationale for the hospice is that the terminally ill can be, and are, abandoned in pain. It is further suggested by the hospice movement that the cancer patient (and other patients with chronic and degenerative diseases) should live his final months as productively and comfortably as possible; to die peacefully and with dignity, and if he chooses to die at home, to assist him in this goal.

Of course, there is no disagreement with these goals and objectives, but is it necessary to structure the concept and call it hospice? As it is with the zeal and righteousness of ethicists, is it to be inferred that the medical profession only pays lip service to the concept? Or that the physician is a figurehead for a group that needs to help the dying, much like the evangelist who needs sinners? Do doctors feel that living and curing have meaning but caring for the dying does not?

Before chemotherapy for patients with cancer, oncology units were places where patients with the diagnosis of cancer came to be nursed and comforted until death. Today, in the hospital setting one can observe the goals of hospice being carried out—not in one concentrated area but within diverse specialties in almost all units, general or specialized. The staff is caring, visiting is liberal, children are welcomed, rooms are made homelike; dieticians, social workers, psychiatrists, occupational and recreational therapists are often full-time and usually available. At the Baltimore Cancer Research Program, major holidays are celebrated jointly with patients, family, and friends. The holiday meal is the central experience and is communal. Patients and family dine together in a solarium. The medical and nursing staff do the serving. This attitude on the part of the staff prevails throughout the year.

There is something wrong with a patient-doctor relationship ending with a transfer to a hospice. The patient now looks at new faces, feels a need for new trusts, a need to adjust to a new environment. A house does not make a home, nor does the hospice concept or building automatically imply the best or most appropriate care for the dying. People make the difference.

Whenever possible, dying at home is to be preferred to dying in an institution. Sampson points out that there are pros and cons to dying at home (32). The patient and his family have an opportunity to cement and repair relationships. Guilt can be assuaged. On the other hand, nursing procedures can be difficult or repulsive. Some patients take too long to die, and some families fear finding the patient dead.

Posing a perspective on hospice can evoke the same counterattack as when one assumes a posture proeuthanasia, much the same as if one comments on motherhood. Simply put, the hospice concept is not new. It is no more or less effective or caring than any accredited medical group or institution. I am apprehensive that the hospice movement will assume the faddish mantle that the "death and dying" fervor carries: such euphemisms as death education, thanatology, healthy dying, peaceful death, and, the worst of all, death with dignity. It should be remembered the birth process is not particularly dignified. It is hoped that hospice does not become the next buzzword with which good health-care personnel are identified.

The hospice concept, not facility, should not be intellectualized because it is not an original one. The approach to the dying person should be to understand the person, not the topic and certainly not the various models of the terminally ill. Those who are experiencing loss and losing need ordinary, calm, unangry, unfrightened human contact, not pseudoscientific thanatologists (33).

No, the hospice movement does not have a corner on the market of palliative care. And, no, the hospice movement is not an alternative to euthanasia. It is euthanasia. "A rose by any other name. . . ."

Is euthanasia good medical practice? Our culture interdicts the right to determine the time and manner of death for those of us who are seemingly in good health. The bioethicists argue that the terminally ill cannot choose, as they are part of the community and therefore do not have that prerogative. Then, who should choose?

Life cannot be measured in dollars and cents, and it is discomfiting to consider finances in the context of the critically or terminally ill patient. Nonetheless, it is a realistic concern if it limits or reduces the resources of the family, the hospital, or the government. In a study of 224 consecutive critically ill patients at the Massachusetts General Hospital, 123 were dead by the end of one month, 31 were home, 70 were hospitalized. By the end of one year 27 of the 224 patients had recovered. Significantly, $515,711 (83%) of the blood charge went to the 164 nonsurvivors, and $101,929 (17%) went to the 62 survivors. (The blood charges were only 21% of the total hospitalization charge) (34). Who shrinks at the sight of the price tag: the patient, the family, or the hospital?

What about the medical practitioner and his personal conflict? His sense of omnipotence is a double-edged sword. It spurs him to work long hours, beyond the call of duty. Saving the patient's life is paramount. Dedication to the task of saving lives, however, supersedes transient human frailties. The ultimate test of the physician rests in the quantity and quality of lives saved (35). Does this mean chemotherapy at the bitter end? Does it mean cardiopulmonary resuscitation for an 80-year-old patient who has been comatose and essentially dead for weeks?

Despite the scientific bent and omnipotence of many physicians there is a movement away from the traditional criteria of permanent and irreversible loss of heart and lung function as death determinants (36). A medical sociologist, Diana Crane, studied over 3,000 physicians, randomly selected from the disciplines of pediatrics, internal medicine, neurosurgery, and pediatric cardiac surgery (37). More than 70% of physicians accepted cessation of brain function as the most valid determinant of death. They felt that ". . . irreversible loss of the capacity for social interaction was a more important consideration than the continuation of the physiological indicator of life, heart beat." Other polls and surveys taken in the general public sphere concur. Whether this is a manifestation of enlightenment or persuasion or social consciousness on the part of most physicians is academic. What is important is that more doctors are becoming sensitive to the melding of the art of medicine with the science of medicine. The result is an increased physician acceptance of the responsibility of treating their patients even to and, perhaps even with a peaceful death. The gift is a very personal two-person relationship in which one partner is permitted to die.

There are demurs to this notion; that committees, families, or the law or some other agency would be better suited. Perhaps, simply by denying death itself by teaching transition, life after death (or life after life), then euthanasia as a concern becomes moot to the disciples of these beliefs.

Committees are cumbersome. Who would comprise a death committee? The awesome responsibility for termination of life cannot be placed on disinterested, objective lay parties, nor can the families or attending physicians be expected to make an emotion-free decision. It would be difficult to create a committee that did not have too many or too few qualifications. The Critical Care Committee of the Massachusetts General Hospital has recommended the establishment of an advisory committee, the Optimum Care Committee. However, they stress that the "Ultimate decision concerning treatment . . . rests with the responsible physician" (38).

Why, then, is it necessary to form a committee? Fulton, in his study, demonstrated that groups terminate life more frequently and sooner than the members of the group would as individuals (39). Further, there is very little about a committee decision in this area that is dignified or humane.

The law: At the moment, only a few states provide, albeit ambiguous and limited, legal protection for the patient or the physician. Perhaps this will be rectified in the near future. There are laws, however, that make active intervention a criminal offense—the law is absolute.

Good medical practice, particularly in the area of care of the terminally ill, should set standards that the law can support (40). The law cannot determine medical procedures, but it can be guided by the establishment of customary standards for the doctor-patient relationship. The doctor and the patient each has his own responsibilities and obligations in the relationship.

The family: Some families can ask for cessation of artificial means of prolonging life for their relative, but almost all fear such a decision would result in a lifetime of guilt. Many families feel they are yo-yos as their relative gets good news, then bad news. Their vigil is all the more burdensome by the guilt they feel for wishing it over.

The patient: If alert, he can request, but without assurance, that his desires will be heeded. He has several options; he can commit suicide, refuse further treatment, or neglect a complicating secondary illness that will result in death. It cannot be overemphasized that the patient is the supreme authority. If he refuses further treatment (surgery, radiation, chemotherapy and blood components and antibiotics), that constitutes the final treatment effort. Just as passive euthanasia is an act of omission, so is his choice for no treatment an active participation in his overall struggle with his illness. Death is as important and useful as life. Death is not an event; it is in fact a process.

The doctor: If one assumes that the decision for a merciful ending is as much a matter of medical judgment as any other part of the patient's medical care, the doctor then cannot abdicate his responsibility. His approach should be the same as at any point in the process of his treating the patient: a consultation with the patient. If the patient is alert, or even semialert, the physician should listen carefully to the patient for an overt or implied request for ending or continuing of therapy or support. If the patient is comatose, the doctor should consult jointly with the family, as he or she would do ordinarily in other medical situations. Again, this would be by listening, not by confronting the family for the decision, thereby leaving them with guilt.

By tender, compassionate concern and listening, the doctor obtains their wishes in an oblique manner. Both family and patient have the opportunity for mourning, resolution, and peace. Thus the doctor truly fulfills his role as healer.

CONCLUSION

Euthanasia or active termination, by an act of either commission or omission, of the dying process should be, and is, a partnership, a cooperative therapeutic endeavor by the patient and his physician. It is the final step in the sometimes meandering path of the disease and the disease-induced dehumanization. Otherwise, the patient is treated without concern for the holistic practice—the art—of medicine. The patient needs realistic personal compassion, not a dutiful, reverent, self-righteous intellectual litany—meaningless words.

Standing to one side of the issue for the moment, it is obvious that the debate itself is fundamentally a confrontation between advocates of situation ethics and those who believe in an absolute morality. Proponents of euthanasia are basically stating that, in certain situations, to terminate the life of a human is not murder, that the essence of a person is not the same thing as a living human animal. The person is a vibrant force in his community, with self-awareness as well as an effect on others. Being self-aware and able to formulate his needs, he retains the right to life and continued attempts to fulfill himself and fulfill others who relate to him. As a corollary, the fetus or the decorticate trauma victim may therefore have organistic qualities that are humanoid, but they are not quite persons. Accordingly, their value to society is in the knowledge, or transplantable organs, they can contribute.

The moral absolutist, on the other hand, embraces the concept of a soul, which, unlike the person, is a quality inherent to the human protoplasm throughout its existence. There is not justification for terminating a being and depriving its soul as a necessary perquisite for continued existence. As was stated in the beginning of this presentation, it is apparent that both positions are based on belief rather than knowledge and that within the convincing logical framework of either system there is little ground for rationally persuading the other of its validity.

So the controversy rages, and the discussion of what to do with the patient gathers more steam, while he, poor fellow, is ignored as he tries to get his wish or word in edgewise. Reinhold Niebuhr offers us a succinct perspective: "The ending of our life would not threaten us if we had not falsely made ourselves the center of life's meaning" (41).

ACKNOWLEDGMENTS

Part of the material contained herein is reprinted with the kind permission of the *Maryland State Medical Journal*, vol. 25, no. 11, November 1976, pp. 66–73 (Euthanasia: Is there an answer? Schnaper N, Schnaper HW, and Schnaper LA) and vol. 26, no. 3, March 1977, pp. 42–48 (Euthanasia: An overview, Schnaper LA, Schnaper N, Fierce AR, and Schnaper HW). Copyrights 1976 and 1977 respectively by the Medical and Chirurgical Faculty of the State of Maryland, Baltimore, Maryland.

The author is grateful for the assistance of Mrs. Patricia L. Harrell.

REFERENCES

1. Schnaper N: Psychosocial aspects of management of the patient with cancer. *Med Clin North Am* 61:1147–1155, 1977.

2. Fletcher J: Ethics and euthanasia. *Am J Nurs* 73:670–675, 1973.

3. Philander C: Quoted in *The Evening Sun*, Baltimore, Oct 26, 1974, p A11.

4. Russell OR: *Freedom to Die: Moral and Legal Aspects of Euthanasia.* New York, Dell Publishing Co, Inc, 1976.

5. Scher EM: Legal aspects of euthanasia. *Albany Law Rev* 4:674–697, 1972.

6. Curran WJ: The Saikewicz decision. *N Engl J Med* 298:499–500, 1978.

7. Relman AS: The Saikewicz decision: Judges as physicians. *N Engl J Med* 298:508–509, 1978.

8. Saunders C: The problem of euthanasia. *Nurs Times* 55:960–961, 1959.

9. Schnaper N, Schnaper HW, Schnaper LA: Euthanasia: Is there an answer? *Md State Med J* 25:66–73, 1976.

10. Fletcher J: Abortion, euthanasia and the care of defective newborns. *N Engl J Med* 292:75–78, 1975.

11. Clouser KO: Panel on death and aging. *South Med J* 62:22–24, 1974.

12. Engelhardt HT Jr: Bioethics and the process of embodiment. *Perspect Biol Med* Summer:486–500, 1975.

13. Jackson DL, Younger S: Patient autonomy and "death with dignity." *N Engl J Med* 301:404–408, 1979.

14. Rachels J: Active and passive euthanasia. *N Engl J Med* 292:78–80, 1975.

15. Shoemaker WC: Interdisciplinary medicine: Accommodation or integration? *Crit Care Med* 3:1–4, 1975.

16. *Time* Magazine, Chicago, Time, Inc., Apr 28, 1975, p 78.

17. Schnaper N: Management of the dying patient, in Lisansky ET, Schocket BR (eds): *Modern Treatment.* New York, Harper & Row, 1969, pp 746–759.

18. Williams G: *The Sanctity of Life and the Criminal Law.* New York, Alfred A Knopf, Publisher, 1957.

19. *The Random House Dictionary*, unabridged edition.

20. Schnaper N and Schnaper HW: A few kind words for the devil. *J Religion Health* 6:107–122, 1969.

21. Talmud, Bereshit Rabbah, 9 and commentary.

22. Talmud, Eccles. vii I.

23. Talmud, Eccles, R, ad loc.

24. *1971 White House Conference on Aging,* US Government Printing Office, December 1971, p 26, nos 13 and 14.

25. Baughman WH, Bruha JC, Gould FJ: Euthanasia: Criminal, tort, constitutional and legislative considerations. *Notre Dame Lawyer* 5:1202–1260, 1973.

26. Rome HP: More about Karen Ann Quinlan. *Psychiatr Ann* 6:97–105, 1976.

27. Kamisar Y: Some non-religious views against proposed mercy-killing legislation. *Minn Law Rev* 6:964–1042, 1958.
28. Williams G: Mercy-killing legislation: A rejoinder. *Minn Law Rev* 43:1–12, 1958.
29. Kutner L: Due process of euthanasia: The Living Will: A proposal. *Indiana Law J* 4:539–554, Summer 1979.
30. Levinsohn AA: Voluntary mercy deaths: Social-legal aspects of euthanasia. *J Forensic Med* 2:57–79, 1961.
31. Wilkes P: When do we have a right to die? *Life Magazine,* New York, Time Life, Inc., Jan 14, 1972, pp 48–52.
32. Sampson W: Quoted in: On dying at home. *Emerg Med,* Feb 1977, pp 137–141.
33. Schnaper N: Death and dying: Has the topic been beaten to death? editorial. *J Nerv Ment Dis* 160:157–158, 1975.
34. Cullen DJ, Ferrara LC, Briggs BA, et al: Survival, hospitalization charges and follow-up results in critically ill patients. *N Engl J Med* 294:982–987, April 29, 1976.
35. Schnaper N, Cowley RA: Overview: Psychiatric sequelae to multiple trauma. *Am J Psychiatry* 133:883–890, 1976.
36. Rome HP: The person who should have died. *Psychiatr Ann* 8:510–515, 1978.
37. Crane D: Consensus and controversy in medical practice: The dilemma of the critically ill patient. *Ann Acad Political Social Sci* 437:109, 1978.
38. Optimum care for hopelessly ill patients: A report of the Critical Care Committee of the Massachusetts General Hospital, special article. *N Engl J Med* 295:362–364, 1976.
39. Fulton R: Coming to terms with death, editorial. *Omega* 5:1–4, 1974.
40. Fletcher GP: Legal aspects of the decision not to prolong life. *JAMA* 23:119–122, 1968.
41. Neibuhr R: *The Nature and Destiny of Man, Vol II, Human Destiny.* New York, Charles Scribner's Sons, 1943, p 293.

22

Is Euthanasia Ever Justifiable?

John C. Fletcher

I use the word "euthanasia" following Kohl (1) to mean active or direct means to end the life of a dying person who requests another, usually a physician, to terminate his or her life in the name of mercy. This form of action is properly called voluntary beneficent euthanasia. One would do it only if requested and only for the sake of the one who suffers. Moral policy that now guides actions with the dying forbids such acts, and the law punishes such acts. Moralists and physicians have made eloquent attacks on this policy, especially in recent years. Therefore, the moral policy should be examined in its major features.

This chapter examines the major consequences of adherence to the moral policy against euthanasia. My thesis is that any moral policy should be followed on the basis of careful examination of the positive and negative consequences that flow from holding it. The reader will see that, although I agree with many of the criticisms of writers who argue for euthanasia, I cannot agree on the basis of the evidence that the moral policy against euthanasia should be changed. The medical care of the dying is undergoing reform that is essential and morally justified, but the policy against euthanasia should remain firm.

To make this argument, I first describe the content of the prevailing moral policy on euthanasia. Second, I discuss the method by which my argument proceeds and some of its assumptions. Finally, the positive and negative consequences of adherence to the policy against euthanasia are projected and analyzed on the basis of the position in ethics that I hold.

MORAL POLICY

I use the term "moral policy" following Callahan (2) to mean the way a particular community chooses to order the moral rules about a particular area of social life. The term "community" is inclusive of a wide variety of human groups and

The author wishes especially to thank Nelson O. Chipchin, a volunteer worker at the Clinical Center, NIH, for library research that contributed to this chapter.

collectivities. A moral policy is a set of moral assumptions or premises that govern specific social practices. A moral policy contains a number of features based on a guide to conduct or a "prescription," as Hare (3) uses the term, that is itself a response to the claims of one or more moral principles. Within the policy there is also a bias toward firmness or looseness of the rules and a recognition of the hierarchy of rules. As Callahan (2) noted, moral policies undergo formation in stages over time. A typical moral problem facing a society occurs when there is dissatisfaction with one or more of the features of a moral policy or with assent to the basic prescription that guides the policy.

Moral policies function to relate the cumulative moral experience of human communities to moral judgments in the decisions of everyday life. An example from another biomedical problem may be useful, that is, abortion. Moral policy on abortion in most of the developed countries has undergone profound change in recent decades. In the United States, there are three rival moral policies on abortion that conflict and contend for ascendency whenever social or legal policy decisions about abortion must be made. Briefly, the policies are proscription of abortion, a list of acceptable reasons for abortion, and permission for abortion on request with a role for the physician in testing reasons. Each option is more responsive to one of the two sides of the conflict between the interests of fetus and mother, and each is responsive to the moral principles that underlie and support the arguments on that side.

In the biomedical fields, especially as these fields interact with the social policy process, there has been a growing tendency to clarify and debate moral policy issues in advance of making fundamental shifts in social policy. The debate of moral policy has taken place in several official commissions and other forums, such as The Commission on the Totally Implantable Artificial Heart, The Commission for the Protection of Human Subjects in Biomedical and Behavioral Research, The Ethics Advisory Board to the Secretary, Department of Health, Education and Welfare, and the newly established President's Commission for the Study of Ethical Problems in Medicine and Biomedical and Behavioral Research. An additional example is the 1975–1976 moratorium on recombinant DNA research that was accompanied by careful study of the ethical and social issues involved before the research was resumed. Through the process of debate, the function and shape of moral policies have been further clarified.

A moral policy contains the basic prescription or guide to conduct in a form that can be communicated when the need arises to express it. The need arises typically when there are specific cases to be considered, when features or the policy are being questioned, and when others need to know what the policy is. As Hare (4) comments, a way to understand the difference between the levels of moral policy and the day-to-day moral judgments that we render in actual decisions is to ask, "What do we want physicians to learn about euthanasia and the care of the dying in their education?" Here, one describes moral policy per se. One would want them to know the basic guide to conduct, the moral rules pertaining to this conduct, the degree of strictness of the rules, the possibility of exceptions, and the leading arguments that challenged the moral policy. On the level of making decisions in the care of patients, the content of decisions cannot be taught as such, unless one abrogates the freedom of the decision maker by insisting that all decisions had to be made in a certain way. In decision making, there is not the clarity and order afforded at the distance of moral policy; yet choices and their results should be in keeping with the policy.

This chapter responds to questions of what ought to be transmitted to physicians in their education, what general guidelines the profession should follow, and what legislatures should take into account as their members consider proposals that would strengthen or change existing policy. In making the argument, I show my preference for an understanding of ethics and the teaching of ethics that runs counter to the case-by-case slogan that so easily leaps to the tongue in debate. In moral education we learn principles that suffice to guide us through the majority of cases. It is only the most unusual cases that require extraordinary consideration or departure from the principles that normally guide our conduct, especially in a setting with as many checks and controls as medicine. Physicians do not, as a matter of fact, spend equal time debating and deliberating carefully over each case. If they did, they could only deal with so few cases at a time that many others would suffer or die as a result. I am in further agreement with Hare (5) that medical ethics should not be shaped by examination of the hardest cases, or even by paying too much attention to singular cases. There is an ethical parallel to the maxim in law that hard cases make bad law. Preoccupation with exceptional cases seduces the mind from the major task of ethics, which is the selection of principles and procedures for application to the greatest number of cases in a specified area. Thus, it makes a great deal of difference that we have reliable facts on where people die, the costs of dying, how many die in the throes of agony, and what kinds of analgesics work effectively.

MORAL POLICY ON EUTHANASIA

Historical studies by Fye (6) and Gruman (7) show that the concept of active euthanasia acquired its modern meaning late in the nineteenth century and was introduced into public discussion by writers outside of medicine who were interested in the implications of Darwinism as applied to the plight of the dying. Active euthanasia had been practiced before that time, but debate about the care of the dying in which the term "euthanasia" was used referred to the state of mind of the dying person at the time of death. So-called spiritual euthanasia pointed to the desired tranquillity of mind of the dying person and how the physician, family, and clergy should work together to bring it about.

Suicide of the dying, called in ancient Greece and Rome the "freedom to leave," was widely practiced in antiquity. Edelstein (8), the leading modern authority on the Hippocratic canon, showed that the section of the oath forbidding the physician to give deadly drugs referred to suicide rather than to murder. The practice of suicide of the sick declined after the second century A.D. because of influences from Judeo-Christian teachings about the value of individual life. The practice of infanticide of defective or unwanted newborns also subsided for the same reasons. Before the seventeenth century, the term "euthanasia" referred to a number of general considerations for an easy death, including the mental and moral attitude a person took toward life and work. After that period, and increasingly into the twentieth century, euthanasia was more related to actions of physicians in the care of the terminally ill.

In contrast to moral policy on abortion, moral policy on euthanasia has remained relatively stable throughout the twentieth century. One of the least
changed aspects of modern medical ethics, when viewed across cultures and
religious traditions, is the restraint of euthanasia. The genocide program of the
National Socialists in Germany was not euthanasia, even though these acts were
referred to as such, since the Nazis were not responding to requests of individual
patients for mercy's sake, but killing in the name of efficiency and racial purity,
as shown by Davidowicz (9).

What is the content of the prevailing moral policy on euthanasia? The first
feature is the basic prescription that guides the policy: it is wrong to kill an
innocent person, even though that person is suffering and requests death in the
name of mercy. There is a general moral rule against the killing of persons that
functions throughout societies. Baier (10) points out that these exceptions are
built into the rule: killing in self-defense, killing an enemy in war, capital punishment, accidental killing (as when the person bent on suicide steps in front of
another's car), and as Baier interestingly puts it, "and possibly mercy killing."
When the moral policy on euthanasia is being taught or debated, it should be
placed in the framework of the general rule about killing persons. When we
learn this rule, we also learn its exceptions, that killing is wrong unless it is one
of these exceptions. One is not considered to be morally educated without know-
ing the exceptions to the rule that have become part of the rule.

The second feature of the prevailing policy is an affirmative stance toward
allowing an individual to die when the evidence shows that death is irrevisible
and attempts to prolong life would increase suffering. Current expressions in
law and professional medical codes of the moral policy on euthanasia hold that
there is a meaningful line between active ending of a dying life and allowing the
individual to die. An example is in guidelines of the Swiss Academy of Medical
Sciences (11):

2. Active euthanasia (or provocation of death) is distinguished from passive eu-
    thanasia. It is recognized that this distinction is not always easy in certain specific
    cases.

    (a) Active euthanasia deliberately curtails life by killing the dying individual.
        It consists of artificially intervening in the vital processes that still subsist,
        in order to hasten the coming of death. According to Swiss Penal Code
        active euthanasia is a punishable intentional homicide. Active euthanasia
        remains punishable even when done at the request of the patient.

    (b) Passive euthanasia is the act of allowing a fatally ill or injured person to
        die, by renouncing measures that would prolong his life. It consists in the
        omission or the discontinuation of medication, as well as of technical mea-
        sures like mechanical respiration, provision of oxygen, blood transfusions,
        hemodialysis, and intravenous feeding.
           It is medically justified to abandon a therapy or limit oneself to alleviating
        suffering if in deferring death one prolongs suffering beyond what is
        bearable and if on the other hand the affliction has taken an irreversible
        turn with a prognostication of death.

The foregoing statement is similar in spirit and content to another moral policy
guideline issued in the United States by the American Medical Association in
1973.

The possibility of making voluntary beneficent euthanasia (mercy killing) an accepted and legitimate exception to the rule against killing persons has been debated more frequently in the twentieth century than at any other time. Those who argue for euthanasia ask that the general rule be further modified to make an exception in certain types of cases for the relief of suffering. Their appeal is, not to self-interest or economic motives, but to moral principles, usually to the principle of freedom.

One can defend moral rules, expecially the moral rule against killing persons, by drawing on imperatives or moral experiences that arise from one or more religious traditions. I have argued this way in the past about the problem of pediatric euthanasia (12), but I now question the efficacy of a moral argument that too directly appeals to theological foundations. The conduct of public debate about moral questions like euthanasia must depend on the likelihood that all parties entertain what they may believe to be an impossible and self-defeating concept, the concept of God as traditionally taught. Many moral persons in a secular society neither belong to religious communities nor feel persuaded to investigate theological claims. I am now working out a more detailed case for these thoughts in essays on genetics, counseling, and religious belief. Although I believe that my argument here is consistent with a reformed theism, especially that one advanced by Hartshorne (13), Ogden (14), and other thinkers inspired by the thought of Alfred North Whitehead, here the reader is not required to adopt a theological point of view to assent to the arguments.

The reader is asked only to examine two claims that have been successfully advanced in the name of human reason. First, we should adopt the overriding principle that we should do what is required by moral rules. This step is called adopting the moral point of view as described by Baier (10), Frankena (15), and other philosophers who have worked toward a rational basis for ethics. My own position in ethics falls roughly under the category of rule-utilitarianism, but this position is often modified in practice by responses to competing ethical claims made from other positions. In this view, to be ethical means to act in a way that best serves to harmonize the interests of all those who will be affected by the action proposed. Further, the most reliable way to act this way in the long run is by submitting self-interest to the tests of following moral rules and assessing the consequences of following the rules in the specific kinds of cases in dispute. The theory is utilitarian in the sense that it estimates the value of actions by reference to their consequences, but the actions are not divorced from the obligation to follow moral rules. The important question for this type of ethical theory is not, "What would be the consequences if Dr. A responded to patient B's request for euthanasia in this particular situation?" Looking at the consequences of acts, while referring to moral rules as rules of thumb or maxims is the main characteristic of another type of utilitarian thought perhaps best represented by Joseph Fletcher (16). In my view, the possibilities for fallacies and self-serving reasoning are significantly reduced if the question is approached, "What would be the consequences if Dr. A followed the moral rule against killing in this situation and if others in Dr. A's situation did likewise?" The reason for caution about situation ethics is that none of us can see the situation as adequately as we ought. We are affected by self-interest to the point of sometimes being blind to where self-interest operates. We need the help of rules that have been adopted under less interested conditions. What may in the short run appear to be in our best interests may in the longer run prove to have been mistaken, and we are relieved that we stayed with a course chosen on moral principle.

In this view, the place of moral rules is obviously very important. To be moral, to paraphrase Baier (10), means to reason in a way that overrules the reasons of self-interest in those cases when if everyone followed self-interest, significant harm would come to everyone involved. To agree to follow moral rules as one's overriding or supreme principle is to seek a level of impartiality and generality that moves a conflict away from the chance that it will be resolved by ruthless force, self-deception, or a fiat based on emotion. Moral rules, such as do not kill, be fair, do not lie, and keep promises are designed to apply to everyone alike, without exception. For this reason, it is in the best interest of all to follow moral rules and to learn how to reason so as not to fall too often into the traps of self-serving reasoning. The power of self-deception and illusion is so great in human affairs that following moral rules is the most reliable procedure that human culture has produced for resolving conflicts of a moral nature. No one is free from self-interest, especially when a matter is in sharp dispute. Rule utilitarianism holds that we should consider first the consequences that follow from the observance of certain moral rules or the entire body of rules commonly accepted in a society. If it could be shown that consistently following a moral policy based on moral rules leads to reprehensible amounts of pain, avoidable suffering, deprivation, or long-term social upheaval, the rule utilitarian is obligated to reassess the ordering of the moral rules and possibly recommend a change in moral policy and practice. No moral policy is inviolable. No application of a moral rule is beyond criticism. We should judge moral policy by the consequences of consistently and faithfully observing it. Moral rules are our greatest safeguard against the dangers of self-deception, but, because moral rules are humanly constructed, the rules must not be elevated to a suprahuman or supernatural position.

The second claim is that we have the freedom to decide to alter the force and applicability of moral rules. We have the freedom to change loyalties. This freedom may be expressed in a number of ways. We may criticize a prevailing moral policy and recommend a change in practice. We may conscientiously object to following a rule and publicly break the rule while accepting the moral and legal consequences. Dr. Hermann Sander (17) acted in this spirit in 1949 when he dictated into the hospital records that he injected 40 cc of air into the vein of a cancer patient on the verge of death. He was tried and later acquitted for the offense. We can express our freedom negatively, rather than positively, by deciding that it is in our interest to cheat, lie, or even kill but then conceal the fact that we have done so to avoid punishment under the rules.

The foregoing examples illustrate individuals acting on their freedom. There are also examples of a wider, more culturally diffused freedom. Moral rules are affected by historical, technological, and cultural change. Whole groups or societies enjoy the freedom to change loyalties. The priorities of the moral rules differ in time and circumstance. Systems of moral rules evolve over time and also change in shape and applicability. An examination of bodies of applied rules, for example, in medical practice and research show differences from society to society, reflecting deeper cultural and religious beliefs that influence the way the moral rules are selected and applied. Moral rules and moral policies are human products, or products of cultural evolution, and for this reason they are subject to the quality of openness and change that characterizes everything human.

On the one hand, because human beings are so capable of fallacies and self-deception, even in the best moments of moral reasoning, it is vital to strive for the greatest degree of objectivity and impartiality when in moral conflicts. One method to achieve this level is to point to the epitome of being moral, namely, to put oneself in the other's place, on both the giving and receiving end of the action. This reciprocity, or ability to see ourselves as both actors and acted on, is at the heart of the special faculty that we call moral. To evaluate euthanasia, we are required to put ourselves in the place of physician, patient, family, and the members of the society who would be affected by the action. Do the consequences that flow from keeping the rule against killing benefit or harm these parties when their interests are treated as equal? If the reader feels that we should not treat each party's interests as equal, he or she has not adopted a moral point of view, namely, one in which moral reasons transcend all other reasons, such as economic, political, social, or technical.

On the other hand, because human beings are free and construct a world that is open toward the future, systems of moral rules are under pressure for change and adaptation to new circumstances and new events. Novelty is a characteristic of the moral dimension of human institutions, just as there is novelty in all other aspects of biological and cultural evolution. Wisdom from the past and human insight into our fallibility makes the objective side of morality necessary. No human being is good enough to be an exception to moral rules. Pressure from the future and its possibilities makes the subjective side of morality necessary. No moral rule is inviolate and unrelated to the consequences that flow from consistent attempts to follow it. Consequences affect our choice of rules. These are the two sides of morality, and an adequate ethical analysis must hold them together. In the end, however, no amount of ethical analysis can deliver the individual from the burden of choice. As Aiken (18) wrote, "decision is king." We have the freedom to alter moral policy on euthanasia, but ought we to do so?

CONSEQUENCES OF MORAL POLICY ON EUTHANASIA

My goal is to evaluate the consequences of consistent adherence to the policy against euthanasia. What will be the procedure, and by what criteria will the consequences be evaluated?

The first step is to describe what those on both sides of the issue state are the consequences for them and those whose interests they represent. For knowledge of consequences, I am dependent on the written history of the dispute and published studies of some of the relevant questions. One should attempt to take as dispassionate a view as possible at this stage of the analysis and simply investigate the substance of the claims on both sides of the issue.

The second step is concurrently to address any empirical questions that may shed light on claims that are made for moral reasons. For example, is it known how many people die in unremitting pain? If there are no extant answers, the analysis should point out where and how answers can be sought. Reliable facts should inform the conduct of debate about moral questions whenever possible. The third step is a moral judgment, strictly speaking.

Because euthanasia is a genuine moral question involving a clash of views about what is and will be good for persons who are dying under certain conditions, a further judgment must be made about whether the consequences of following the rule contribute to a greater opportunity for good than evil for those whose interests are most affected. A greater opportunity for good than evil includes what can be empirically known about benefits or deficits, but all genuine moral issues require a judgment beyond the facts, based on beliefs about what it means to be ethical or to act for the best. My own view is that we increase the opportunity for good when we act to harmonize the variety of interests and values that contend in a moral issue like euthanasia. Good is the strength of unity in diversity and its opposite, diversity in unity. Evil is either of two kinds. Intolerable conflict is evil because it destroys the unity that exists between the parts in a system. Monotony or excessive opposition to change is evil because it destroys variety and its power to promote the need for unity. Conflict in itself is not evil, because clashes of values, persons, and duties eventually enrich human experience with the resolutions that they inspire. Evolution at all levels is toward a richer, more complex existence. However, the two evils mentioned can inhibit or even destroy evolution. The kind of harmony that I am defining as good does not lack conflict or movement, but it resists solutions that have aspects of violence, coercion, or avoidance of the issue.

NEGATIVE CONSEQUENCES

Cruelty and Depersonalization

Many writers have pointed to cases in which they considered it cruel or depersonalizing to allow a patient to continue living in unremitted agony or a simply vegetative existence when death is inevitable in a short period. Rachels (19) argues that maintaining the bare difference between active and passive euthanasia contributes toward situations where it is patently cruel to allow defective newborns to die through dehydration and infection rather than by a swift, painless injection. Though not finally advocating euthanasia, Freeman (20) comments on the same problem.

Fletcher (21) describes the consequences of excessive prolongations of life as transforming the dying individual into a monster comparable with the severely defective infant. Lying behind this term is his understanding of the relationship between quality of life and exercise of the rational and critical faculties. The theme of the effect of depersonalization on the dying and the living is woven throughout the work of a widely read tract by Mannes (22) that appeals for "the right to choose death when life no longer holds any meaning . . . (as) the last human right."

What is the empirical status of these claims? How frequently would one actually meet with cruelty, in the sense of allowing excessive, avoidable pain and depersonalization of the dying?

There is little doubt that until quite recently, and probably even now, society in the broadest sense is not being well served in medical care of the dying. Robert Butler (23), Director of the National Institute of Aging, wrote in 1978, "currently, less than one percent of the hospitals in the United States have any type of program related to the care of the dying." Just under 2 million Americans died in 1976. Of this number, 980,000 died in hospitals, and 420,000 died in nursing homes, according to Ryder and Ross (24). Therefore, the chance that significant change or improvement of the care of the dying has occurred is slight. A report of the Comptroller General of the United States (25) in 1978 found 59 organizations that used the term "hospice" in their purposes, but they differed widely in depth of experience and numbers of patients served. In Great Britain, where the hospice concept began in earnest, there are 40 special units for the care of the dying, with only 10 inside the National Health Service, according to Ford (26).

Saunders (27), whose personal and professional experience in the care of the dying exceeds any other living person, laments over continually meeting "patients who give us histories of weeks and months of unrelieved pain, anorexia, vomiting, incontinence, and other forms of physical distress." Serious research into the relief of pain and discomforts of terminal illness has recently increased, in part because of the successes in Great Britain's hospices.

Many persons, and possibly many physicians and nurses, share a misconception that an incurable disease like cancer means a painful experience that always ends in an agonized death. Turnbull (28) and Aitken-Swan (29) in Great Britain and Oster and colleagues (30) in the United States conducted studies showing that between 25% and 50% of cancer patients die with no pain or negligible pain. A painful death from cancer is not inevitable, but pain is a considerable problem that doubtless contributes to the felt need for euthanasia. This fact is illustrated by a study of Parkes (31) that showed that the degree of success in relieving pain is much less in home and hospital-based care than in the St. Christopher's hospice, a specialized unit for relieving symptoms of terminal illness. Parkes found that about 20% of the hospital patients died with unrelieved pain that was severe and continuous. About the same percentage had comparable pain before admission to the hospital. Of those who died at home 10% began with severe pain, but this proportion rose to 50% before death itself. In the hospice unit the percentage of patients with severe pain fell from 36% to 8%.

The state of the art in the relief of pain of terminal illness by drugs has been reported by Twycross (32), based on his own careful research with various analgesics. West (33) summarized the state of the art in managing pain in terminal illness by pointing to the need for further research, but he emphasized also that "the failure to make full use of the knowledge we already possess explains much of the unrelievable pain that those with a terminal illness still have to endure." The probability that a patient will die with severe and uncontrollable pain, a condition close to the center of the argument for euthanasia- would appear to be greatly reduced if the patient is under the care of a physician who follows practices of pain relief based on doses given on an individual basis planned after careful assessment of the patient. Much more research needs to be done on pain and pain management. Chronic pain can dominate the thinking of an individual and lead to the conclusion that life is not worth living. But this conclusion need not occur because of pain alone, although it may occur for other reasons.

The other reasons are likely linked to the depersonalization of dying. There are reasons to believe that the avoidance of death and the dying in hospitals, so characteristic when Kubler-Ross (34) began her early studies, has been in part remedied through the impact of education and research on the attitudes of physicians. Published studies (35, 36) of physician attitudes on revealing the diagnosis to the cancer patient show a complete reversal in a 20-year period, probably reflecting also more openness to discussion of death. Yet, the site of dying is linked to experience of depersonalization, with the chances of depersonalization being greater in hospitals. Hinton (37) interviewed four groups of 20 dying patients and their families in settings of an acute hospital, a Foundation Home (nursing home), and a hospice. Patients were least depressed and anxious in the hospice setting, and they preferred the more frank communication about dying in that site. Martinson and colleagues (38) found considerably less depression and alienation in parents and siblings of children dying of cancer who were cared for at home as compared with those who died in the hospital. The problem of continuation of life-support systems or other treatment that is sometimes linked to depersonalization of irrelevant prolongation of life is greatly lessened if home or hospice is the site of dying. Research needs to be done on effects of overcoming fear of depersonalization in those hospitals that have developed special care units or staff teams for the dying, for example, Royal Victoria Hospital (Montreal) and St. Luke's Hospital (New York).

The phenomenon of depersonalization of the dying and their families is not necessary, but it is mostly linked to the rapid growth of the hospital as the site of dying and to the nursing home as site of long-term care. In 1946 just half of the deaths in the United States occurred at home or at the scene of accidents. By 1976 this figure had dropped 30%. The health-care system of today, according to a report of a Subcommittee on Terminal Illness of the National Institutes of Health (39), is geared to episodic, acute, and curative interventions, mostly of a sophisticated nature. The needs of a patient for whom there is no reasonable hope of cure, and the needs of the patient's family, are distinctly different. The patient needs help with uncontrolled physical symptoms and social-psychological problems of separation from family and friends. The culture of the typical acute care unit is not conducive to meeting these needs. The family may have limited access to the dying patient in such settings. Seen in a historical perspective, the reform of the medical care of the dying has gradually been emerging just to transform the legitimate and accurate charges of cruelty and depersonalization. The psychiatrist Parkes (40) reports that requests for euthanasia are related to uncontrollable pain, fear of dying, and depression. According to Parkes, each can be directly addressed but does not prevent the occasional suicide. He suggests that the dying patient who is depressed be asked about the urge to commit suicide, so that the underlying physical and emotional cause can be met and relieve the problem. He notes that family members who fear that telling the patient will result in suicide are responding from fear rather than reason, but these relatives often press physicians for a policy of concealment. He recommends that the physician open up the subject of the feelings of the family, so that the need for concealment can be transformed.

On any kind of empirical assessment of the scope of the problems of relievable pain and avoidable depersonalization in terminal illness, there is little doubt that the incidence is significant. These consequences, however, do not stem so much from following the moral policy on euthanasia as from the kind of research that has been most rewarded, the great growth in hospitals as the site of dying, and the diffusion of expensive, high technology for the care of the acutely ill. An open question remains as to whether the health-care systems can be successfully reformed to diffuse the successful hospice principles and methods to dying persons. One moral question to be addressed is whether the great remainder of the unmet needs of the dying justifies the introduction of euthanasia for those who will never enjoy the benefits of reformed medical care of the dying.

Deprivation of Freedom

Flew (41) and Morison (42), among others, point to a negative consequence of the policy against euthanasia, in that the unique human freedom to choose is restricted. Flew argues that the burden of proof for depriving a person of liberty is always on those who would do so.

How many people would take advantage of this denied choice if given the privilege? A Gallup (43) poll found in 1973 that 53% approved this statement: "When a person has a disease that cannot be cured, do you think doctors should be allowed by law to end the patient's life by some painless means if the patient and his family request it?" In 1950 only 30% approved this same question. Assuming that this response has not changed a great deal, one should assume that the number of persons whose freedom to choose euthanasia is being restrained is significant, perhaps several thousand.

Is this restraint of freedom translated into self-destruction? Specifically, does restraint of euthanasia contribute to the high suicide rate among the elderly? Reviews of suicide by Frederick (44) and Shulman (45) show that the highest rate of suicide over the longest period is found in the elderly. The over-65 age group comprises 18% of the population and commits 23% of the suicides. The rate of successful suicides is highest in the elderly group, and they have the lowest rate of attempted suicide. The presence of serious physical illness is clearly one of the contributing causes of suicide in the elderly. Does the knowledge that euthanasia is not a realistic possibility, along with the fear of becoming depersonalized by a prolonged period of dying, help to make suicide more plausible? I know of no specific study to answer this question, but one is clearly needed. Only one study in Canada, by Kraus and colleagues (46), bears indirectly on attitudes of the elderly toward euthanasia and suicide. Elderly applicants to long-term care institutions ($N = 115$) and elderly residents of the community ($N = 141$) were questioned on their potential interest in active euthanasia, and a series of questions were asked that presupposed different customs about euthanasia. The respondent was asked to imagine that he or she had a very serious illness with no hope of recovery and with much pain and suffering. The choices that were available were:

1. Carrying on as best they could
2. An injection that caused death painlessly and quickly
3. A lethal pill that could be taken at any time
4. Other options to be supplied by respondent

Of the respondents, 19% and 23%, respectively, said they would want a lethal injection, and 10% and 9%, respectively, said they would want a lethal pill. The majority in both groups, 56% and 46%, said that they would carry on as best they could. The remainder suggested either that they would carry on but reject life-prolonging procedures or that they were vague about an answer.

This study is indirect evidence because the respondents are not actually in the situation described. The study does not tell us what they would do. But the report does suggest that there may be a relationship in a certain number of cases between restraint of euthanasia and readiness to commit suicide in the elderly.

An indirect source on which to estimate the use of the freedom to choose euthanasia is to ask about the number of persons who have taken advantage of the provisions of the California Natural Death Act, passed in 1976. Although the act as legislated contains some compromises that may make it difficult to use or understand, the evidence to date suggests that it is rarely used. According to its provisions, the patient who is certifiably terminally ill can execute instructions to the physician to withhold treatment or life supports that prolong life. These instructions remain in effect after the patient becomes legally incompetent. Since the legislature provided no funds for an evaluation of actual use of the legal directive, there is no definitive information. Some reports do provide provisional data. Towers (47) wrote a substantial report on the status of the new act in 1978 and concluded that the major impact was probably symbolic in that death was more openly discussed in patient-physician relations and in public. Klutch (48), an official of the California Medical Association, conducted a survey of 168 physicians who had ordered at least 100 copies of the form. He received 112 replies. The respondents reported that 67 patients had made use of the directive. The respondents agreed that the act had not changed the way they had been practicing medicine but that the act had also been a positive force in the discussion of terminal illness with patients and families. Humphrey (49) quotes one of the drafters of the act in 1979 as estimating that it had been used "only 30 or 40 times in two years." One can conclude that possession of the document does not imply use. Exactly why the act is not being used needs more study and documentation; yet the four years' experience does lend support to the notion that legal possession of the right to choose euthanasia would not entail that large numbers of persons would use it.

In summary, the facts that are available suggest that there are persons who would use the freedom to choose euthanasia and that these persons comprise a significant number, probably highest in the elderly. On occasion, it seems, the restraint of euthanasia contributes to reasoning that results in suicide. If the legal right to practice euthanasia were granted, there would be no logical reason to suppose that large numbers of people would use it, especially if economic conditions supported a type of medical care that resulted in a high rate of interaction between patients and physicians.

Responding to Flew, there is a further moral question beyond these facts, about the justification for restricting the freedom to choose.

Economic Burden

There is no published argument for euthanasia solely on the basis of economic reasons. The economic burdens of terminal illness are usually listed by proponents of euthanasia among the causes of suffering that afflict the dying and their

Table 1. Costs of Terminal Illness

Economic		Social	
Direct	*Indirect*	*Direct*	*Indirect*
Hospital	Costs of	Mortality of	Pain
Physician services	deferred	bereavement	Loneliness
Drugs	plans,	Morbidity of	Fatigue
Transportation	education	bereavement	
Appliances		Behavior	
Home nursing care		problems in	
Funeral		children	
Burial			
Lost income of			
decedent			
Lost income of			
family, friends			

families. Russell (17) refers to the economic ruin that can devastate families following a costly terminal illness.

The ethical implications of the costs of terminal illness were reviewed by the author (50) in an article. Table 1 illustrates the types of costs of terminal illness. The social costs also have economic implications. There are good reasons to believe that the costs of the final year of life are a significant economic and social problem in the United States. Expenditures for health totaled $192 billion in 1978. In 1974, Mushkin (51) estimated that 22% of all hospital expenditures, except psychiatric, were for terminal illness. Since at least 40% of all health expenditures in 1978 were for hospitals (52), a figure of $17 billion for only hospital care of terminal illness can be derived. Much more research needs to be done in both the economic and social costs of dying, especially in comparing costs of dying at home, hospital, or hospice.

There are three reasons for believing that any legal proposal for euthanasia would not result in substantial reduction of costs. First, all euthanasia bills authorize action only for a patient who requests it and is certified by physicians to be in an irreversible state. Action would come at the end of the trajectory of the whole illness, and the greatest part of the expenditure will have been made. Second, the proposals do not affect the economic costs of supporting incompetent patients who could not request euthanasia. Third, the proposals do not include the costs of any monitoring system that would likely be needed to ensure the voluntary aspects of any legal system of euthanasia.

Does following the policy against euthanasia increase the total burden of suffering when one accounts for the often desperate economic measures (53) families must use to meet the costs of the last year of life? It is possible that such is the result for some families, but, on the assumption that willingness to use euthanasia is not synonomous with unwillingness to use the health-care system, with all its concomitant expenses, it is not reasonable to conclude that the policy against euthanasia contributes substantially to the economic causes of suffering.

Involuntary Euthanasia

Does the policy against voluntary beneficent euthanasia actually contribute to the incidence of acts of involuntary euthanasia? This question is the opposite of one of the classic questions about the consequences of capital punishment. Does the existence of capital punishment deter homicide and reduce violence? One can turn the question around with the policy against euthanasia and ask if one effect is encouragement of the killing of suffering patients in secret. I am drawn to exploring this possibility by following the logic of Flew's (41) argument:

> . . . there are, and for the foreseeable future will be, people afflicted with incurable and painful diseases who urgently and fixedly want to die quickly. The first argument is that a law which tries to prevent such sufferers from achieving this quick death, and usually thereby forces other people who care for them to watch their pointless pain helplessly, is a very cruel law. . . . In such cases the sufferer may be reduced to an obscene parody of a human being, a lump of suffering flesh eased only by intervals of drugged stupor. . . .

How many persons who care for patients and watch their pointless pain respond to helplessness by taking matters into their own hands and, without further consulting with the patient or family, perform an act that kills the patient? Mercy may be the motive, but the act is involuntary.

The twelve cases of euthanasia tried in American courts before 1973, cited by Veatch (54), except for one case in which a man strangled his 6-month-old son with Down's syndrome with a lamp cord, had enough features of a motive of mercy to convince juries to acquit seven cases, convict three on lesser charges, and to fail to indict one. The man in the Down's syndrome case was convicted of murder and given a life sentence that was later commuted to 6 years. The thirteenth and most recent case, in 1978, involved a nurse, Mary Rose Robaczynski (55), who was charged with murder for disconnecting the respirators of four patients. In court, she admitted disconnecting three patients who she believed to be dead. However, she did not consult with or request permission from a physician or the families for her action. Charges were dropped because of a consistently hung vote by a jury confused by Maryland's statute on the definition of death. The jury was not asked to make a judgment about her professional conduct in making unilateral decisions without consultation and consent but only about whether she killed a patient.

Robaczynski's conduct raises questions about the frequency of the so-called invisible act, which can be understood as involuntary euthanasia. Glaser and Strauss (56) reported observational studies and interviews in six hospitals in the Bay area of San Francisco in 1965. Two kinds of invisible acts were discussed, but no indications were given for frequency. In certain cases of patients who lingered long in dying, physicians, nurse, family, and even the patient were involved in decisions to speed up dying, but all were committed to a policy of secrecy to avoid publicity. In some cases, however, neither family nor patient was involved in the decision. There are no published studies, to my knowledge, on the incidence of decisions to hasten death by overdose or premature dose of narcotics or other measures.

Acts of involuntary euthanasia would probably be reduced if a form of voluntary euthanasia were available and the need for secrecy were overcome. There may be many more invisible acts that are not reported and prosecuted than cases that reach the courts. Why has there only been one euthanasia case in American courts since 1973? One answer may be that physicians are more conservative in managing the last days of life and prolonging life to avoid prosecution. Another, and a more likely answer, is the growing use of categorization of patients in intensive care, as is done at Beth Israel Hospital (57) and Massachusetts General Hospital (58).

POSITIVE CONSEQUENCES

Besides defending the moral policy against euthanasia by appeal to virtues, ideals, or principles, those who argue on the other side of the issue also point directly or indirectly to positive consequences that they believe have resulted from keeping faith with the policy. Beauchamp and Childress (59) and Veatch (54) review these consequences by type. Each can be examined here in some detail.

Protection of Vulnerable Persons from Abuse

If a policy of euthanasia were enacted, what kinds of persons may be most abused? Opponents of euthanasia single out the misdiagnosed, those in whom euthanasia just preceded a life-saving advance in therapy, the incompetent, and those who act out underlying but resolvable problems in either requesting or administering euthanasia.

The Misdiagnosed

The case of Helen Blanchfield (60) illustrates the potential for abuse of misdiagnosed persons. In 1976, Blanchfield was informed by an oncologist, Dr. Lewis Dennis, that she had multiple myeloma of the bone marrow, and she began chemotherapy. Dennis reportedly told her that she had "between one month and a year to live" and advised her to set her affairs in order. She resigned her job, mortgaged her home, and her son and daughter-in-law moved in with her. She made funeral arrangements and became very depressed. After six months of chemotherapy and deepening depression, a friend suggested a second opinion. Blanchfield pursued that goal at Sloan-Kettering Cancer Center. No evidence of multiple myeloma was found, and a new diagnosis of dysgammaglobulinemia was made. Blanchfield returned to private life and sued Dennis, winning a settlement of $800,000, which is now being appealed. If an option for euthanasia had been available, possibly Blanchfield may not have followed the advice of her friend.

The exact number of misdiagnoses in supposed terminal illness will likely never be known, although the single reports that do exist could be collated. The reported numbers are likely to be small, but one would expect to find variations within the strata of the practice of medicine and types of hospitals. Williamson and colleagues (61) reported that evaluation in one community hospital showed that more than one-half of the abnormal laboratory findings were either ignored or inadequately handled. One would expect misdiagnosis of hopeless illness to be more frequent in that setting.

Advances in Research

To what extent have lives been saved by introduction of new, life-saving therapies that might have otherwise been lost to euthanasia? Kamisar (62), a critic of legal proposals of euthanasia, wrote of the precarious nature of the decision that a patient is incurable, because of the possibility that a new cure could be made available through medical research. This line of criticism can lead to a positive claim that lives have been saved that may have otherwise been lost. To answer the question with accuracy, one would have to know something about the frequeny with which persons would use euthanasia. The earlier review of this question showed that a certain number of persons are disposed to use euthanasia, perhaps several thousand. If this presumption is correct, there would be a finite number of mistakes made by choosing euthanasia prematurely. Lives would be lost.

Other lives might be lost as a result of depression of medical research if euthanasia were successfully argued and legalized for the majority of cases of dying. The reader has only to imagine the difficulty of constructing a sensible rationale to invite a dying person to participate in a test of toxicity of a new drug or later to test the therapeutic value of the agent when the physician-investigator was also obligated to tell the patient that euthanasia was one option among others. The prevention of adventitious deaths is the hallmark of modern medicine, as Fox's (63) work illustrates on the evolution of medicine, and the same motivation nurtures medical research. Death at the end of the life cycle is not fought with the tenacity represented by the pact between the patient-volunteer and the physician-investigator in medical research in diseases that cause death prematurely. A truly fair euthanasia option should be made only to adults at every point in the life cycle, since it would be clearly unfair to offer euthanasia only to the very old person dying of a number of causes. An across-the-board euthanasia option would probably chill motivation to do research on cures of preventable lethal disease because it would beg the question of the value of doing such research at all if one would choose death from the same hands of the physician who also wanted to do research to prevent death from that disease. At this level, the euthanasia issue raises questions about the validity of the orientation of activism and meliorism from which physicians conduct medical research in the lethal diseases. Although one may not hold out hope for the patient who is currently dying of the disease, the justification can be made that participation in research now may benefit others in the future. If elective euthanasia is as preferable or more preferable than participating in research, why do the research at all? If the answer is that the future benefit to others who will be threatened by the disease would be chosen by enough persons to allow research to continue, the proponent of euthanasia has already predicted some adverse consequences to medical research. On this basis, one would have to add to the list of persons made vulnerable by euthanasia some of those who will suffer from diseases in which research may lead to cure.

Incompetence

A third group of vulnerable persons are the incompetent dying, those who may be at risk from an attempt to extend the argument for voluntary euthanasia to a logical next step, namely, euthanasia made available by a legal process based on the grounds that "if they could speak for themselves they would undoubtedly choose euthanasia." The incompetent dying include infants, children, the comatose, retarded, mentally infirm, and others who have been declared legally incompetent. Veatch (54) described a shrinking circle of incompetence due to a trend to value the rights of older minors and the mentally infirm. In the interest of space, only two groups of persons who could be especially vulnerable are discussed here to demonstrate that the numbers are significant.

Jonsen and Lister (64) estimated that 12 of every 1,000 live-born infants die of disease or distress that neonatal intensive care units attempt to meet. Despite improvements in these units, many of these infants will continue to die in the future. Infants who might be more at risk for euthanasia in these units, provided there were a floor of euthanasia for competent adults, are those born with defects that might have been detected earlier with prenatal diagnosis. Some parents may feel euthanasia to be their second chance for abortion and insist on pediatric euthanasia. On the assumptions that the efficacy of prenatal diagnosis will increase and that the supply will not meet the demand, there may be many times more such vulnerable infants in the future.

A larger group of more vulnerable persons is found at the other end of the life cycle in the increasing number of elderly persons with a chronic mental disorder who are institutionalized in nursing homes. Glasscote (65) reported on the more than 100% increase between 1965 and 1973 in the number of mentally ill nursing home residents more than 65 years of age, although the number of residents of that age in all types of psychiatric hospitals decreased by 30% to 40%. The increase was from 96,000 to 194,000. In the steadily growing number of elderly persons, the mentally infirm would be especially vulnerable to an extension of voluntary euthanasia. Mushkin and colleagues (66) forecast that expenditures for nursing home care in the year 2000 could be as high as $56.9 billion but in any case would not fall below $31.2 billion in the year 2000 prices. The weight of such expenditures could lend an additional warrant to an extension of the euthanasia argument.

I stress that these predictions of vulnerability assume the wedge of a change in moral policy against euthanasia. Some critics of abortion, especially Ramsey (67), use the wedge argument to forecast an increase of euthanasia of newborns or even other adults on the basis that permitting abortion increases the chances for successful argument for euthanasia and the ensuing deeds. The wedge argument against abortion can at least be examined empirically for its accuracy in forecasting. Even though the numbers of legal abortions have greatly increased since 1973 in the United States there has been a decrease in the reported cases of euthanasia when compared with the seven-year period before 1973. There is no information on unreported successful or unsuccessful attempts to do euthanasia. Further, although British surgeons began in the early 1970s to select infants with spina bifida and meningomyelocele for nontreatment (68), pediatric euthanasia such as directly hastening death by injections is not practiced in Great Britain. There is no necessary connection between abortion and euthanasia when examined in the light of recent historical experience. One could also assume that there is no necessary connection between an increasing opportunity to do euthanasia and its being done, unless the moral policy against it were changed.

Indirect Appeal for Help
A fourth group of vulnerable dying are those who request euthanasia as an indirect means of appealing for help with a resolvable problem or who could be given euthanasia by persons who are themselves troubled by guilt or rage

toward the dying person and redirect it in a supposedly beneficial act. The problem of self-rejection by the dying and the guilt of caretakers of the dying has been described extensively in the psychiatric literature, as reviewed by Parkes (40). One can gain perspective on this problem without moving to a scenario in which euthanasia is legalized. In the current setting of medical care of critically ill patients, there are often requests by patients or family for death with dignity, which means suspension of attempts to prolong life or withdrawal of life supports already administered. Jackson and Younger (69) report ambivalence and confusion in six recent cases of patients or family members who requested death with dignity from their physicians in a critical care unit. If the physicians had simply responded to the patient's autonomy, they would have not only overlooked deeper psychological and medical realities, but they would have made serious errors in clinical judgment. Physicians were confronted with ambivalence, depression, an identification of a hidden problem, fear, confused perceptions in the family, and confused perceptions in the medical staff of a patient's concept of death with dignity. Each patient presented a complex problem and could have been severely abused by a literalistic approach to the current ethical practice of allowing patients to die. If such is the case in the current scene, one might expect an even greater degree of ambivalence and confusion if euthanasia became a reality.

The entire spectrum of these four vulnerable groups constitutes a large number of persons, many times larger than the number of persons who may be disposed to use euthanasia under moral and legal sanctions. Do the needs and interests of these persons for protection from potential harm outweigh the needs and interests of those who believe that they could benefit from euthanasia? Although the number of vulnerable persons who would actually be at risk of mistakes, errors, and misjudgments in the context of permissible euthanasia is smaller than the total number of persons who make up these groups at any given time, it is apparent that if one looks only at the numbers, the vulnerable ones would still be greater than those who would actually make a claim while dying that euthanasia would benefit them. Does the fact that the numbers are larger constitute a claim that has weight in morality? Ought we to keep the policy because we might protect more people? The answer to this question is not simple, for the simple prevention of euthanasia is not manifestly good if the conditions that give rise to the appeal for euthanasia are not met, understood, and relieved. Only to prevent the practice of euthanasia while not addressing the causes would appear to be mere statistical morality.

Reform of Medical Care of the Dying

Viewed from an evolutionary perspective, medical care of the dying in the twentieth century is being gradually reformed to embody both the singular dedication to the dying of the work of religious orders of the past and modern scientific principles of medical care of the dying and their families. Commitment to the care of the dying is not new, as shown by the history of the medieval hospice and the various orders of men and women whose work brought solace and comfort to the dying. Stoddard (70) described the rise of the modern hospice movement in Great Britain, Europe, and the United States, a seedbed for the new forms of research and development of care of the terminally ill that can and are being applied in many other settings.

In the evolution of modern medicine, as described by Fox (63), the goal became the prevention of adventitious death, and the modern hospital and its staff measured competence by the ability to forestall or defeat death. However, it became increasingly difficult in the hospital to care for those whose death occurred at the end of the life cycle or whose disease defied the cutting edge of medical research. The fact that the hospital separates the patient from the family can encourage a more rapid recovery of a patient who is surrounded by the expert help of the hospital staff rather than an anxious family, but it does not help a patient who will not recover or the family to accomplish the tasks of dying. Also, a scientific and medical approach to the dying calls for different methods of drug administration, symptom relief, and ongoing evaluation of the patient's condition.

Adherence to the moral policy against euthanasia was one force among several that contributed to the social and political pressure to provide a reformed medical care of the terminally ill. Although sentiment and support for euthanasia rose and fell at various points during the century, at no point were the arguments for euthanasia so persuasive as to permit it morally or legally. The argument to maintain the policy had to depend, in some measure, on an implicit promise to address the conditions of pain, depersonalization, and gross economic burdens that lent validity to the appeal for euthanasia. If little or nothing could have been done positively to remedy these conditions, it is likely that the policy against euthanasia would have been weakened by the evidence of suffering and gradually modified, for it would have been doubly cruel not only to perpetuate such conditions but to do so in the name of morality. The steady rise of interest in reformed medical care of the dying and its results reinforced the moral policy against euthanasia.

What are the reformed principles of medical care for the terminally ill, and what is the evidence that the majority of cases of dying persons could benefit from their application?

The NIH Subcommittee report (39) formulated these principles for terminal care:

1. The patient and the family, not the disease, are the unit of care.
2. Treatment of symptoms, including psychological and social, of terminal illness is of prime importance in patient comfort.
3. Follow-up of survivors (bereavement care) has benefit and should be included in all programs of terminal care.
4. Home care as well as institutional care must be a part of the program for the terminally ill and must be available 24 hours a day.
5. Terminal care requires a multidisciplinary approach involving physicians, nurses, social workers, dieticians, clergy, volunteers, etc. . . .
6. Regular medical evaluation is required to determine if disease-oriented treatment would be of value to the patient and to provide necessary management of symptoms.

The evaluation research that has followed efforts to deliver terminal care in accordance with these principles has been meager because of the energy required to begin new programs, but what has been published is encouraging. In addition to the research of Parkes (31), Hinton (37), and Martinson (38) cited earlier, the recent publication of a major collection of patient reports, studies, and discussions edited by Saunders (71), substantially enlarges the empirical basis of evaluation of reformed care of the dying. The early cumulative evidence is that adaptation of the hospice principles significantly reduces chronic pain, increases closeness in the family, and reduces depression.

No studies exist with large numbers comparing the costs of hospital care with other settings capable of applying home care or hospice care. Reports from St. Christopher's Hospice (72) and the Palliative Care Unit of the Royal Victoria Hospital of Montreal (73) indicate significant savings when compared with the standard general hospital approach to care. In the United States, the Health Care Finance Administration of the Department of Health, Education and Welfare has inaugurated the Medicare and Medicaid Hospice Demonstration Program to study costs and use of services on an outpatient and home care basis. Prohibitions against paying for certain costs will be waived for participating hospice organizations in the project. Much more should be learned about the comparative costs issue from this study.

The state of the art of reformed medical care of the dying is much more developed in Great Britain. However, the diffusion of the principles of medical care of the dying and new forms of institutionalizing the principles are developing rapidly in both Great Britain and the United States. The ethical problem now facing policymakers is how the most fitting approach to experiments to test the delivery of terminal care can be formulated. Currently, eight organizational approaches to reformed terminal care are being used:

1. A hospital with a home care program
2. A palliative care unit in a hospital
3. A home care and outpatient program
4. A freestanding hospice with physical facilities and home care program
5. A hospital with a team of experts who work with dying patients and families; dying patients are not separated from others
6. A hospital whose leadership attempts to reeducate staff and establish a reformed approach in the whole hospital
7. A nurse-directed home care program; physicians serve as consultants to nurse
8. A hospice attached to a teaching hospital that is also equipped with a home care program

Each of these approaches has its strengths and weaknesses. Each will be used in different ways, and, for purposes of policymaking in this field, it is too early to make any more than educated guesses to guide the evaluation, research, and planning that will be needed to make later decisions about which approaches are best suited to particular locales. The probabilities are, however, that the eighth model will be best suited in the United States to channel both ancient and modern tributaries into the care of the terminally ill in metropolitan areas and to foster the research and development necessary to diffuse advances in this area to smaller communities. The total cost of building and equipping a national system of freestanding hospices would be significantly greater than adapting space and methodology in the setting of a teaching hospital, where the patient's interests could be reinforced by staff of a separate hospice unit and also served in a home care program.

To summarize, convictions that arose in part from the moral policy against euthanasia were translated into concrete actions to alleviate suffering of the dying and their families. To this extent, efforts to implement hospice principles are one of the consequences of the moral policy itself. A simple thought experiment that imagines a bill before Congress to legalize euthanasia concurrently with a bill before the same body to fund cost comparisons of hospice and hospital care will leave the reader with a picture of the relationship between euthanasia and hospice care.

Legal and Legislative Developments

Another set of consequences, represented by legal and legislative developments, can be examined that are alternatives to euthanasia. These public policies are not direct consequences of only the moral policy against euthanasia, but they are not completely unrelated. The policy against euthanasia should be seen as a moral limit beyond which no legal or legislative remedy has been allowed to proceed. Also, to the extent that legislation and court decisions encourage social directions and embody principles drawn from morality, these activities clearly have drawn on the policy against euthanasia while creating a wider latitude of freedom to intervene in the dying process without the penalty or blame that is attached to euthanasia.

Veatch has reviewed extensively the legislative (74), legal (54), and public policy options (75) that bear on the issue of euthanasia and the decision-making process with respect to dying persons. In the interests of space, only the most prominent trends are noted here:

1. Legislatures and courts have increasingly strengthened the right of competent individuals to refuse any medical treatment for whatever reason they desire, with the exception of prisoners, if the treatment is offered for their own good. All life-prolonging treatments are included in this statement.
2. These bodies have increasingly strengthened the right of guardians or family to make decisions for incompetent patients with respect to refusal of life-prolonging treatment, as long as stipulations of due process are followed.
3. These bodies have increasingly moved to protect physicians who participate in such decisions from charges of homicide for following the instructions of the patient, family, or guardian.

These trends follow a fundamental cultural shift in the attitudes of physicians, lawyers, legislators, and the public, as noted by Crane (76), from an absolutist application of the sanctity of life principle to a modified position based on a desire to avoid the harms of unreasonable prolongation of life. Although there are many complex and as yet unresolved questions of due process in cases of children and incompetent individuals, a clear direction has been set by courts and legislatures of relativization of the earlier absolute to preserve life at all costs. The appeal for euthanasia was a protest against the consequences of the absolutist position, but the moral policy against euthanasia has guided the general outlines and limits of the legal remedies. A postmodern attitude about death, as noted by Fox (63), is more open to cessation of treatment for the irreversibly dying, while remaining opposed to euthanasia.

DISCUSSION

I have attempted to weigh the claims of those on both sides of the euthanasia debate in terms of consequences about which something tangible can be known. The reader must judge whether I take the validity of the appeal for euthanasia seriously.

If the moral policy were changed, certain good results would ensue. A significant number of persons, largely elderly persons, would not commit suicide, because they would believe that euthanasia would be a better choice. An unknown number of involuntary acts of euthanasia would be prevented because they would be unnecessary, and the patient and family would have the benefit of concurring in the decision. Furthermore, and probably most important, a significant number of persons who are now being restrained by the policy could exercise their freedom to choose. Although there would be much more debate about whether making this option available was a good in itself, for the purposes of this discussion a new exercise of freedom should be weighed in the balance of its own merits.

If the moral policy against euthanasia remains unchanged, another set of good consequences will continue to ensue. A significant number of vulnerable persons will be protected from mistakes, misjudgments, or malevolence that would occur if euthanasia were permitted. Medical research on lethal diseases can continue with the participation of more of those who are currently afflicted. New forms of medical care especially designed for the terminally ill and their families will be slowly but increasingly offered in a variety of institutional forms. On the basis of evidence that has accumulated in the past 10 years, these forms of care address in a significant way almost all the underlying causes of the appeal for euthanasia. Further, new directions in legal and legislative reasoning will expand freedom to intervene in the dying process by withholding life-prolonging treatment on request of the patient, with due process in cases of incompetent patients, and by decisions of the physician in consultation with family and patient.

Which set of consequences has the greatest potential for benefiting the greatest number of dying persons and their family members in the greatest number of ways? Which set of consequences has the possibility of bringing about the greatest degree of harmony in a diverse society to prevent the greatest degree of violence and to bring about the greatest amount of needed change? An examination of the consequences persuades me, and should, it is hoped, persuade the reader that there is a strong case against euthanasia.

The case against euthanasia is not an absolutely closed case, however. The strength of the appeal for euthanasia is to remedy cruelty and dehumanization. If the promise of reformed medical care of the dying is blocked by intransigence, competition from other medical sectors, or political opposition, the case for euthanasia remains open, and the evidence of suffering will gradually make it more plausible.

Finally, I should respond to the moral issue raised by Flew as to the justification for restraining the freedom of those who would freely choose euthanasia. The justification is based on an examination of consequences that shows that maintaining the moral policy will result in more good and restrain more evil, produce more harmony and resolve more conflict, and restrain the killing of innocent persons while meeting much of the suffering that gives rise to the request for euthanasia. The interests of many more persons will be served in the long run by maintaining the moral policy while nurturing the many ways in which society has already responded to the compassionate insights in arguments for euthanasia. The evidence of consequences points to a moral basis for an appeal to those who espouse Flew's position to join in the struggle to make justice in medical care of the dying more universal. For without an extension of justice, there is not so strong a case to justify the continued restraint of freedom of those who would choose euthanasia if they could. For the future, legislatures should be pressed to provide leadership for reform of medical care of the dying, rather than legalization of euthanasia.

REFERENCES

1. Kohl M: *Beneficent Euthanasia*. Buffalo, NY, Prometheus Books, 1975, p 130.
2. Callahan D: *Abortion: Law, Choice and Morality*. New York, Macmillan, 1970, p 341.
3. Hare RM: *Freedom and Reason*. Oxford, Oxford University Press, 1977, p 4.
4. Hare RM: Can the moral philosopher help? in Spicker SF, Engelhardt HT (eds): *Philosophical Medical Ethics: Its Nature and Significance*. Boston, D Reidel Publishing Company, 1975, p 58.
5. Hare RM: *Language of Morals*. Oxford, Oxford University Press, 1977, p 1.
6. Fye WB: Active euthanasia: An historical survey of its conceptual origins and introduction into medical thought. *Bull Hist Med* 52:492, 1978.
7. Gruman GJ: Death and dying: Euthanasia and sustaining life (historical perspectives), in Reich WT: *Encyclopedia of Bioethics*. New York, Free Press, 1978, p 261.
8. Edelstein L: *The Hippocratic Oath: Text, Translation, and Interpretation*. Baltimore, Johns Hopkins Press, 1943.
9. Davidowicz LS: *The War Against the Jews: 1933–1945*. New York, Holt, Rinehart and Winston, 1975.
10. Baier K: *The Moral Point of View*. New York, Random House, 1965, p 99.
11. Swiss Academy of Medicine: Guidelines concerning euthanasia. *Hastings Cent Rep* 7:30, 1977.
12. Fletcher JC: Abortion, euthanasia, and care of defective newborns. *N Engl J Med* 292:75, 1975.
13. Hartshorne C: *The Logic of Perfection*. Lasalle, Ill, Open Court Publishing Co, 1962.
14. Ogden SH: *The Reality of God*. New York, Harper and Row, 1967.
15. Frankena WK: *Ethics*, ed 2. Englewood Cliffs, NJ, 1973, p 113.
16. Fletcher J: *Situation Ethics*. Philadelphia, Westminister Press, 1966.
17. Russell OF: *Freedom to Die*. New York, Human Sciences Press, 1975, p 104.
18. Aiken HD: *Reason and Conduct*. New York, Alfred A Knopf, Inc, 1962, p 87.
19. Rachels J: Active and passive euthanasia. *N Engl J Med* 292:78, 1975.
20. Freeman J: Is there a right to die—quickly? *J Pediatr* 80:904, 1972.
21. Fletcher JC: The "right" to live and the "right" to die, in Kohl M (ed): *Beneficent Euthanasia*. Buffalo, NY, Prometheus Books, 1975, p 46.
22. Mannes M: *Last Rights*. New York, New American Library, Inc, 1975, p 9.
23. Butler RN: A humanistic approach to our last days. *Dallas Med J* 64:509, 1978.
24. Ryder CF, Ross DM: Terminal care: Issues and alternatives. *Public Health Rep* 92:22, 1977.
25. Comptroller General of the United States: Report to Congress, Hospice Care: A Growing Concept in the United States. HRD-79-50, 1979.
26. Ford G: Terminal care in the National Health Service, in Saunders CM (ed): *The Management of Terminal Disease*. London, Edward Arnold Publishers, Ltd, 1978, p 169.

27. Saunders CM: Editorial note, unrelieved relievable distress, in Saunders CM (ed): *The Management of Terminal Disease.* London, Edward Arnold Publishers, Ltd, 1978, p 65.

28. Turnbull F: Intractable pain. *Proc R Soc Med* 47:155, 1954.

29. Aitken-Swan J: Nursing the late cancer patient at home. *Practitioner* 183:64, 1959.

30. Oster MW, Vizel M, Turgeon LR: Pain of terminal cancer patients. *Arch Intern Med* 138:1801, 1978.

31. Parkes CM: Evaluation of family care in terminal illness, in Pritchard LR, et al (eds): *The Family and Death.* New York, Columbia University Press, 1977.

32. Twycross RG: Relief of pain, in Saunders CM (ed): *idem,* p 65.

33. West TS: Management of pain in the terminally ill, in Ng LK (ed): *Proceedings of a National Conference on Pain, Discomfort, and Humanitarian Care,* National Institutes of Health, 1979 (in press).

34. Kubler-Ross E: On death and dying. *JAMA* 2:174, 1972.

35. Oken D: What to tell cancer patients. *JAMA* 175:1120, 1961.

36. Novack DH, et al: Changes in physicians' attitudes towards the cancer patient. *JAMA* 241:896, 1979.

37. Hinton J: Comparison of places and policies for terminal care. *Lancet* 1:29, 1979.

38. Martinson IM, et al: Home care for children dying of cancer. *Pediatrics* 2:106, 1978.

39. National Institutes of Health: Report of the sub-committee on terminal illness. Interagency Committee on New Therapies for Pain and Discomfort, 1979 (unpublished).

40. Parkes CM: Psychological aspects, in Saunders CM (ed): *idem,* p 56.

41. Flew A: The principle of euthanasia, in Beauchamp TL: *Ethics and Public Policy.* Englewood Cliffs, NJ, Prentice-Hall, 1975, p 409.

42. Morison R: Death: Process or event? *Science* 173:694, 1971.

43. Gallup: Approval of mercy killing rises. *Am Med News,* Aug 13, 1973, p 11.

44. Frederick CJ: Current trends in suicidal behavior in the United States. *Am J Psychother* 32:181, 1978.

45. Schulman K: Suicide and parasuicide in old age: A review. *Age Ageing* 7:201, 1978.

46. Kraus AS, et al: Potential interest of the elderly in active euthanasia. *Can Fam Physician* 23:123, 1977.

47. Towers B: The impact of the California Natural Death Act. *J Med Ethics* 4:96, 1978.

48. Klutch M: Survey results after one year's experience with the Natural Death Act. *West J Med* 128:329, 1978.

49. Humphrey D: Natural Death Act: Few benefit. *Los Angeles Times,* Jan 8, 1979.

50. Fletcher JC: Ethics and the costs of dying, in Milunsky A (ed): *Genetics and the Law* (in press).

51. Mushkin SJ: Terminal illness and incentives for health care use, in Mushkin SJ (ed): *Consumer Incentives for Health Care.* New York, Prodist, 1974, p 183.

52. Department of Health, Education and Welfare: *Health: United States.* No (PHS) 78-1232, 1978, p 379.

53. Cancer Care, Inc: *The Impact, Costs, and Consequences of Catastrophic Illness on Patients and Families.* New York, 1973.

54. Veatch RM: *Death, Dying and the Biological Revolution.* New Haven, Conn, Yale University Press, 1976, p 79.

55. Saperstein S: Unhooked system, nurse says. *Washington Post,* Mar 20, 1979, p C3.

56. Glaser BG, Strauss AL: *Awareness of Dying.* Chicago, Aldine Publishing Company, 1965, p 198.

57. Rabkin MT, Gillerman JD, Rice NR: Orders not to resuscitate. *N Engl J Med* 295:364, 1976.

58. Clinical Care Committee, Massachusetts General Hospital: Optimum care for hopelessly ill patients. *N Engl J Med.* 295:362, 1976.

59. Beauchamp TL, Childress C: *Principles of Biomedical Ethics.* New York, Oxford University Press, 1979, p 110.

60. Weiser B: It wasn't cancer. *Washington Post,* Jan 18, 1980, p A1.

61. Williamson JW, Alexander M, Miller GE: Continuing education and patient care research. *JAMA* 201:938, 1967.

62. Kamisar Y: From euthanasia legislation: Some non-religious objections, in Gorovitz S, et al (eds): *Moral Problems in Medicine*. Englewood Cliffs, NJ, 1976, p 410.

63. Fox R: Medical evolution, in Fox R (ed): *Essays in Medical Sociology*. New York, John Wiley & Sons, 1979, p 499.

64. Jonsen AR, Lister G: Infants and ethics. *Hastings Cent Rep* 8:15, 1978.

65. Glasscote R, et al: *Old Folks at Homes*. American Psychiatric Association, Washington, DC, 1976, p 23.

66. Mushkin SJ, et al: Cost of disease and illness in the United States in the year 2000. *Pub Health Rep* 93:544, 1978.

67. Ramsey P: Reference points in deciding about abortion, in Noonan JT (ed): *The Morality of Abortion*. Cambridge, Harvard University Press, 1970, p 60.

68. Lorber J: Selective treatment of mylomeningocele: To treat or not to treat? *Pediatrics* 53:307, 1974.

69. Jackson DL, Younger S: Patient autonomy and "death with dignity." *N Engl J Med* 301:404, 1979.

70. Stoddard S: *The Hospice Movement*. Briarcliff Manor, NY, Stein and Day Publishers, 1978.

71. Saunders CM: *The Management of Terminal Disease*. London, Edward Arnold Publishers, 1978.

72. St. Christopher's Hospice: Forty First Newsletter, Analysis of Nursing Costs, 51-53 Lawrie Park Rd Lond SE 26, March, 1978.

73. Palliative Care Service, Royal Victoria Hospital: Report to McGill University. Montreal, October, 1976.

74. Veatch RM: Death and dying: The legislative options. *Hastings Cent Rep* 7:5, 1977.

75. Veatch RM: Death and dying: Euthanasia and sustaining life: Public policies, in Reich WT (ed): *Encyclopedia of Bioethics*, vol 1, New York, The Free Press, 1978, p 278.

76. Crane D: *The Sanctity of Social Life: Physicians' Treatment of Critically Ill Patients*. New York, Russell Sage Foundation, 1975, p 206.

Part 4

OTHER TREATMENT AND METHODS OF RESEARCH

23

High-Dose Methotrexate with Rescue: An Effective Treatment for Refractory Neoplasm

Isaac Djerassi

Keith Mills

Henry G. Ohanissian

Jung Sun Kim

High-dose methotrexate with citrovorum factor rescue (HDMTX-CF) is still a frontier modality in chemotherapy. The full scope of its clinical value and of its antitumor activity is yet to be defined. Unpredictable and catastrophic toxicity has been a major obstacle to its orderly development. Therefore, the basic tenet of this approach, namely, the dose escalation of methotrexate (MTX) on successive treatments until tumor response is observed, remains the least widely studied aspect of methotrexate therapy.

Although the clinical trials reporting tumor responses far outweigh those describing failures, the incidence and duration of the remissions reported are quite inconsistent. This is, however, to be expected when using this modality in purely clinical settings. More often than not, dose schedules and procedures whose details were selected to comply with basic knowledge and practical reasons are modified to fit the facilities or the working schedule of the investigators. These modifications are usually on the "safe side," meaning limited MTX dosage or undue and excessive citrovorum factor (CF) rescue–all with an inevitable impact on effectiveness or safety. The best clinical results were obtained by experienced investigators who tried to reproduce prior observations before engaging in freehand modifications. The basic reason for the contrasting observations in this field is, beyond doubt, the lack of attention given to the mechanisms responsible for the therapeutic advantage of using both MTX and CF.

The following discussion, therefore, focuses on the rationale, concepts, and hypotheses that led to and still guide the development of the HDMTX-CF approach to chemotherapy. Careful consideration and analysis of this information may resolve at least some of the misconceptions complicating its further use.

In 1947 Sidney Farber (1) successfully used the folic acid antagonist Aminopterin to induce remissions in children with acute lymphocytic leukemia. By the end of the next decade cancer chemotherapy was an established treatment modality, and a folic acid antagonist, Amethopterin (methotrexate), was responsible for the first chemotherapeutic cure of a malignant tumor—chorioepithelioma (2). Despite the extensive basic studies of the mechanism of action of antifols and of CF, the clinical usefulness of these compounds during the 1950s remained quite limited. Even in acute leukemia, MTX assumed a modest position among the effective agents, well behind steroids and 6-mercatopurine.

A second wave of progress in the field of antifols was started in the 1960s with the introduction of the HDMTX, followed or not by CF rescue (3–5). Remarkably, no controversy complicated the pioneering work in this field from 1963 until 1972. The few periodic reports on this modality were viewed as a pharmacological curiosity consistent with the scientific temperament of its main proponent. Early confirmation and extension of these observations by Bertino (7,8) also failed to encourage widespread studies of HDMTX. Not until 1971 did Sidney Farber and his associates initiate the first study in osteogenic sarcoma (9). The dramatic responses of the first few patients with recurrent and terminal disease, treated by Jaffe, occurred while osteogenic sarcoma was still considered the most hopeless of all solid tumors (10). In May of 1972, Farber and Jaffe, soon joined by Frei, initiated the adjuvant study of HDMTX in osteogenic sarcoma, thereby focusing attention on this form of chemotherapy ever since (11). The combined efforts of Bertino (12), Frei (13,14), Goldman (15), Chabner (16), and, of course, those of Jaffe (10,11), Rosen (17,18), and Isaacoff (19), supported by imaginative and meticulous work in Europe by Kotz and Salzer (20), Wilmanns and Sauer (21) started finally filling in the gaps of knowledge in this area. This information was especially pertinent to the occasional and unpredictable failures to prevent toxicity with CF. Based on this new knowledge, a safe dose schedule for CF rescue was recently developed (22), allowing for large-scale and cooperative studies of HDMTX, previously considered impractical.

SIGNIFICANCE OF THE HIGH-DOSE METHOTREXATE–RESCUE APPROACH

A major source of the disagreement concerning the potential of HDMTX was the premature expectation of a dose schedule suitable for routine care of patients with various tumors. The lack of a single and universally effective dose schedule detracted from the central contribution of this research, namely, the introduction into chemotherapy of considerations based on the known mechanisms of action of a drug and bringing clinical pharmacology into the actual treatment of the patients. Another contribution of these studies was the concept of the rescue of normal tissues from the effects of a drug while retaining its antitumor activity. The intellectual impact of these concepts is already felt in recent studies on thymidine for MTX rescue (14) and for rescue or enhancement of the effects of 5-fluorouracil (5-FU) (23). Similarly, a rational approach, founded on basic pharmacology, was recently announced for the combined use of MTX and of 5-FU (24). The HDMTX-CF rescue thus signaled a new era in the field of chemotherapy, making the transition from the old "blind" attack on all growing cells to a sophisticated manipulation of the DNA synthesis of cancer cells while minimizing interference with normal dividing tissues.

POINTS OF CONTENTION CONCERNING HIGH-DOSE METHOTREXATE

Recent literature on HDMTX does, indeed, contain diverging data and conclusions. Remarkably, however, clinical effectiveness in a variety of tumors has been reported from almost all major cancer centers in this country. A 29% response rate in patients with terminal and unresponsive breast cancer was observed at the M. D. Anderson Institute in Houston (25). The addition of HDMTX to the CMF regimen for breast cancer patients resulted in the more effective super CMF at the Sidney Farber Institute in Boston (26). At the same institution, HDMTX was of value also in the treatment of oat cell cancer of the lung (27). Bertino and his associates at Yale found that head and neck tumors respond to this treatment (8,28). His findings were recently fully confirmed and expanded by the Harvard group (29). At Roswell Park Memorial Institute in Buffalo, Freeman observed favorable responses in pediatric non-Hodgkin's lymphoma (30). A most recent report from the Sloan-Kettering Memorial Hospital indicated a high degree of effectiveness in cancer of the bladder (31). The results of Rosen in osteogenic sarcoma (18,32), again at the Sloan-Kettering Memorial Hospital in New York, confirmed and surpassed those of Jaffe in Boston (11).

In contrast to these observations made by experienced investigators in some of the most prestigious cancer research institutions in this country, devoted fully to the study of HDMTX, a smaller number of publications reported negative findings such as in cancer of the lung (33,34).

Characteristically these observations were made by cooperative groups or by individual investigators during their first clinical experience with this form of chemotherapy.

An observation frequently quoted to revive doubts in the biological activity of HDMTX is a claim by investigators at the Mayo Clinic. A regimen including HDMTX for adjuvant therapy of osteogenic sarcoma produced favorable results in 50% of the patients, but their simultaneous untreated controls apparently did just as well (35). This observation, right or wrong, was communicated via the grapevine before publication and was somehow interpreted to mean that HDMTX is ineffective against this tumor. This logic overlooked the numerous reports from centers in this country and abroad documenting major objective responses in primary or recurrent osteogenic sarcoma (9,17,20). The controversy about the value of adjuvant chemotherapy in osteogenic sarcoma is an issue beyond the scope of this discussion. It may suffice to mention that the 50% survival at the Mayo Clinic of untreated osteogenic sarcoma patients is well surpassed by the latest 80% survivals in New York (31) and in Vienna (36).

Another major point of contention is the need for really high doses of MTX and for progressive escalation of the amounts given to a patient. The first point is addressed to the existence of a dose-effect relationship when using MTX. The ineffectiveness of the conventional daily 5 to 10 mg or of the 30 mg/m² of MTX twice weekly for MTX-resistant leukemia, non-Hodgkin's lymphoma, osteogenic sarcoma, breast cancer, and oat cell lung cancer is well known. The effectiveness of higher doses in those tumors has been repeatedly confirmed (4,5,27,30,37–39). This alone establishes the dose-effect relationship. The HDMTX pulse, at least in the hands of investigators fully devoted to its study, seems endowed with antitumor activity absent with conventional doses.

The second question of how high a dose is high enough for a specific tumor, however, remains unanswered at this time. Without directly challenging the threshold principle (40), different investigators have limited their maximal doses of MTX to different predetermined values. Bertino obviously feels comfortable only within 3 g/M² body surface and benevolently leaves what he calls "industrial doses" to others (41). Frei, on the other hand, ventures as high as 7.5 g of MTX/M² body surface area. The unfortunate consequences of these self-imposed limits is that whenever these doses fail, the validity of the whole approach is questioned, especially by those unaware of the concepts under investigation. One obvious reason for the self-imposed limits on dose escalation of MTX was the risk associated at that time with higher doses. Another and equally effective reason was and still is the cost and availability of the drug. The fail-safe equimolar CF rescue (22) may resolve the disagreement on upper limits of escalation by allowing new and safe studies of a cooperative nature. The cost of such treatments will be easily reduced to levels competitive with other drugs, once the need for industrial doses is well established.

The biological antitumor activity of HDMTX-CF is, therefore, well established in patients untreatable with conventional doses of MTX (40,42). The dose-effect relationship is proved beyond contention by the same studies.

The need for escalation is mainly in question when doses higher than these acceptable at various centers are concerned. Consistently effective rescue and better understanding of the mechanisms involved in the therapeutic advantage of HDMTX-CF are likely to resolve any remaining differences of opinion.

WORKING CONCEPTS IN THE STUDY OF HIGH-DOSE MTX-CF

The early studies on HDMTX were in fact an exploration on the clinical level of the mechanisms of action of MTX and of resistance to antifols. The practicality of specific dose schedules of MTX, with or without CF rescue, for routine treatments was never emphasized.

Unfortunately, almost all clinical investigators in the "post osteogenic sarcoma era" viewed HDMTX-CF as a new "drug" to try for treatment of specific tumors, emphasizing side effects, overall clinical benefit, costs, and logistics of the treatment when used in routine care. The primary concern of the original studies on HDMTX-CF, namely, the problem of resistance to antifols, was largely overlooked in regard to both theoretical and practical implications.

Remarkably, the investigators who helped develop or apply these concepts, including, but not only, Bertino, Frei, Rosen, and Jaffe, were its most successful clinical investigators. For this reason, the following discussion emphasizes the initial hypothesis for HDMTX-CF and its subsequent evolution and modification as a result of accumulated clinical and experimental observations.

1. The first hypothetical premise and the origin of all studies on HDMTX-CF was that resistance to antifols (i.e., methotrexate) is never absolute. It was seen instead as a variable tolerance to such agents (3,4,43). The working hypothesis proposed that this resistance tolerance could perhaps be overcome by increasing the number of MTX molecules entering the cell. This first and most important assumption was based on the mechanism of failure to respond to antifols, suggested by the work of Bertino, namely, the increased cell levels of dihydrofolic acid reductase lead to resistance to antifols. This enzyme is the one responsible for the conversion of folic acid into CF or folinic acid. We interpreted this to mean that failure to neutralize all of the enzyme could occur either because of an excess of enzyme or because of insufficient MTX molecules entering the cell. In either case, resistance could perhaps be overcome by forcing more molecules into the cell.

2. A second major assumption at the start of these studies was that saturation of cells with MTX can be achieved by passive diffusion of the drug when the active transport mechanism of the cell is not sufficient (4,43).

3. Because of the stoicheometric and irreversible (44) binding of MTX to the intracellular dihydrofolic acid reductase, a short-lasting high intracellular concentration was considered possibly sufficient to cause cell death later, during the S phase of mitosis. This particular concept was corrected recently, following Goldman's (15) demonstration of the importance of an excess of free intracellular MTX to maintain complete enzyme saturation.

4. The response to small amounts of MTX depends on the efficiency of the active transport mechanism of the cell for this agent. The efficacy of the high doses was considered, instead, dependent on the extent of passive diffusion (permeability) of the cell membrane to MTX.

5. It was noted that the rate and extent of passive diffusion is determined by the concentration of the agent (C) and the time allowed for it to occur (t). The amount of MTX entering the cell passively was expected, therefore, to vary according to the product of $C \times t$ (3,4,43).

6. Various cell types require different amounts of intracellular MTX to saturate all the variable amounts of dihydrofolic acid reductase. It was anticipated, therefore, that different $C \times t$ will be required to achieve the MTX concentrations needed in cells with different amounts of enzyme and different permeability to the drug under passive diffusion, in order to prevent completely folic acid reduction.

7. The variable requirement for intracellular MTX by various cancer cells and meeting it by increasing the dose of MTX was more recently formulated as the "dose threshold" principle (40,45). The sum total of this principle is that different tumor cell types, and even the same type of tumor in individual patients, can achieve adequate intracellular concentrations of MTX under various high values of $C \times t$. Anything below a specific $C \times t$ value is completely ineffective. Tumor response is not observed until the $C \times t$ surpasses the threshold value for the tumor cell under study. Since the time

factor in the C × t cannot be extended freely without risking serious toxicity (4,40), the drug concentration, determined by the dose of MTX, remains the practical variable. In other words, the effective dose of MTX varies from one tumor to another and even from one patient to the next. This effective dose must be determined for each patient by gradually escalating the dose on consecutive treatments. Failure to respond to small (1 to 2 g/M^2) or moderate doses (6 to 7 g/M^2) of MTX may be followed by tumor reduction when really high doses (12 to 20 g/M^2) are administered. The dose escalation of MTX on consecutive treatments was derived from these observations and was recommended as a means to determine and then use the optimal threshold dose of MTX for each type of tumor in individual patients.

8. The "shifting threshold" principle (40,45) is a corollary of the concepts discussed above. It is based on observations of initial response to a specific dose of MTX, followed by eventual relapse, despite maintenance with periodic treatments with the same dose. When higher doses of MTX are administered, a new regression of the tumor is again seen. These observations are consistent with the expected behavior of large numbers of cells when exposed to toxic agents. Slight variations of permeability to the MTX most likely account for the survival of some cells. The surviving cells are then cloned to produce tumors resistant, or tolerant, to the same dose of the agent. Higher doses, however, can overcome the cells selected by the previous treatments, and tumor destruction occurs again. The threshold has shifted to a higher dose. The "anticipatory dose escalation" was derived from these observations. Since each relapse and reinduction of remission is associated with substantial morbidity and mortality, maximal duration of single remissions was sought and achieved by escalating the MTX dose beyond the level needed for the initial response, usually to a maximum consistent with tolerable and acceptable side effects. The rationale for anticipatory escalation is most commonly overlooked, and dose escalation beyond the initial level for response is among the most frequently questioned features of the original (3,42) HDMTX-CF treatment schedules.

9. The "pulse" approach to MTX, and subsequently to almost all intensive chemotherapies, evolved from the early observations of toxicity following HDMTX (4). Frequent infusions of even moderate amounts of MTX were found to be cumulatively toxic. The same, or higher, doses on the other hand, were well tolerated when longer recovery periods were allowed between treatments. Substantial experience led to the selection of 28 days as a safe interval between MTX infusions without CF rescue (3) and 21 days for HDMTX-CF schedules (42). Biochemical changes indicating liver or kidney toxicity, even though asymptomatic, usually reverted to normal by the end of the selected intervals. On the other hand, treatments superimposed on damage caused previously, and before completion of the repair, led to prohibitive cumulative toxicity (4). Hence the extended periods between MTX pulses. A corollary of the pulse approach is the use of maximal doses of MTX, as with the anticipatory escalation approach, in order to achieve maximal tumor destruction per treatment and allow extension of the intervals without losing the therapeutic advantage gained.

CONCEPTS USED IN DEVELOPING THE CITROVORUM FACTOR RESCUE

Soon after the introduction of the antifols by Farber (1), synthetic CF (tetrahy-drofolic acid = folinic acid) was shown by Burchenal to reverse toxicity due to Aminopterin in animals (46) and in patients with acute leukemia (47). Unfortunately, it also neutralized completely the antitumor effect of the antifol. This same study introduced also the notions that citrovorum factor (CF) must be given simultaneously with the antifol and at least in equimolar concentrations (doses) in order to be effective. Goldin's work in mice a few years later showed that CF can protect animals from MTX and offer a therapeutic advantage even when administered 48 hours after the antifol (48). This observation, however, was neither confirmed nor followed by other studies. The equimolar and simultaneous use of CF remained an unquestioned dogma.

The work on HDMTX was originally started as a clinical-pharmacological study of resistance to MTX alone. CF rescue had no place in the original study design. The incidental observation (3) that liver enzymes increase at the fourth day following the infusion of high doses of MTX (5 to 15 mg/kg of body weight) led to the successful use of CF for rescue of normal tissues. The delayed injury of the liver suggested the possibility of using delayed CF rescue. Indeed, CF given 48 hours after the MTX prevented the liver damage (3). Since practically all MTX was expected to be excreted by this late hour, a small dose of CF was used and was found effective. The dose differential concept for the use of CF was thus formulated. CF was shown to be effective without giving it simultaneously and in equimolar doses with MTX.

The possibility that the successful rescue from MTX without loss of antitumor activity could be due to the differences in the cytokinetics of normal and tumor cells was considered (3,4,40,43). The short (24 to 36 hours) doubling time of the sensitive normal cells (hemopoietic and intestinal mucosa cells) was contrasted with the relatively prolonged (4 days) doubling time of leukemia cells. A short-lasting presence of CF could thus protect almost all the vulnerable normal cells while sparing only a fraction (25%) of the leukemic population. A simple calculation, supported by clinical observations, soon demonstrated that CF rescue could not be used in acute leukemia (49) or non-Hodgkin's lymphomas (37) in remission when MTX was given at long intervals. The concept was revised and became more useful later when dealing with more slowly dividing solid tumors (40,42). The major point of these considerations, consistently overlooked today, is that CF cannot be used in acute leukemia or non-Hodgkin' lymphomas unless given in minute amounts and in short pulses and unless the interval between MTX treatments is very short (three to seven days). The short intervals between treatments are needed to achieve the 10^2 decrement of tumor cells in acute leukemia, which is the minimal reduction needed for remission induction. Despite the CF rescue, however, such treatments are usually toxic and hazardous.

The differential cytokinetics concept remained the best explanation for the CF rescue advantage until the early 1970s (40,42). At this time, experience with toxic patients with solid tumors showed that tumors may regress despite prolonged CF administration covering almost all the tumor cells' doubling cycle.

The dose differential between MTX and CF was then reconsidered as the crucial mechanism for the therapeutic advantage. Until then, the uptake of CF by normal and by tumor cells was considered to be always optimal. This certainly appeared correct as long as leukemias and lymphomas were the model tumors.

The high resistance of most solid tumors to MTX and the initial failure of moderately high doses to affect them led to the development of dose schedules (6,42) using infusions of up to 18 to 24 g of this agent. Tumor response to such doses reemphasized the role of passive diffusion of MTX for saturation of cells with poor active transport for it. The administration of small doses of CF (15 to 25 per course) to such patients could not possibly equal the passive diffusion of the many grams of MTX. The rescue of the MTX-resistant tumor cells by the small doses of CF most likely was achieved, if at all, via the active transport mechanism. Since these tumors were MTX-resistant, however, their transport mechanism for MTX and, therefore, for CF was presumably poor. The result was that MTX was forced into the tumor cells by passive diffusion, leaving them to be rescued by their inadequate active transport for both CF and MTX. At the same time, the sensitive normal tissues, with known excellent active transport for both CF and MTX, were being salvaged by the low doses of the former.

This dose differential concept of the therapeutic advantage of CF rescue is best supported by the observations that MTX-sensitive or mildly resistant tumors such as leukemias and non-Hodgkin's lymphomas are more readily rescued by CF and, therefore, are better treated with more modest doses of MTX (5 to 30 mg/kg) that can be tolerated without CF rescue. Highly MTX-resistant tumors, on the other hand, may respond to massive doses of MTX without interference from small doses of CF, even on prolonged administration.

Passive transport of CF was considered recently for the rescue of patients who fail to respond to the usual small doses of CF. Patients clearly headed for catastrophic MTX toxicity despite treatment with the usual small doses of CF were rescued fully with massive doses of CR (50). More recent and current observations on patients with closely monitored MTX serum levels have indeed shown that 2 g of citrovorum per dose, every six hours, can spare all normal tissues, even when the MTX present in an adult patient far exceeds the 2 g of citrovorum (50,51). Smaller doses of 0.5 or 1 g of CF may fail under such circumstances. Passive diffusion of the CF, which by definition is noncompetitive with the diffusion of the MTX, may explain this phenomenon.

The equimolar rescue is the most recent advance in understanding the events responsible for the therapeutic advantage of CF rescue (22). The studies of Wilmanns and Sauer (21) indicated that rescue of the hemopoietic tissues must be achieved within 36 hours following MTX treatment in order to avoid bone-marrow depression. Indeed, huge doses of MTX (up to 100 g per treatment) were administered without any side effects when CF concentrations were made, at great effort, to exceed those of the MTX within 24 hours (51). After this study, however, it became apparent that at 36 hours almost all adult patients, treated with HDMTX and proper alkalinization and hydration, usually have less than 10 to 12 mg of MTX in their total extracellular space. The usual 20- to 25-mg dose of CF therefore exceeds the MTX of almost all occasions and ensures an equimolar rescue before serious hemopoietic damage has occurred. Adjusting the CF dose at that time (36 hours) to exceed (by a factor of 4 times) the total MTX still present, led to complete elimination of all side effects in all patients otherwise eligible for HDMTX (22). A correction of our early interpretation of the dose differential effect of MTX and CF is, therefore, due. At lower doses, when the active transport is the only mechanism for the two agents to enter the cells, Burchenal (46,47) was at least partially correct—the CF concentrations must equal, and probably exceed, that of MTX. At very high concentrations, CF and MTX enter the cells by passive diffusion independently of each other. Low CF concentrations in the presence of high MTX beyond the thirty-sixth, and certainly beyond the forty-eighth hour, is dangerous.

TOXICITY ASSOCIATED WITH HIGH-DOSE METHOTREXATE

The introduction of continuous infusions of MTX in high doses (3,4) elicited new toxic effects of this antifol. Skin rash and hepatotoxicity were added to the previously known alopecia, bone marrow depression, mucositis, and renal damage. Leukoencephalopathy and pulmonary damage were considered more recently as additional rare complications. Severe and prolonged bone-marrow depression, extensive buccal and intestinal ulcerations with production of thick mucous, and severe renal failure became the most common causes of irreversible toxic reactions. Analysis of the 10 years' experience with a variety of dose schedules of MTX, with or without CF rescue, showed in 1975 an overall mortality close to 10% (40). At least 30% of the remaining patients required at one time or another massive support with platelet and granulocyte transfusions. A survey of patients treated in other centers after the introduction of urine alkalinization (13) and forced hydration still showed a 6% mortality rate (53).

The substantial incidence of morbidity and mortality following HDMTX-CF rescue justifiably restricted it to investigational use only. The demonstration of its effectiveness in osteogenic sarcoma, however, led to widespread studies of this modality in a variety of tumors in centers around the world, often with catastrophic results. The failure of CF to ensure consistent rescue of the patients led to consideration of effects of MTX on RNA and protein synthesis, possibly independent of folinic acid. Alternative rescue approaches were, therefore, pursued, including studies of thymidine (54), bacterial carboxipeptidases (55), and asparaginase (56).

The recent demonstration of the effectivensss of massive CF rescue in patients who fail to respond to the previously established doses suggested strongly that the previous failures may have been due to interference with the transport of the CF into the sensitive normal cells, rather than to esoteric metabolic effects of MTX, bypassing folinic acid synthesis. Severe toxicity from HDMTX is usually associated with renal failure. Frei emphasized the role of renal infarction with precipitated crystalline MTX leading to complete obstruction of the renal tubules. Although in our experience anuria usually occurred several days after the highest intrarenal concentrations of the drug and could not, therefore, be due to simple mechanical obstruction, prevention of intratubular precipitation of the MTX by vigorous alkalinization of the urine markedly reduced renal failure (13). In fact, urine alkalinization remains at par with equimolar rescue (22) as the most critical new step in avoiding MTX toxicity.

PHARMACOKINETICS OF METHOTREXATE AS PART OF THE TREATMENT WITH HDMTX

Toxicity from MTX correlates better with the duration of the infusion than with the total dose of drug administered (4,40). Studies of MTX clearance following standard 6-hour infusions showed that the rate of clearance varies among patients with otherwise normal renal function. Occurrence of toxicity correlated well with the serum drug concentration uncleared at 48 hours after treatment (16). Since few, if any, patients who show less than 10^{-6} M concentrations of MTX at that time ever become toxic, routine determination of serum MTX at 48 hours after the infusion became an essential part of this chemotherapy. Whenever, for unknown reasons, the serum MTX concentrations exceed 10^{-6} M at 48 hours, CF administration is continued by most investigators beyond the initially prescribed number of doses. Although this adjustment of the CF rescue often fails to ensure the safety of HDMTX, the practice of following closely the serum MTX concentrations eventually led to understanding of the time factor involved in matching the concentrations of MTX and CF and made possible the equimolar rescue.

DOSE SCHEDULES OF CF AND EQUIMOLAR RESCUE

The doses of CF used in the early studies of HDMTX were selected empirically in accordance with the dose-differential principles described above. The first and intuitive adjustment of the CF doses, according to the dosage of MTX, was made with the original description of what is today considered a very high dose of MTX (42). This description recommended to increase the CF from 6 mg per dose when 1 g of MTX was used to as high as 24 mg per dose after 18 g of MTX. It also prescribed 6 doses only for the smaller amounts of MTX and 12 doses for the more substantial doses. This recommendation was first questioned and then neglected by many new investigators who used instead a fixed amount of CF (usually 15 mg per dose).

Recently Frei and his associates reconsidered the matter and found less toxicity with the higher dosages of CF (14). Similar findings were reported also by Rosen (57). The paramount importance of the timing for CF rescue in order to protect the bone marrow effectively was emphasized by Wilmanns and Sauer (21). Chabner (58), on the other hand, demonstrated that, at least in vitro, bone marrow is rescued only when the CF concentration exceeds that of MTX. These observations led us to the recent development of the equimolar rescue (22).

The equimolar approach to rescue consists of adjusting the concentration of CF in the extracellular fluids of the patient to exceed that of MTX by the thirty-sixth-hour after the infusion of the antifol.

At that time the total amount of MTX still present in the extracellular fluids of the patients is calculated. This is done more easily when the serum concentration is expressed in micrograms per milliliter of serum instead of molarity. For example, a 10^{-6} M concentration represents the presence of 0.5 micrograms (µg) of MTX per milliliter of serum or 5 mg/liter (1,000 ml). The MTX is well distributed and in equilibrium between the various compartments (intravascular and intercellular) of the extracellular fluids. This total fluid space is about 20% of the patient's body weight or about 12 liters for an average adult weighing 60 kg. The amount of MTX per liter of serum multiplied by the total volume, in liters, of fluids yields the total amount of extracellular MTX. The following formula can be used for this calculation:

$$\frac{Serum\ (\mu g) \times 1,000 \times body\ weight\ (kg) \times 20}{100}$$

or

$$MTX\ (\mu g) \times body\ weight\ (kg) \times 200 = extracellular\ MTX\ (mg)$$

Since only the transport into the cell is relevant and the efflux of free MTX at 36 hours is not likely to affect significantly the extracellular concentrations, a dose of CF is then administered, calculated to equal or surpass the MTX concentration. Taking into consideration the rapid urinary clearance of CF and the time required for achieving equilibrium between the intravascular and the intercellular compartments, a dose of CF in excess of the calculated total amount of MTX is obviously needed to produce rapidly equimolar concentrations of the two agents. Empirically, a dose of CF four times greater than the total MTX present was found to be satisfactory. Future studies on CF clearance and distribution may suggest a better basis for determining the equimolar CF doses. Because of the expected individual variations, however, an excess of CF will still be needed until very rapid assays for CF become available.

CLINICAL AND EXPERIMENTAL OBSERVATIONS AS BASIS FOR CONCEPTS ON HDMTX-CF

The hypotheses and the concepts discussed above were substantiated or modified at this center in the course of extensive clnical trials from 1963 until the present. Substantial clinical and laboratory-experimental information was provided by others, especially since the stimulating observations in osteogenic sarcoma.

The redefinition of acquired MTX resistance to antifol tolerance was established with the first reports in this field (3,4). Children with acute lymphocytic leukemia who relapsed while receiving conventional and even moderately high doses went into remission when treated with higher doses given by continuous intravenous infusions (Tables 1 and 2). Tumors inherently resistant to antifols, for which conventional MTX was no longer considered, were shown to respond consistently to infusions of higher doses (5 to 30 mg/kg) (5,6,42). End-stage non-Hodgkin's lymphoma responded to MTX alone (Table 3). Sequentially used HDMTX and other agents produced 6 long-term, unmaintained survivors in a group of 12 children with generalized disease (37). Acute myelogenous leukemia, considered unresponsive to MTX even today, was successfully treated by Bertino using HDMTX and CF rescue (7).

The MTX dose-threshold concepts were derived from the studies on resistance tolerance to MTX in leukemia and lymphoma and were further substantiated by the work on lung cancer (6,42) and other solid tumors starting in 1969 (40). The type of observations that established the need for dose escalation of MTX

Table 1. Remission Introduction with 18-Hour Infusions of Methotrexate in Children with Acute Lymphocytic Leukemia Resistant to Conventional Doses of MTX

Patient	Age (yr)	Initial WBC	% Blasts	Previous Therapy	Duration of Treatment (days)	Duration of Complete Remission (days)	No of Platelet Transfusions	No of Platelet-Concentrates Used	Relapse at End of Study
1	14	4,400	98	MTX, [a]P[b], 6 MP, [b]CTX, VCR[a], HU	42	165+ (off study)	86	525	No
2	10½	1,600	95	MTX, [a]P, VCR	36	101	13	73	No
3	3	26,500	85	MTX, [ab]VCR, 6 MP, [b]P, [a]HU	50 (34 days to partial remission)	26	22	82	Yes
4	9½	3,000	40	MTX (im), [a]P, 6 MP, [a]VCR, [a]HU	25	20	4	21	Yes
5	3	385,400	90	MTX[a] (continuous infusion), P, VCR	36	72	9	31	Yes
6	7	1,150	98	MTX, [a]6 MP, [ab]P	31	74+ (off study)	8	35	No

7	14	750	100	MTX (only 2 weeks) 6 MP[a], [b]P	16	97+ (off study)	30	210	No
8	10½	1,000,000	98	6 MP, VCR, P	25 (to partial)	128 (off treatment after 100 days)	11	61	No
9	9½	5,000	10	MTX, [a]P, 6 MP, [a]VCR	20 (from partial relapse)	30+ (off study)	0	0	No
10	3	4,500	13	MTX, [a]VCR[b], [b]P, [a]HU	12 (from partial relapse)	80 (expired)	10	39	No

[a]Relapsed while receiving the drug for maintenance.
[b]Failed to respond after adequate trial on first or subsequent treatment.
MTX = Methotrexate.
P = Prednisone.
6 MP = 6-Mercaptopurine.
VCR = Vincristine.
HU = Hydroxyurea.

Table 2. Reinduction of Remission with High-Dose Methotrexate in Patients Tolerant to Smaller Doses

Patient	% Blasts at Partial or Complete Relapse	% Blasts after Treatment	Treatment
1	42	10	25 mg/kg, once a week × 2
2	95	30	5 mg/kg, 4-hour infusion 2 days a week × 2
	34	7	5 mg/kg, rapid IV once a week × 3
3	21	4	30 mg/kg, 4-hour infusion once a week × 3 with citrovorum factor
4	15	2	30 mg/kg, 4-hour infusion 3 consecutive days with citrovorum factor
5	22	5	30 mg/kg, 4-hour infusion once a week × 2
6	9	2	10 mg/kg, rapid IV once a week × 3
7	11	3	6 mg/kg, 4-hour infusion 8 mg/kg, rapid IV

until the response is elicited is illustrated in Figure 1. The response of tumors to a higher dose of MTX after failure of lesser, although unconventional doses, as shown in Figure 1, is a common observation in such patients.

The desirability of anticipatory escalation, discussed above, was suggested by observations such as shown in Table 2 and was further substantiated in patients with solid tumors (Fig. 2). The relationship of tumor response to the dose of MTX was suggested by extensive observations of this nature. In vitro and animal studies confirmed this dose-effect relationship repeatedly and most recently (59,60).

The different sensitivity of various solid tumors to MTX reflected in the threshold concept is illustrated in Figure 3. For example, cancer of the pancreas and of the ovaries may respond to doses of MTX lower than needed for tumors of the lungs or osteogenic sarcoma. Melanoma or colon cancer, after an initial and very modest response to moderate doses may require exceedingly high amounts of MTX (50 or more grams per infusion) for further response. Head and neck cancer on the other hand was shown by others to respond to modest doses (8,28,29).

The early concepts for the use of CF were supported mainly by its relatively consistent clinical success. The reduction of the effectiveness of HDMTX in patients with rapidly growing tumors (acute leukemia or lymphomas) by CF was well established in our clinic (37,40,43). These observations strongly supported the differential cytokinetics concept, especially when more slowly growing solid

Table 3. Remission Introduction with High-Dose Methotrexate in Children with Otherwise Unresponsive Non-Hodgkin's Lymphoma

Patient	Stage	Histology	Presenting Sites	Leukemic Conversion	Response	Survival (yr)	Cause of Death
1	IV_L	PDL	Thymus, bone marrow	Yes	C.R.	37/12	Progressive CNS disease, gram (−) sepsis
2	IV_L	UNC	Skin, mediastinum, bone marrow	Yes	C.R.	18/12	Progressive disease, leukopenia, gram (−) sepsis
3	IV_L	UNC	Mediastinum, bone marrow	Yes	C.R.	13/12	Leukopenia, gram (−) sepsis candidasis, drug-related death
4	IV_L	PDL	Mediastinum, bone marrow	Yes	C.R.	11/12	Progressive disease, leukopenia aspergillosis
5	IV	U	Pelvis, lymph nodes	No	P.R.	9/12	Progressive disease
6	II_E	PDL	Mediastinum, chest wall	No	C.R.	9/12	CNS toxoplasmosis, cerebral necrosis
7	II	PDL	Mediastinum	No	C.R.	7/12	Progressive disease, leukopenia, gram (−) sepsis
8	IV_L	H	Abdomen. CNS, lymph nodes	Yes	C.R.	7/12	Progressive disease
9	IV_L	H	Abdomen, pleura, bone marrow, CNS	Yes	P.R.	6/12	Progressive disease
10	IV	U	Parotid gland, abdomen, CNS	No	C.R.	5/12	Progressive CNS disease

H = Histiocytic.

PDL = Poorly differentiated lymphocytic.

U = Undifferentiated.

UNC = Unclassified.

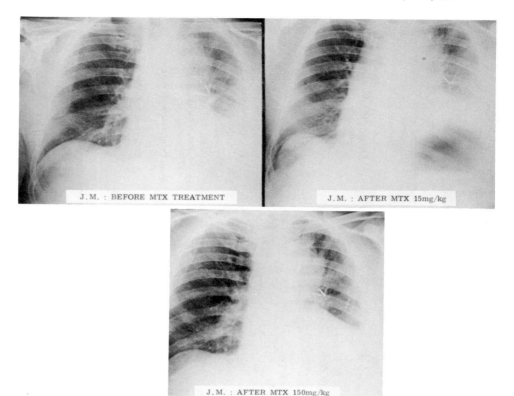

Figure 1. Effects of high-dose MTX on adenocarcinoma of the lung.

tumors appeared to respond better to HDMTX-CF. The dose-differential concept for the use of CF, as initially conceived or as interpreted later, again appears supported by numerous clinical observations. There is little doubt that large and potentially lethal doses of MTX are routinely survived by patients receiving miniscule amounts of CF. Obviously, the total doses of the two drugs need not be equal. The role of passive diffusion of CF and the need for equimolar concentration of MTX and CF to rescue bone marrow, and other sensitive normal tissues, within 36 hours after treatment, although consistent with the most recent clinical observations (22,52) and with in vitro studies (58), warrants further study on both the clinical and laboratory levels.

The early initiation of CF rescue (2 hours after MTX) in the lung cancer dose schedule (6,41), which was adapted by Jaffe for osteogenic sarcoma and by others in many subsequent studies, was based on the early dose-differential principle. The latter assumed that CF, being a physiological compound with high and preferential affinity for the active transfer mechanism, will be incorporated by the normal cells even in the presence of overwhelmingly higher concentrations of MTX. A study comparing quantitatively the effectiveness of CF rescue started at 2 hours versus 36 or 48 hours after the infusion of MTX has not been carried out even in this clinic. Such a study may well resolve the question of the need for early initiation of small doses of CF.

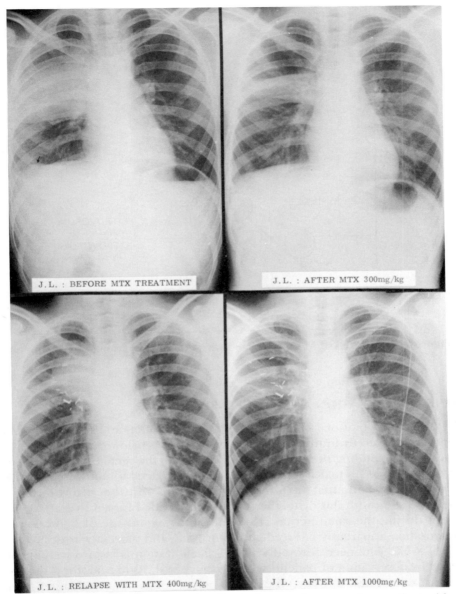

Figure 2. Response of two dose levels of high-dose methotrexate in a patient with osteogenic sarcoma.

The concepts about the therapeutic advantage provided by the CF rescue in the HDMTX-CF modality remain, by and large, hypothetical. They are supported above all by their empiric clinical success. As the most recent work with the so-called equimolar rescue shows, substantial advances in regard to both safety and effectiveness with the HDMTX-CF modality may be derived from further in-depth studies of the clinical pharmacokinetics of both MTX and CF.

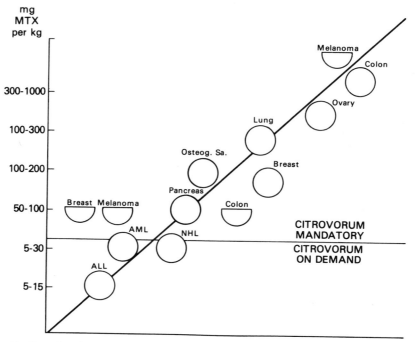

Figure 3. Dose levels of MTX associated with clinical response in various tumors.

URINE ALKALINIZATION AND FORCED HYDRATION

The isoelectric point of MTX is about 5.5. Precipitation and crystal formation will, therefore, occur in the urine whenever its pH is below this value. Frei and associates (13), finding precipitated MTX crystals in the renal tubules of patients succumbing to MTX toxicity recommended prophylactic administration of alkali before, during, and after the infusion of MTX. In a further effort to prevent renal infarction with this drug, they also recommended forced hydration of the patient during the same period (13). The simultaneous use of hydration and alkalinization apparently reduced both morbidity and mortality associated with HDMTX-CF. The need for and value of alkalinization is impressively demonstrated by observation of patients whose urine pH shifts to acid, for a variety of reasons, during the infusion of MTX. Their urine suddenly changes from a dark, but clear, fluid to a "muddy" white-yellowish excretion. Prompt intravenous administration of additional alkali restores the original appearance within minutes. Undue persistence of such acid urine obviously could lead to renal infarction with MTX. These observations are responsible for the emphasis on urine pH stability and close monitoring as discussed below.

The role and value of forced hydration alone is less well established, since it has always been studied in conjunction with alkalinization. The combined use of both, however, modified the previous HDMTX-CF dose schedules in more ways than just reducing toxicity. The more consistent, and possibly the more rapid, clearance of the MTX by the kidneys resulted in a reduction of the $C \times t$ value for these treatments. Reduction of the antitumor effectiveness is, therefore, to be expected. The experience in this center strongly suggests that 30% to 50% higher doses of MTX are needed to reproduce the antitumor effects of previously studied dose schedules when alkalinization and hydration are used. The effect of the higher doses is to restore the $C \times t$ value to its former level, compensating by an increase of the drug concentration (C) for the shorter time (t) during which the drug is present around the cells. Studies designed specifically to clarify this aspect of rapid MTX clearance are urgently needed. Alkalinization alone may suffice to prevent kidney damage and toxicity and make smaller doses of MTX more effective.

BASIC DOSE SCHEDULES FOR HDMTX-CF

The first observation of antitumor activity of HDMTX-CF in osteogenic sarcoma was made using a specific dose schedule developed during studies on lung cancer as a model tumor (6,42). These reports were followed by widespread trials of HDMTX-CF in osteogenic sarcoma and in other tumors in this country and abroad. Almost all centers engaging in such studies, however, modified theMTX or the CF doses as well as other details of the procedure. In almost all instances this resulted in inconsistent clinical effectiveness or in preventable toxicity. Lack of familiarity with the theoretical considerations discussed in the previous sections is perhaps the main reason for the tendency to modify freely the original and effective dose schedules. Remarkably, Jaffe (10) and Rosen (17,18,32), who determined in their own early work the validity of the threshold concept and the need for escalation of MTX up to effective doses, obtained the best results. Their subsequent modifications of the initial method contributed to, instead of detracted from, the proper development of this treatment approach.

The central theme of the studies on HDMTX and the novelty of this approach was the discovery that short infusions of large amounts of MTX without CF rescue, previously considered very dangerous, can usually be given with impunity. Although the potential value of CF was described at the same time (3,4), it remained incidental to this work until lung cancer replaced acute leukemia as the model tumor for the studies on resistance to antifols (6,42). Over 1,000 infusions of MTX in doses ranging from 2 to 30 mg/kg of body weight, without any CF rescue, were studied from 1964 to 1969 in children with acute leukemia (49) and non-Hodgkin's lymphoma (37), treated for remission maintenance. CF rescue during this phase of the work was used only on the rare occasions when ominous toxic signs appeared or when very frequent (every 3 to 7 days) administration of MTX was needed for studies on remission induction. This experience clearly showed that up to 30 mg/kg of MTX (1.2 to 2.0 g in adults) can be used safely under optimal conditions, without CF rescue, in patients with excellent kidney function and minimal, if any, tumor load. The same doses, however, could be lethal in very sick patients with extensive disease. CF rescue was used in such patients mainly when remission induction with MTX was unavoidable. Only a few (one to four) small doses of CF could then be given without canceling all the effectiveness of the treatment. Often such low CF rescue failed to prevent extreme toxicity. The possible value of HDMTX alone for remission mainte-nance was, therefore, emphasized in contrast to using this approach for induction of remission.

When lung cancer was chosen as the model tumor for studies on solid tumors (6), a major escalation of the MTX doses was carried out to reach effectiveness according to the threshold concepts. Only then did CF become a compulsory step in the HDMTX-CF treatment. Lost on the early observers of the osteogenic sarcoma studies was the fact that CF was not necessarily needed, nor indeed was it desirable, for the optimal effects in acute leukemia and non-Hodgkin's lym-phoma. Emphatic statements to this effect (37,40,43) remained largely unno-ticed. The mere term "CF rescue" by that time had become inseparable from the high dose of MTX. Accordingly, recent studies of HDMTX-CF in lymphoma, although generally positive, fall short of the potential of HDMTX in this disease, because of extensive rescue with 8 to 12 doses of CF. Freeman and associates recently noticed and avoided this misunderstanding (30). Two basic dose sched-ules for HDMTX must, therefore, be distinguished as follows:

Moderately High-Dose Methotrexate without Citrovorum Rescue

Rapidly growing tumors, relatively sensitive or moderately resistant to MTX, cannot be treated successfully with doses of MTX that require substantial and prolonged rescue with CF. Typically, this principle applies to acute leukemia and non-Hodgkin's lymphoma. Such patients, when in remission can tolerate well up to 30 mg of MTX/kg of body weight without using CF rescue at all. The same doses used for remission induction are generally quite toxic. The main potential value of these dose schedules is, therefore, for remission maintenance in these diseases. A recommended procedure for administration of these doses of MTX is the four-hour infusion (3). About 60% of the total dose is given in a rapid intravenous injection, followed by slow infusion of the remaining drug over four hours. Up to 15 mg/kg of MTX can thus be given on each of two consecutive days without need for CF rescue. Up to 30 mg/kg can also be ad-ministered, preferably as a single four-hour infusion. An interval of 21 days, at least, between maintenance treatments was found necessary to avoid cumulative and irreversible renal and hepatic damage (4). Whenever other agents are used to supplement sequentially the infusions of MTX (40,61), the latter should be spaced at 28-day intervals. Treatments with this dose range of MTX for remission maintenance can be started with the rather low 5 mg/kg dose of MTX in a single infusion. Two equal infusions are then given on the next cycle on two consecutive days. The dose for each infusion is escalated on subsequent cycles until 15 mg/kg (total of 30 mg/kg for the two-day treatment) is reached or undue toxicity occurs. In the latter event, the MTX dose is decreased to 10 mg or even back to 5 mg/kg for two or three months when escalation is again attempted. Often the second attempt at increasing the MTX dose is uneventful. The reason for this latter observation is not established, although the possibility of gradually developing better tolerance by the mucosal cells is rather compelling. This same observation is another reason for the gradual escalation of MTX in the schedules later developed for solid tumors. Hydration and alkalinization were not, and are not, used in this clinic for treatment of children with acute leukemia or lymphomas in remission. Their MTX serum levels are usually less than 5×10^{-7} (0.1 to 0.3 μg/ml of serum) 24 hours after a single infusion. They are usually equally low 24 hours after the second dose.

When moderately high doses of MTX (5 to 30 mg/kg) are used as a last resort for the induction of remission in these leukemia or lymphoma patients, alkalinization and moderate hydration should be used. One to three doses of CF can then be given 24 hours after the infusion, especially on the second and subsequent treatments, which are given three to seven days apart. Toxicity is practically unavoidable with such treatments, despite the short coverage with CF.

High and Massive Doses of Methotrexate with Citrovorum Factor Rescue

The moderately high doses of MTX (up to 30 mg/kg) usually without CF rescue, which were studied previously in leukemias and lymphomas, were found in 1969 to be either ineffective or extremely toxic in patients with advanced lung cancer. According to the concepts leading to and derived from the previous studies, a dose escalation of the MTX was carried out until consistent antitumor effects were observed. Since the high risk of MTX doses greater than 30 mg/kg was already known, CF rescue was introduced as an inseparable element of each HDMTX treatment. Numerous trials of various dose-frequency schedules in lung cancer patients led to the description of a preferred dose schedule for this tumor type (42). A gradual dose escalation of both MTX and CF, on consecutive treatments, was the basis for this schedule. The full dose of MTX for lung cancer according to it was 300 mg/kg or 18 g per adult patient with an average weight of 60 kg. The CF was escalated from an initial 6 mg to 24 mg per dose. The interval between MTX administrations was shorter initially (10 and 14 days), reaching 3 weeks after the administration of 6 or more grams of MTX. This dose schedule was used unchanged by Jaffe and Farber for their initial, and quite successful, studies on recurrent osteogenic sarcoma (9,10). Doses of MTX ranging from 300 mg/kg were subsequently used by many investigators, often with substantial modifications and all under the denomination of high-dose MTX. The massive doses of MTX (40) consisting of as much as 1 g of MTX/kg resulted from two advances in this field. First, alkalinization and hydration, while increasing the safety of HDMTX-CF, apparently reduced the effective $C \times t$ of previous treatments. Maintaining the incidence of objective tumor responses in our tumor model (lung cancer) required MTX doses higher than the previously optimal 300 mg/kg. Second, the increased safety offered by the massive CF rescue (50) and by the recent equimolar rescue (22) made it possible to pursue safely the threshold and shifting threshold principles in resistant tumors with massive doses of MTX. The information thus gathered substantiated the rationale of the high MTX, if not the practicability of the massive doses.

It has been our contention that specific and different dose schedules of MTX may eventually be found to be optimal for various tumor types. Such optimal dose schedules, however, can only be determined by intensive and large-scale studies, once the overall biological activity and usefulness of HDMTX-CF are determined in pilot studies as those carried out at this time by numerous investigators.

A dose schedule and procedure used successfully in this clinic for pilot studies of antitumor activity in parallel with studies of pharmacological nature is therefore outlined below.

An individual clinical trial of HDMTX-CF is always designed to determine the threshold of MTX sensitivity of the tumor under treatment. Because of individual variations of such sensitivity, even among patients with the same type of malignancy, the initial doses of MTX are limited to moderate levels (15 to 50 mg/kg or 1 to 3 g of MTX per 60 kg adult patient). The MTX doses are increased by increments of 100% (6, 12, and 24 g, respectively) for the following three treatments. The intervals between are determined by the tumor response, the renal function 7 to 10 days after the MTX, by the bone-marrow function, and by the urgency of the clinical symptomatology due to the tumor load. For example, in the absence of tumor response after 1 to 3 g of MTX, but in the presence of adequate creatinine clearance and normal blood counts, a second treatment (3 to 6 g of MTX) can be given 7 to 10 days after the first. A third treatment with the next dose level can be considered again, assuming conditions have not changed after 10 to 14 days. Decreased renal function or suppressed blood counts at this time would be an indication for extending the interval by at least 7 to 10 more days. The once-a-week treatments, feasible in young patients with osteogenic sarcoma (62), are rarely possible in older patients with extensive tumor load. The approach described above is the only practical and safe approach for such patients. A three-week interval between treatments becomes mandatory after the third or fourth dose (12 or 24 g of MTX).

Each treatment starts with a creatinine clearance determination. Full MTX dosage is used whenever the clearance is greater than 60 ml/min. Reduced dosage (50% of total) is considered for patients with clearance raging between 40 and 60 ml/min. Use of HDMTX-CF in patients with creatinine clearance of less than 40 ml/min is only considered under special circumstances, acknowledging the substantial risks involved.

The second and most critical step in carrying out each treatment is to ensure aklalinization of the urine immediately before the infusion of MTX. Sodium bicarbonate (88 mEq) is infused by rapid injection, and urine specimens starting 30 minutes later are tested and must have a pH greater than 7.0 before the infusion of MTX is initiated. Oral intake, except for plain water, is stopped with the first alkalinization for at least 12 hours, in order to avoid inadvertent, and possibly very dangerous, acidification of the urine during this critical period. The MTX, dissolved in 500 to 1,000 ml of 5% dextrose in water, according to total amount of drug, is administered, starting with rapid (10 to 15 minutes) infusion of 40% of the total dose (not exceeding 4 g) and following this with a drip infusion of the remaining amount of drug over 6 hours. Sodium bicarbonate (44 mEq for adult patients) is infused rapidly again every 2 hours during the infusion of MTX (three doses). The ph of all urine specimens is determined during the first 24 hours, and additional bicarbonate is rapidly infused whenever found to be less than 7.0. At the end of the MTX infusion, moderately forced hydration is initiated by administering 1,000 ml of 5% dextrose in 0.3% normal saline with added 44 mEq of sodium bicarbonate and 30 mEq of KCl, unless otherwise indicated by serum potassium levels, in a 6-hour infusion repeated four times during the first 24 hours. The same 1,000 ml of fluids is given in 8 hours, three times a day during the second and third days for a total of 10 bottles during the first 72 hours after the MTX. Fruits and juices, as well as acid-containing foods, are specifically avoided. Serum MTX levels are determined 24 and 36 hours after the start of the MTX infusion and daily thereafter. The EMIT system (SYVA, Palo Alto, Cal.) provides a suitable MTX assay because of its simplicity and prompt availability of the results.

CF rescue is started 2 hours after completion of MTX administration. Whenever the MTX dose is 3 g or less (15 to 50 mg/kg), each single dose of CF is limited to 15 mg given intravenously by rapid injection of infusion every 6 hours for a total of 12 doses. Whenever the MTX dose is 6 g or more, the individual dose of CF is increased to 25 mg every 6 hours for 12 doses. A critical measurement of the CF dose is carried out on the basis of the thirty-sixth-hour serum MTX level. The rapid EMIT assay allows adjustments of the CF dosage to be implemented within 30 to 60 minutes, according to the principles of the equimolar rescue described above. Whenever, for logistic reasons, the second MTX determination can only be carried out at 40 to 48 hours after the start of the MTX infusion, the CF dosage is adjusted in the same fashion as ideally done at 36 hours. With such late correction, risk of bone-marrow suppression reappears but is substantially smaller than without CF adjustments at all. Whenever the total MTX in the extracellular fluids exceeds 500 mg, the CF dose can be kept constant at 2 g every 6 hours regardless of the MTX concentration. CF doses of 2 g per infusion in our experience have fully protected patients who had retained 5 or more g of MTX for periods greater than 72 hours. There is little doubt that 2 g of CF per dose creates concentrations sufficient to protect normal cells by passive diffusion, independently of the active transport that is blocked by the excess of MTX. Doses of 1 g of CF can fail under such circumstances, as observed repeatedly in our clinic. Persistence of small amounts of MTX in the patient's serum can occur in older patients and on repeated MTX treatments despite adequate pretreatment creatinine clearance. The detection of 0.1 to 0.2 μg of MTX per ml of serum (2 to 4×10^{-7} M) for as long as a week after treatment is not uncommon and can result in severe bone-marrow suppression and late impairment of renal or hepatic function. Accordingly, continued administration of small amounts of CF (10 mg every 6 hours) often by mouth, is used in this clinic until the MTX concentration is less than 0.1 μg (10^{-7} M).

The dose schedule of HDMTX-CF above is designed mainly for exploring the biological activity of HDMTX-CF in solid tumors unresponsive to more conventional doses of MTX. Its main feature is the open-end dosage of MTX that, if desirable, can be escalated just as safely to 36 to 50 g per infusion. The practicability of these latter massive doses for routine treatments is, however, questionable, especially on a continual basis.

This dose schedule, however, is the most effective and safest initial schedule whenever the use of this modality is first considered. Accumulated experience with it in any specific tumor type may well suggest modifications more suitable to the clinical objectives under more routine circumstances.

CAUSES FOR CONFLICTING CONCLUSIONS REGARDING EFFECTIVENESS OF HDMTX-CF

Failure of HDMTX-CF to affect tumors that have been successfully treated with it by others are usually traced to the following errors or misunderstandings:

1. A vague definition of high dose. Doses of MTX as varied as 500 mg or 50 g have been all considered a high dose.

2. Closed versus open-ended escalation of MTX. Reluctance to escalate the MTX dose beyond a predetermined safe dose has led to opposing conclusions. The most common upper limits used by others are 3 and 7.5 g of MTX per M^2 body surface. Tumors whose threshold of sensitivity for MTX happens to be below such doses are proclimed responsive. Other tumors that may be biologically even more suitable for HDMTX-CF, although starting to respond only at higher MTX doses (12 g/M^2 or 18 g or more per single adult dose) are pronounced unresponsive. The problem with this closed escalation is that it conflicts with the most basic of the reasons for using HDMTX-CF to start with. Our discussion of the concepts and rationale for HDMTX-CF clarifies the need for open-ended escalation until objective tumor response is elicited or further trials are considered unsafe or beyond practicability.

3. Inadequate follow-up is a major reason for variable conclusions. The dosage of MTX is fully dependent on rapid evaluation of the effectiveness of the previous treatment. A measurable lesion is most helpful in this respect. Infrequent measurements, however, are a common cause for erroneous conclusions. The maximal effect, if any, of HDMTX-CF on most solid tumors occurs 7 to 10 days after each treatment. A tumor with a substantial number of growing cells, unless massively destroyed, may regrow to its original size in three weeks when the patient usually returns for further treatment and a follow-up measurement is first taken. In order to determine accurately the sensitivity of the tumor to HDMTX-CF, and the need or advisability for further dose escalation, a measurement of the observable lesion on the very same day of treatment and 7 to 10 days later is essential. Failure to do so may lead to erroneous conclusions and abandonment of a potentially useful treatment.

4. Maintenance with the minimal effective dose. This common error is due to lack of familiarity or of appreciation, of the shifting threshold concept. Part of this misunderstanding is also the expectation of cumulative effect from repeated but equal treatments. Because of the pulse nature of the HDMTX-CF and the inevitable regrowth of the tumor during the interval, real cumulative effect of marginally effective treatment is impossible. Net antitumor gain can only occur if the regrowth fraction is smaller than the one destroyed by each treatment. Early response of a tumor to a moderate dose of MTX as determined by the close follow-up mentioned above is a strong indication for escalation of the MTX dose to levels known to be consistently and continually effective in the same tumor type.

5. The use of CF rescue for moderate (less than 30 mg/kg) MTX doses, when treating rapidly growing tumors with marginal but existing active transport for folates, is another major and common error usually committed when treating acute leukemias and non-Hodgkin's lymphomas.

CONCLUSION

HDMTX was conceived, developed, and studied in an effort to clarify clinically the mechanisms of resistance to antifols. Premature and widespread clinical trials resulted from its successful application to the treatment of osteogenic sarcoma. Its wide range of antitumor activity is easily missed without constant consideration and application of the information already available concerning the mechanisms of action and resistance to antifols. No single dose schedule of HDMTX-CF is currently available for use in trials as a new drug. In this sense HDMTX-CF is still a developing modality. The newly added safety with the use of equimolar rescue does now justify an intensified study of its clinical value.

REFERENCES

1. Farber S, Diamond LK, Mercer RD, et al: Temporary remission in acute leukemia in children produced by folic antagonist 4-amethopteroylglutamic acid (aminopterin). *N Engl J Med* 238:787–793, 1948.
2. Li MC, Hertz R, Spencer DB: Effect of methotrexate (amethopterin) therapy upon choriocarcinoma and chorioadenoma. *Proc Soc Exp Biol* 93:361, 1956.
3. Djerassi I, Abir E, Royer GL Jr, et al: Long-term remissions in childhood acute leukemia: Use of infrequent infusions of methotrexate; supportive roles of platelet transfusions and citrovorum factor. *Clin Pediatr* 5(8), 1966.
4. Djerassi I, Farber S, Abir E, et al: Continuous infusion of methotrexate in children in acute leukemia. *Cancer* 20:233–242, 1967.
5. Djerassi I, Royer G, Treat C, et al: Management of childhood lymphosarcoma and reticulum cell sarcoma with high-dose intermittent methotrexate and citrovorum factor. *Proc Am Assoc Cancer Res* 9:18, 1968 (abstract).
6. Djerassi I, Rominger CJ, Kim JS, et al: Methotrexate-citrovorum factor in patients with lung cancer. *Proc Am Assoc Cancer Res* 11:21, 1970 (abstract).
7. Hryniuk WM, Bertino JR: Treatment of leukemia with large doses of methotrexate and folinic acid: Clinical-biochemical correlates. *J Clin Invest* 48:2140–2155, 1969.
8. Cappizzi RL, DeConti RC, Marsh JC, et al: Methotrexate therapy of head and neck cancer: Improvement in therapeutic index by the use of leucovorin "rescue." *Cancer Res* 30:1782–1788, 1970.
9. Jaffe N, Farber S, Traggis D, et al: Favorable response of metastatic osteogenic sarcoma to pulse high-dose methotrexate–citrovorum administration (HDMC): Children's Cancer Res Fndn and Harv Med Schol, Boston, Mass. *Proc Am Assoc Cancer Res* 13:27, 1972 (abstract).
10. Jaffe N, Farber S, Traggis D, et al: Favorable response of metastatic osteogenic sarcoma to pulse high-dose methotrexate with citrovorum rescue and radiation therapy. *Cancer* 31:1367–1373, 1973.
11. Jaffe N, Frei E, Traggis D, et al: Adjuvant methotrexate and citrovorum factor treatment of osteogenic sarcoma. *N Engl J Med* 291:994–997, 1974.
12. Bertino JR: The mechanism of action of the folate antagonists in man. *Cancer Res* 23:1286, 1963.
13. Frei E III, Jaffe N, Tattersall MHN, et al: New approaches to cancer chemotherapy with methotrexate. *N Engl J Med* 292:846–851, 1975.
14. Howell SB, Krishan A, Frei E: Cytokinetic comparison of thymidine and leucovorin rescue of marrow in humans after exposure to high-dose methotrexate. *Cancer Res* 39:1315–1320, 1979.
15. Goldman ID: Analysis of the cytotoxic determinants for methotrexate: A role of "free" intracellular drug. *Cancer Chemother Rep* 6:51–61, 1975.

16. Stoller RG, Hande KR, Jacobs SA, et al: Use of plasma pharmacokinetics to predict and prevent methotrexate toxicity. *N Engl J Med* 297:630–634, 1977.

17. Rosen G, Suwansirikul S, Kwon C, et al: High-dose methotrexate with citrovorum factor rescue and adriamycin in childhood osteogenic sarcoma. *Cancer* 33:4, 1974.

18. Rosen G: Symposium on Osteogenic Sarcoma. Vienna University, 1979.

19. Isacoff WH, Eliber F, Tabbarah H, et al: Phase II clinical trial with high-dose methotrexate therapy and citrovorum factor rescue. *Cancer Treat Rep* 62:1295–1304, 1978.

20. Kotz R, Arbes H, Hackel H, et al: Ergebnisse der Chemotherapie in der Nachbehandlung von malignen Knochentumoren. *Orthop. Praxis* 11:1021, 1976.

21. Sauer H, Schalhorn A, Wilmanns W: The biochemistry of the citrovorum factor rescue effect in normal bone marrow cells after high-dose methotrexate. *Eur J Cancer* 15:1203–1209, 1979.

22. Djerassi I, Mills K, Ohanissian H, et al: Elimination of the hazards of high-dose methotrexate (HDMTX) with improved citrovorum factor rescue (CF). *Am Soc Clin Oncol* 21:361, 1980 (abstract).

23. Martin DS, Nayak R, Sawyer RC, et al: Enhancement of 5-FU chemotherapy with emphasis on the use of excessive thymidine. *Can Bull* 30(6):219–224, 1978.

24. Bruckner HW, Schreiber C, Waxman S: Interaction of chemotherapeutic agents with methotrexate and 5-fluorouracil and its effect on de novo DNA synthesis. *Cancer Res* 35:801–806, 1975.

25. Yap HY, Blumenschein GR, Yap BS, et al: High-dose methotrexate for advanced breast ca. *Cancer Treat Rep* 63:757, 1979.

26. Henderson IC, Canellos GP, Blum RH, et al: Prolonged disease-free survival in advanced breast ca (BC) treated with "super CMF"–Adriamycin: An alternating regimen employing high-dose methotrexate (M) with citrovorum factor (CF) rescue. *Proc Am Soc Clin Onc* 20:327, 1979 (abstract).

27. Skarin AT, Green H, Canellos GP, et al: High-dose methotrexate with citrovorum factor rescue (HDMTX-CF) alternating with combination chemotherapy (M-CAV-CMc) in small cell lung ca (SC lung). *Proc Am Soc Clin Oncol* 20:328, 1979 (abstract).

28. Bertino JR, Mosher MB, DeConti RC: Chemotherapy of cancer of the head and neck. *Cancer* 31:1141, 1973.

29. Ervin TJ, Miller D, Foley G: Improved survival in patients with advanced squamous carcinoma of head and neck responding to preoperative high-dose methotrexate-leucovorin. *Proc Am Assoc Can Res* 21:141, 1980 (abstract).

30. Brecher ML, Thomas PRM, Sinks LF, et al: Updated results on the treatment of childhood non-Hodgkin's lymphoma (NHL). *Proc Am Soc Clin Oncol* 20:438, 1979 (abstract).

31. Yagoda A, Watson RC, Whitmore WF: Phase II trial of methotrexate in urinary bladder cancer. *Proc AACR* 21:427, 1980 (abstract).

32. Rosen G, Nirenberg A, Juergens H, et al: Osteogenic sarcoma; 3-Year disease-free survival in excess of 80% with combination chemotherapy, including effective high-dose methotrexate with citrovorum rescue. *J Natl Cancer Inst* (in press).

33. Minna J, Pelsor F, Ihde D, et al: High-dose methotrexate (HDMTX)-citrovorum factor rescue (CFR) treatment of adeno and large cell carcinoma of the lung. *Proc Am Soc Clin Oncol* 18:289, 1977 (abstract).

34. Ettinger DS, Stanley KE, Nystrom JS: High-dose methotrexate (HDMTX) with citrovorum factor (CF) rescue in inoperable non-oat cell bronchogenic carcinoma (NOBC). *Proc Am Soc Clin Oncol* 20:347, 1979 (abstract).

35. Edmonson JH, Green SJ, Ivins JC, et al: Post-surgical treatment of primary osteosarcoma of bone—comparison of high-dose methotrexate vs. observation: Preliminary Report. *Proc Am Soc Clin Oncol* 21:476, 1980 (abstract).

36. Kotz R, Leber H, Plattner E, et al: Experiences with HDMTX protocol at the orthopedic University Clinic of Vienna. *Chemioterapia Oncologica II* (2), 205, 1978.

37. Djerassi I, Kim JS: Methotrexate and citrovorum factor rescue in the management of childhood

lymphosarcoma and reticulum cell sarcoma (non-Hodgkin's lymphomas). *Cancer* 38:1043–1051, 1976.

38. Fisher RI, DeVita VT, Hubbard SM, et al: ProMACE-MOPP combination chemotherapy: Treatment of diffuse lymphomas. *Proc Am Soc Clin Oncol* 21:468, 1980 (abstract).

39. Skarin A, Canellos G, Rosenthal D, et al: Therapy of diffuse histiocytic (DH) and undifferentiated (DU) lymphoma with high-dose methotrexate and citrovorum factor rescue (MTX/CF) Bleomycin (B), Adriamycin (A), Cyclophosphamide (C), Oncovin (O), and Decadron (D) (M-BACOD). *Proc Am Soc Clin Oncol* 21:463, 1980 (abstract).

40. Djerassi I, Kim JS, et al: High-dose methotrexate with citrovorum factor rescue: A new approach to cancer chemotherapy, in *Recent Advances in Cancer Treatment* edited by HJ Tagnon and MJ Staquet, Raven Press, New York, 201–225, 1977.

41. Bertino JR, Pitman SW: Effectiveness of high-dose methotrexate in head and neck tumors. *Chemioterapia Oncologica*, Anno II, n. 2, Giugno 1978 (Firenze).

42. Djerassi I, Rominger CJ, Kim JS, et al: Phase I study of high doses of methotrexate with citrovorum factor in patients with lung cancer. *Cancer* 30:22–30, 1972.

43. Djerassi I: High-dose methotrexate (NSC-740) and citrovorum factor (NSC-3590) rescue: Background and rationale. *Cancer Chemother Rep* Part 3, 6(1), 1975.

44. Werkheiser WC: The biochemical, cellular, and pharmacological action and effects of the folic acid antagonists. *Cancer Res* 23:1277–1285, 1963.

45. Djerassi I: Working concepts of high-dose methotrexate (HDMTX) and citrovorum factor (CF) rescue. *Chemioterapia Oncologica II,* 111, 1978.

46. Burchenal JH, Babcock GM, Broquist HP, et al: Prevention of chemotherapeutic effects of 4-amino-N^{10}-methylpteroylglutamic acid on mouse leukemia by citrovorum factor. *Proc Soc Exp Biol* 74:735, 1950.

47. Burchenal JH, Babcock GM: Prevention of toxicity of massive doses of 4-amino-N^{10}-methylpteroylglutamic acid (A-methopterin) by citrovorum factor. *Proc Soc Exp Biol Med* 76:382–384, 1951.

48. Goldin A, Mantel N, Greenhouse SW, et al: Effect of delayed administration of citrovorum factor on the anti-leukemic effectiveness of aminopterin in mice. *Cancer Res* 14:43–48, 1954.

49. Djerassi I: Methotrexate infusions and intensive supportive care in the management of children with acute leukemia: Follow-up report. *Cancer Res* 27:2561–2564, 1967.

50. Djerassi I, Kim JS, Nayak N, et al: New "rescue" with massive doses of citrovorum factor for potentially lethal methotrexate toxicity. *Cancer Treat Rep* 61:4, 1977.

51. Djerassi I, Ohanissian H, Kim JS, et al: A new approach to massive methotrexate-citrovorum rescue: A non-toxic dose schedule for methotrexate resistant tumors in poor risk patients. *Proc Am Assoc Cancer Res* 20:398, 1979 (abstract).

52. Djerassi I, Mills K, Ohanissian H, et al: Elimination of the hazards of high-dose methotrexate (HDMTX) with improved citrovorum factor rescue (CF). *Proc Am Soc Clin Oncol* 21:361, 1980 (abstract).

53. Von Hoff DD, Penta JS, Helman IJ, et al: Incidence of drug related deaths secondary to high-dose methotrexate and citrovorum factor administration. *Cancer Treat Rep* 61:745–748, 1977.

54. Ensminger WD, Frei E III: The prevention of methotrexate toxicity by thymidine infusion in man. *Cancer Res* 37:1857–1863, 1977.

55. Chabner BA, Johns DG, Bertino JR: Enzymatic cleavage of methotrexate provides a method for prevention of drug toxicity. *Nature* 239:395–397, 1972.

56. Bertino JR: Rescue techniques in cancer chemotherapy: Use of leukovorin and other rescue agents after methotrexate treatment. *Semin Oncol* 4:203–216, 1977.

57. Nirenberg A, Mosende C, Mehta BM, et al: High-dose methotrexate with citrovorum factor rescue: Predictive value of serum methotrexate concentrations and corrective measures to avert toxicity. *Cancer Treat Rep* 61:779–783, 1977.

58. Chabner BA: Presentation at NIH task force on high dose methotrexate, 1978.

59. Hoglind JA: Evaluation of the utility of high-dose methotrexate (MTX) protocols against a drug-resistant tumor. *Proc Am Assoc Can Res* 21:299, 1980 (abstract).

60. Zaharko DS, Fung WP, Yang KH: Relative biochemical aspects of low and high doses of methotrexate in mice. *Cancer Res* 37:1602–1607, 1977.

61. Djerassi I, Suvansri U, Kim JS: Long remissions in acute lymphocytic leukemia: Pulse methotrexate and a 4-drug combination. *Proc Am Assoc Cancer Res* 13:94, 1972 (abstract).

62. Jaffe N, Frei E III, Traggis D, et al: Weekly high-dose methotrexate-citrovorum factor in osteogenic sarcoma. *Cancer* 39:45–50, 1977.

24

Is High-Dose Methotrexate with Rescue More Effective than Lower-Dose Methotrexate Alone?

Arthur C. Louie

Franco M. Muggia

Marcel Rozencweig

INTRODUCTION

Methotrexate is one of the oldest and most extensively studied of the currently available anticancer drugs. Since the first report of the successful use of aminopterin in childhood acute leukemia by Farber (1), folic acid antagonists have had an important place in both cancer treatment and the biochemical pharmacology of antineoplastic drugs.

In spite of nearly 15 years of clinical trials, controversy persists over the proper role for high-dose methotrexate with citrovorum factor rescue (HDMTX-CF) in the treatment of cancer. The persistence of this controversy illustrates the weaknesses inherent in a clinical trials literature dealing with an attractive concept but composed almost exclusively of small nonrandomized pilot studies. The debate is not over the issue of whether methotrexate given in high doses with CF rescue is an active treatment against cancer. Sufficient clinical evidence exists showing that high-dose methotrexate is indeed active against many forms of cancer. The central issue of the debate lies in establishing what clinical circumstances make the use of high-dose methotrexate appropriate.

In this chapter, we argue that the high-dose methotrexate "package," which requires facilities for infusion therapy, hydration, urinary alkalinization, measurement of methotrexate levels, and the detection and aggressive treatment of unpredictable and potentially lethal toxicities, is not sufficiently superior to conventional-dose methotrexate to justify its routine use for patients with any disease. High-dose methotrexate with citrovorum factor rescue is indeed a kind of therapeutic Mount Everest. The fact that we have the technical means for delivering massive doses of methotrexate in relative safety does not justify using this form of therapy simply because it exists. We review the rationale for high-dose methotrexate treatment and base our conclusions regarding its clinical use on an analysis of clinical results (see "Materials and Methods").

Goldin's experiments (2–4) with aminopterin in L1210 leukemia showed that the biological effects of antifolates could be reversed with citrovorum factor and that these reversal effects could be manipulated to produce apparent but modest improvements in therapeutic response in animals. Although subsequent clinical trials have used markedly higher doses and distinctly different rescue regimens, these important observations are cited as the experimental rationale for the improved therapeutic index of high-dose methotrexate. By 1960 several groups (5–6) reported using methotrexate in relatively large doses on infrequent schedules for children with acute leukemia. In 1966 Djerassi (7) noted that methotrexate could be given in high doses to patients with acute leukemia without apparent severe toxicity, and it is this observation that led to the use of higher doses of methotrexate with the addition of citrovorum factor rescue in methotrexate treatment regimens.

In Djerassi's experiments, patients with acute lymphocytic leukemia in remission were given relatively high doses of methotrexate as part of several different maintenance regimens. Citrovorum factor was added to one of these regimens to reduce the toxic effects encountered with methotrexate. Using this treatment, he could administer 525 mg/M^2 daily of methotrexate for two consecutive days with tolerable toxicity. In later anecdotal reports Djerassi described the successful retreatment of patients relapsing after methotrexate maintenance with even higher doses of methotrexate.

The use of methotrexate with citrovorum factor rescue after 1966 is marked by the extreme variability of methotrexate treatment regimens. No single regimen appears clearly superior to all others, but the very large number of treatment regimens, each with slight variations on the dose and duration of methotrexate infusion, time interval before rescue, and dose and duration of citrovorum factor, pose obstacles in comparing clinical results.

Drug toxicity depends on dose, duration of administration, and efficiency of elimination of methotrexate from the body. Chabner and Young (8) demonstrated that suppression of DNA synthesis following exposure to methotrexate is directly related to plasma drug concentration. It follows that the duration of this period of suppression is directly related to the persistence of methotrexate in plasma above the minimum level required for suppression of DNA synthesis. In addition to its effect on DNA synthesis, precipitation of methotrexate in the renal tubule reduces renal function, which delays methotrexate excretion, further exacerbating methotrexate toxicity (9–11).

Citrovorum factor competes with methotrexate for entry into the cell and, once inside the cell, restores the pool of reduced folates, allowing resumption of DNA synthesis (12,13). The prevention of methotrexate toxicity requires monitoring of MTX blood levels and adjustment of the dose and duration of CF rescue accordingly (14–16). Additional measures to minimize methotrexate nephrotoxicity include adequate hydration (17,18) and alkalinization of the urine (19). Although the last two measures improve methotrexate solubility in the urine, their effect on treatment efficacy is unknown. In spite of the sophisticated and expensive supportive measures mentioned above, up to 10% of patients develop significant toxicity and drug-related complications (20,21). The drug-related fatality rate may be as high as 5% in published series (21,22).

It should be clear from the discussion above, that high-dose methotrexate treatment involves increased practical complexity, patient inconvenience, and considerably higher cost both for the drug and for its proper administration and that the use of citrovorum factor rescue does not entirely prevent severe and sometimes catastrophic methotrexate toxicity. All these problems can be accepted if it can be shown that HDMTX-CF has significantly better efficacy than conventional-dose methrotrexate.

We present data from an extensive review performed by the Cancer Therapy Evaluation Program of the Division of Cancer Treatment, National Cancer Institute, which specifically compares the antitumor activity of high-dose methotrexate with moderate- and low-dose methotrexate regimens. The data are presented in terms of response rates (RR) obtained from the literature. Unfortunately, there are no data suggesting a survival advantage in a population treated with HDMTX-CF versus a concurrent untreated control or versus a conventional-dose methotrexate regimen without rescue. We show that the response rates reported for high-dose methotrexate are quite similar to those reported for moderate-dose with rescue and conventional-dose methotrexate without rescue in most types of cancer.

MATERIALS AND METHODS

Data were collected from the general medical and oncologic literature. Studies were excluded where assessment of the antitumor effect of methotrexate was obscured. This usually occurred when methotrexate was used simultaneously with surgery or radiation therapy or when methotrexate was used as part of a drug combination with other drugs known to be efficacious.

High-dose methotrexate is defined as any dose in excess of 500 mg/M^2 given by bolus injection or prolonged IV infusion. Moderate-dose methotrexate is defined as any dose in the 100 to 500 mg/M^2 range given with CF rescue. Conventional or low-dose methotrexate is defined as a dose less than 100 mg/M^2, usually given without CF rescue. Studies in which dose escalations led to treatment of some patients with low doses and other patients with moderate doses of methotrexate were assigned according to the treatment received by the majority of patients.

Complete response is defined by the complete disappearance of all measurable disease. Partial response indicates greater than 50% reduction in the size of all measurable tumor unless otherwise noted.

CLINICAL TRIALS

Brain Tumors

Methotrexate given in high doses (>1 g/M^2) by either bolus injection or 20-hour infusion penetrates the cerebrospinal fluid (CSF) and achieves levels equal or greater than 10^{-6} M (8,23). In addition, the clearance of methotrexate from this

Table 1. Antitumor Activity of Single-Agent Methotrexate

	Conventional-Dose MTX w/o CF Rescue					Moderate-Dose MTX w/ CF Rescue					High-Dose MTX w/ CF Rescue				
	Eval Pt	CR	PR	RR	Ref	Eval Pt	CR	PR	RR	Ref	Eval Pt	CR	PR	RR	Ref
Brain															
Pediatric											23	1	12	57%	24–27
Adult											6	0	0	0%	28
Breast	237	1	81	35%	29–40						57	2	14	28%	27,42,43
Childhood solid tumors											36	1	1	5%	44–47
Gastrointestinal	127	0	19	15%	33,34,36–38,48	18	0	5	28%	49	34	0	6	18%	27,50
Genitourinary															
Bladder	39	1	5	15%	51,52	16	1	7	50%	53					
Testicular	10	0	4	40%	54										
Other											1	1	0	100%	55
Gynecologic															
Ovary	16	0	4	25%	37	2	0	0	0%	56	19	0	3	16%	56,57
Cervix	34	0	6	18%	33,58,59	39	0	8	20%	60–62					

Gestational trophoblastic	247	148	40	76%	63–74	38	34	0	90%	61,62	2	0	1	50%	27
Other															
Head and neck	259	26	74	39%	33,35,37,38, 76–84	163	4	62	38%	60,85,92, 132	160	5	68	46%	27,86,92–98, 132
Luekemia															
ALL	107	20	17	35%	5,101–103	34	26	4	98%	89,99	1	0	0	0%	46
AML/AMoL	76	8	4	16%	102,103	10	1	2	30%	89	6	0	3	50%	27,46
CML/blast crisis	3	2	0	66%	102										
Lymphoma															
Hodgkin's	18	1	1	11%	29,105–106										
Non-Hodgkin's	27	3	7	37%	29,105–106						80	31	26	71%	108–113, 27
Burkitt's	19	6	4	53%	107										
Lung															
Non-small cell	173	3	32	20%	33,35,37,114– 116	22	0	6	27%	60,114, 117	126	1	20	17%	27,117– 123,27
Small cell						2	0	1	50%	60	2	0	0	0%	
Melnoma	26	0	2	8%	29,35,37,38						93	8	6	15%	27,124–126
Myeloma															
Osteosarcoma											20	2	3	25%	127–129
Soft-tissue sarcoma	32	8	5	41%	130						34	0	10	29%	27,110,131

compartment is considerably slower than from the serum (8). As shown in Table 1, the data for treatment of brain tumors (24–28) are extremely limited. No data were found for treatment with conventional or moderate-dose MTX. The majority of cases reported deal with pediatric neoplasms. If patients treated with combination therapy and intrathecal MTX therapy are excluded, only 1 complete response and 12 partial responses are seen among 23 pediatric patients. Responses have been reported in medulloblastomas and pontine gliomas. For adult gliomas, Shapiro (28) was unable to detect any activity in 6 patients treated.

Breast Cancer

The cumulative activity for single-agent conventional-dose methotrexate in 237 patients, the majority with advanced or recurrent breast cancer, is 1 complete and 81 partial responses for a combined response rate of 35% (29–40). For moderate-dose methotrexate the data are difficult to find. The Southeastern Cancer Study Group (41) reported the preliminary results of a randomized trial in which moderate-dose MTX-CF (125 mg/M^2 P.O. q6h × 4) was compared with weekly oral methotrexate (15 mg/M^2 P.O. q6h × 4) and weekly IV methotrexate (60 mg/M^2). They found no difference among the three regimens and combined the data together from all three groups. Five partial responses were observed in 17 patients, and responses were defined as tumor regression greater than 25%.

HDMTX-CF treatment was reported by Henderson (42) to produce 3 partial responses among 19 patients. Isacoff (27) treated 17 patients with refractory advanced breast cancer in a phase II study and found 1 complete and 4 partial responses. These responses lasted only a median of two months. Twenty-seven patients were treated by Yap (43) with 1 complete and 7 partial responses. The results in 57 patients all with advanced breast cancer, all treated with methotrexate at doses greater than 2.5 gm/M^2, are 2 complete and 14 partial responses for an overall response rate of only 28%.

Childhood Solid Tumors

No data are available for the treatment of childhood solid tumors with either conventional or moderate-dose methotrexate. With high-dose methotrexate only 2 responses (5%) were seen in 36 patients (44–47). A complete response was reported in 1 patient with Ewing's (46) sarcoma and a partial response in 1 patient with rhabdomyosarcoma (44).

Gastrointestinal Tumors

Methotrexate has only minimal activity in colon cancer when used at conventional doses. Cumulative data from six studies (33,34,36–38,48) involving 127 patients showed only 19 partial responses for a response rate of only 15%. Moderate-dose methotrexate was used by Cheng (49) to treat 18 patients with pancreatic cancer. Five partial responses were observed, but toxicity was severe in 3 patients, with 2 patients dying of treatment-related complications. Not included in Table 1 is the Southeastern Cancer Study Group study (41), which also entered patients with colorectal cancer into the randomized three-arm study already mentioned in the section on breast cancer. Again, no significant differences were found among the three treatment options, and the data were combined. Only 3 partial responses were seen in 27 patients. Isacoff (27,50) treated patients with a variety of GI malignancies using high-dose methotrexate. Six partial responses (18%) were observed in 34 treated patients. Five of these responses occurred in patients with colon cancer, and 1 response was seen in a patient with bilary tract cancer. Thus, with the possible exception of pancreatic cancer, methotrexate at any dose appears to have only marginal activity for gastrointestinal tumors.

Genitourinary Tumors

There is scanty experience with methotrexate in the treatment of patients with genitourinary cancers. Overall 39 patients (51,52) with bladder cancer were treated with relatively low doses of methotrexate with 1 complete and 5 partial responses for an overall response rate of 15%. Included in this is Gad-El-Mawla's series (51) of bladder cancer from Egypt, which contains a significant number of patients with squamous cell tumors of the bladder. Turner (53) treated 16 patients with advanced bladder cancer using 200 mg of methotrexate given intramuscularly. This moderate-dose treatment produced 1 complete and 7 partial responses (50%) with the complete response lasting 20 months and the partial responses lasting an average of 4 months. Similarly in one institution the same group of researchers found HDMTX-CF of borderline effectiveness, but an appreciable response rate was obtained with conventional-dose methotrexate (137). There is evidence of activity of conventional-dose methotrexate in testicular cancer (54) but no data for higher-dosage regimens, and there is a single case report of a complete response to high-dose methotrexate in a patient with metastatic carcinoma of the penis (55).

Gynecologic Tumors

There are very few data on the use of low-dose methotrexate in ovarian cancer. Sullivan et al. (37), in a broad phase II study, reported treating 16 patients with advanced ovarian cancer, with 4 objective responses, using 5 mg of methotrexate given in 24 hours either in divided oral doses or by continuous infusion. Barlow and Piver (56) reported treating two ovarian cancer patients with moderate-dose methotrexate. No objective response was noted, but one patient did have stabilization of disease. As part of the same study Barlow also treated 11 patients with high-dose methotrexate and observed 2 partial remissions. Eight patients with measurable ovarian cancer were treated by Parker (57) using methotrexate at a dose of 3.0 gm/M^2. HDMTX-CF was felt to be ineffective because only one partial response (13%) was seen.

Response rates are comparable for treatment of carcinoma of the cervix using conventional-dose and moderate-dose methotrexate. In three series collected by Condit (33), Roy (58), and Haffner (59) only 6 responses were seen in 34 patients treated (18%). An almost identical rate of response is found after treatment with moderate-dose methotrexate. Mills (60) reported 3 partial responses in 10 patients after treatment with MTX/CF at a dose of 100 mg/M^2 by four-hour infusion, and Nikrui (61,62) reported only 5 partial responses among 29 patients using a two-hour infusion of 200 mg/M².

It is well known that trophoblastic malignancies respond to methotrexate (63–74). In 12 series collected from the literature (63–74) 76% of patients responded to methotrexate given at conventional doses. Goldstein (74) treated 38 patients with moderate-dose methotrexate, 1 to 2.5 mg/kg IM given every other day for four doses and observed 34 complete responses (90%).

Head and Neck Cancer

Head and neck tumors are clearly responsive to methotrexate given at any dose level. In a collected series of 13 studies (33,35,37,38,76–84) involving 259 patients treated with relatively low doses of methotrexate, without rescue, an overall response rate of 39% was achieved. This includes 26 complete responders and 74 partial responders. Moderate doses of methotrexate were administered in seven studies (60, 85–92) to 163 patients with 4 complete and 62 partial responses achieved. The overall response rate was 38%. High-dose methotrexate (27, 86,92–98, 132) was used with very similar results in 160 patients. Only 5 complete responses were observed among 73 patients with objective response, for a 46% response rate. The apparent decrease in the complete response rate seen with moderate and high-dose MTX is probably due to the selection of patients with somewhat more advanced or refractory disease in later studies.

In 1977 Beuchler (86,87) reported the results of a trial in which patients were randomized to receive methotrexate with or without BCG. Methotrexate was given at a dose of 15 mg/kg. In the final phase of the study patients were given escalating doses of methotrexate—up to 7 g total dose. Methotrexate given alone at a dose of 15 mg/kg produced only 1 complete and 2 partial responses in 12 patients (RR = 25%). On the escalating-dose regimen only 1 partial response was seen among 8 patients. Response duration was generally quite brief. The study reported by Vogler (41) for the Southeastern Cancer Study Group and already mentioned in the sections on breast and gastrointestinal cancers is not included in the table because the responses from all three treatment groups are reported together. They found no difference in response rate among moderate-dose oral methotrexate with CF rescue, low-dose oral methotrexate, and low-dose IV methotrexate. Eleven partial responses among 26 treated patients were found, but responses were defined by 25% or greater tumor regression.

The recent study by Woods et al. (92,132) is one of the few attempts to directly compare low versus moderate versus high-dose methotrexate. In this study patients with advanced squamous cell carcinomas of the head and neck were randomized to receive weekly methotrexate at 500 or 5,000 mg/M². All patients, including those at the lowest dose level, were given citrovorum factor. Patients not achieving a response at one dose level were crossed over to receive the next higher dose. Low-dose methotrexate produced 1 complete and 5 partial responses among 23 patients; moderate-dose methotrexate produced partial responses in 7 of 27 patients; and the high-dose methotrexate group had 1 complete and 9 partial responses among 22 patients. The differences in response rates were not significant (P> .05). On crossover from conventional-dose to moderate-dose methotrexate 4 of 9 patients responded. Six of 15 patients crossed over from moderate-dose to high-dose methotrexate responded. Not unexpectedly, they found more severe toxicity among patients receiving the higher-dose treatments. Four cases of fatal drug toxicity were encountered, and the authors concluded that there was no overall advantage to using high-dose methotrexate as initial drug treatment for patients with head and neck cancer.

Leukemia

Folic acid antagonists have an important place in the history of leukemia treatment (1). Relatively few studies have used methotrexate as a single agent, and as a consequence an unambiguous response rate is difficult to determine from studies reported in the literature.

Condit (5) reported the use of relatively large doses (5 mg/kg) of methotrexate without rescue in three patients, all of whom achieved transient complete remission while on treatment. Perrin et al. (101) gave methotrexate at 3 mg/kg every two weeks to 14 children with acute leukemia and reported 12 of 14 patients achieving remissions that lasted an average of 4.4 months. Huguley et al. (102) used a different dose and schedule of methotrexate (1.25 to 3.75 mg P.O. q6h × 20 doses) to treat 24 adult patients with a variety of leukemias. Nineteen patients with acute myelocytic or monocytic leukemias were treated, with 6 complete and 2 partial remissions. Only 2 patients with adult acute lymphocytic leukemia (ALL) were treated with no objective responses observed, and three patients with chronic myelogenous leukemia in blast crisis were treated with 2 complete responses observed. The largest study of conventional-dose methotrexate treatment of leukemias was reported by Frei et al. (103) for the Acute Leukemia Group B (now CALGB). They treated both children and adults with leukemias with methotrexate followed by 6-mercaptopurine or 6-mercaptopurine followed by methotrexate or a combination using both drugs together. When the results obtained using methotrexate alone are analyzed prior treatment with 6-mercaptopurine did not affect response to subsequent methotrexate treatment. Eighty-one children with acute lymphocytic leukemia were treated, with 16 complete and 5 partial responses. Only 9 children with acute myelogenous leukemia (AML) were treated, with 1 complete and 1 partial response achieved. Treatment of 48 adult patients with acute myelogenous leukemia produced only 1 complete and 1 partial response, and 7 adults with acute lymphocytic leukemia were treated, with 1 complete remission reported.

Moderate-dose methotrexate appears active for acute lymphocytic leukemia, but only a limited number of clinical reports are available for analysis. The combined results from two separate studies show 30 of 34 patients achieving an objective response, all but 4 of the responders achieving a complete response (89,99). Very few patients with AML have been studied with methotrexate treatment. Although responses have been reported (1 complete and 2 partial) the number of patients described in the literature is too small to evaluate drug efficacy.

Clinical experience with high-dose methotrexate for leukemias is even more limited (27,46), and responses have been seen in AML. A role for high-dose methotrexate in the prevention of central nervous system (CNS) leukemia is being explored by the CALGB (100).

Lymphomas

Responses have been observed in lymphomas after methotrexate treatment used at both conventional doses and high doses with rescue (105–107). The treatment of Hodgkin's disease using conventional doses of methotrexate reveals only 1 complete and 1 partial response among 18 patients treated (29,105,106). For the non-Hodgkin's lymphomas 27 patients were treated in three series (29,105,106), with 3 complete and 7 partial responses for a 37% response rate. High-dose methotrexate has produced 31 complete and 26 partial responses among 80 patients in the collected results of seven series (27,108–113). Comparisons are very difficult to make among these studies because of the marked differences in natural history among the different histologic types of non-Hodgkin's lymphomas and the frequent lack of histologic subclassification among these studies. Again, prevention of CNS disease is a consideration in the use of high-dose methotrexate in current chemotherapy regimens (104,110).

Lung Cancer

Methotrexate at any dose appears only marginally active in non-small cell lung cancer. There are insufficient data to evaluate the activity of methotrexate for small cell lung cancer.

The cumulative results from seven series that treated non-small cell lung cancer patients with conventional-dose methotrexate shows only a 20% response rate with 3 complete and 32 partial responses among 173 patients (33,35,37, 38,114–116). The largest study in this group was performed by Selawry et al, (116), who randomized patients to receive methotrexate at 0.6 mg/kg or 0.2 mg/kg twice weekly or placebo twice weekly for four months. The placebo group had 2 partial responses among 34 patients. The 0.2 mg/kg group did slightly better with 4 partial responses in 37 patients. The 0.6 mg/kg group had a 21% response rate with 10 partial responses among 48 patients.

The clinical experience with moderate-dose methotrexate and citrovorum factor rescue is comparable with conventional-dose methotrexate. Mills (60) treated six patients with 100 mg/m² of methotrexate by four-hour infusion given weekly and observed two partial responses. Djerassi (119) in his phase I study reported no responses among three patients given methotrexate at 100–800 mg doses.

High-dose methotrexate appears to perform no better than more conventional-dose treatment. Djerassi (117) reported 10 partial responses in 11 patients treated with HDMTX/CF. Three patients suffered severe toxicity on treatment. Subsequent reports from a variety of investigators (27,117–123) have not confirmed such high response rates. Minna et al. (118,120) found only 1 partial response among 35 patients treated. Tornyos et al. (121) treated 13 patients with metastatic squamous cell carcinoma, with no objective responses. Only 1 partial response and 4 patients with stable disease were reported by Ettinger (123) among 28 patients with inoperable non-oat cell lung cancer given high-dose methotrexate.

Melanoma

Only marginal activity has been reported for methotrexate treatment of malignant melanoma. Sullivan (37) treated 12 patients with 5 mg of methotrexate per day for 5 to 10 days and noted only 2 partial responses. The group at UCLA (124) reported treating 22 patients with disseminated melanomas using high-dose methotrexate (50 to 250 mg/kg). Pain relief was noted at 50 mg/kg, and objective responses were seen at the 200 mg/kg dose. Five complete and 3 partial responses were achieved, with the best results occurring in patients with skin, lymph node, and bone metastases. Isacoff (27) studied another 20 patients, 8 treated previously with chemotherapy, and achieved 3 complete and 2 partial responses. Median response duration in this group was four months. Prior chemotherapy seems to reduce the chances for response to methotrexate. Fisher (125) treated 23 patients, all with melanomas refractory to DTIC or methyl CCNU, and observed no objective responses. Similarly, Karakovsis (126) observed only 1 partial response in 28 patients.

Osteosarcoma

High-dose methotrexate has been extensively used for the treatment of osteosarcoma, especially in the adjuvant setting. A search of the literature, however, shows no series of patients treated with either conventional-dose or moderate-dose methotrexate. The activity of high-dose methotrexate used as a single agent in patients with measurable disease is approximately 25% (127–129). Jaffe (128) reported treating 10 patients with six-hour infusions of high-dose methotrexate (50 to 500 mg/kg, q2 to 3 wk). Two complete and 2 partial responses were observed, but partial response was defined by tumor regression greater than 25%. He observed various and unpredictable toxicity in spite of rescue. Three patients who progressed were subsequently treated with 24-hour infusions of high-dose methotrexate, and one of these achieved a partial response. Ambinder (129) in a phase II study, treated 7 patients with advanced osteosarcoma using six-hour infusions of methotrexate (25 to 250 mg/kg). No objective responses were seen, but 1 patient had stabilization of disease for 23 months. Data based on necrosis of primary tumors (134) are difficult to interpret (133). Favorable results in adjuvant trials contrasted with historical controls must be viewed as possibly related to other factors, and not the chemotherapy. The results achieved with HDMTX-CF must retrospectively be viewed with a particularly critical eye because (1) negative studies have appeared (135), (2) the addition of HDMTX-CF to other regimens has not improved previous results (135), and (3) most important, a recent randomized study indicates no better results than concurrent untreated controls (136).

Soft-Tissue Sarcoma

Wiltshaw (130) reported treating 32 patients with a variety of soft-tissue sarcomas, with 2.5 to 10 mg of oral methotrexate given in divided doses for 2 to 15 days. Eight complete and 5 partial responses were observed for a 41% response rate. High-dose methotrexate has been used by Pitman (110) and Isacoff (27) for sarcomas. Four of 18 patients in Pitman's series responded to weekly high-dose methotrexate (1 to 7.5 gm/M², IV push), and 5 of 15 patients treated by Isacoff had partial remissions. There appears to be no advantage to high-dose methotrexate in this disease.

DISCUSSION

Methotrexate has been in clinical use for more than 25 years; high-dose regimens for nearly 15 years. What emerges after all this time is a body of literature composed almost entirely of small nonrandomized studies. Although clinical observations from small groups of patients often provide the seminal ideas to important experimental issues, some clinicians, in their fervor to achieve good results and to make exciting theories work, have more clouded than clarified the methotrexate issue. It is not surprising that optimistic reports based on small series of patients, sometimes evaluated by nonstandard criteria, have proved difficult to reproduce in larger, more carefully designed trials. Another source of confusion can be traced to the rapid introduction of HDMTX-CF into drug combinations and multimodality treatments where the contribution of methotrexate to the final clinical result is completely obscured. The confusion that has resulted from trying to interpret these trials has perpetuated the debate over the proper role of high-dose methotrexate in cancer treatment.

High-dose methotrexate has attracted attention precisely because it has such a clear and plausible rationale. Pharmacologic advances during the last decade have given us the technical means for delivering massive doses of methotrexate in relative safety. But both the drug and the means for its administration have proved to be expensive and cumbersome. Although citrovorum factor rescue prevents methotrexate toxicity in the majority of patients, unpredictable and occasionally catastrophic toxicity continues to be a problem even in the hands of the experienced investigators. In this instance, combination chemotherapy should be further discouraged because of the hazards of unforeseen drug interactions.

In Table 1 we present data on the activity of methotrexate when used by itself for the treatment of cancer. Where adequate data are available, methotrexate used in conventional doses appears as active as high-dose methotrexate with citrovorum factor rescue. Minimal differences in antitumor activity are found in methotrexate treatment of breast cancer, gastrointestinal tumors, gynecologic tumors, head and neck cancer, lung cancer, melanoma, and soft-tissue sarcomas over a very wide range of doses. The routine use of high-dose methotrexate for these tumors is not justified. For the remaining tumor types there are insufficient data to permit comparison between high- and low-dose methotrexate. In the absence of sufficient data the most reasonable initial course of action continues to be use of the more convenient and less expensive conventional-dose regimens. Djerassi's observations (14) and the recent report by Woods et al. (92) suggest that responses can still be achieved with higher doses of methotrexate after failure of initial lower-dose regimens. Thus, higher doses of methotrexate may be used if lower-dose treatment proves inadequate, but this approach has limited the practical implications.

In conclusion, HDMTX-CF remains an attractive concept. In spite of its promise, there is no proof for either enhanced antitumor selectivity or efficacy. Other issues such as correlation of efficacy with toxicity, other methods of biochemical modulation, and optimal scheduling in relation to specific disease circumstances remain important topics for study. It continues to be an alternative to conventional-dose methotrexate, but its cost, inconvenience, and potential for severe toxicity require common sense criteria for its use. We have shown HDMTX-CF to be comparable in antitumor activity with conventional-dose MTX in a variety of tumors. Treatment superiority of HDMTX-CF for special circumstances (CNS disease) and osteosarcoma must be confirmed in randomized studies. In all other instances, we conclude that initial therapy with conventional-dose methotrexate is preferred where use of high-dose methotrexate might be considered. Treatment with higher doses of methotrexate may be considered for resistant tumors.

REFERENCES

1. Farber S, Diamond LK, Mercer RD, et al: Temporary remission in acute leukemia in children produced by folic acid antagonist, 4-aminoptero-glutamic acid (aminopterin). *N Engl J Med* 238:787–793, 1948.

2. Goldin A, Mantel N. Greenhouse SW, et al: Effect of delayed administration of citrovorum factor and the antileukemic effectiveness of aminopterin in mice. *Cancer Res* 14:43–48, 1954.

3. Goldin A, Mantel N, Greenhouse SW, et al: Factors influencing the specificity of action of an antileukemic agent (aminopterin): Time of treatment and dosage schedule. *Cancer Res* 14:311–314, 1954.

4. Goldin A, Venditti JM, Humphreys SR, et al: Factors influencing the specificity of action of an antileukemic agent (aminopterin): Multiple treatment schedules plus delayed administration of citrovorum factor. *Cancer Res* 15:57–61, 1955.

5. Condit PT, Eliel LP: Effects of large infrequent doses of A-methopterin on acute leukemia in children. *JAMA* 172:451–453, 1960.

6. Perrin JCS, Mauer AM, Sterling TD: Intravenous methotrexate (aminopterin) therapy in the treatment of acute leukemia. *Pediatrics* 31:833–839, 1963.

7. Djerassi I, Abir E, Royer GL Jr, et al: Long term remissions in childhood acute leukemia: Use of infrequent infusions of methotrexate: Supportive roles of platelet transfusions and citrovorum factor. *Clin Pediatr* 5:502–509, 1966.

8. Chabner BA, Young RC: Threshold methotrexate concentration for in vivo inhibition of DNA synthesis in normal and tumorous target tissues. *J Clin Invest* 52:1804–1811, 1973.

9. Tattersall MHN, Parker LM, Pitman SW, Frei E III: Pharmacology of high dose methotrexate (NSC-740). *Cancer Chemother Rep* Part 3 6(1):25–29, 1975.

10. Stoller RG, Jacobs SA, Drake JC, Lutz RJ, Chabner BA: Pharmacokinetics of high dose methotrexate (NSC 740). *Cancer Chemother Rep* Part 3 6(1):19–24, 1975.

11. Isacoff WH, Eilber F, Block J: Clinical pharmacology of high dose methotrexate. *Proc AACR* 17:190, 1976, (abstract) 758.

12. Bertino JR: "Rescue" techniques in cancer chemotherapy: Use of leucovorin and other rescue agents after methotrexate treatment. *Semin Oncol* 4:203, 1977.

13. Sirotnak FM, Donsbach RC, Moccio DM, Dorick DM: Biochemical and pharmacokinetic effects of leucovorin after high dose methotrexate in a murine leukemia model. *Cancer Res* 36:4679–4686, 1976.

14. Djerassi I: High dose methotrexate (NSC 740) and citrovorum factor (NSC 3590) rescue: Background and rationale. *Cancer Chemother Rep* Part 3 6(1):3–6, 1975.

15. Levitt M, Mosher MB, DeConti RC, et al: Improved therapeutic index of methotrexate with "leucovorin rescue." *Cancer Res* 33:1729–1734, 1973.

16. Nirenberg A, Mehta B, Murphy ML, et al: Serum methotrexate levels: The risk of clinical toxicity following high dose methotrexate with citrovorum factor rescue. *Proc AACR* 17:124, 1976.

17. Jaffe N, Traggis D: Toxicity of high dose methotrexate (NSC-740) and citrovorum factor (NSC-3590) in osteogenic sarcoma. *Cancer Chemo Rep* Part 3 3(6):31–36, 1975.

18. Nirenberg A, Mosende C, Mehta BM, et al: High dose methotrexate with citrovorum rescue: Predictive value of serum methotrexate concentrations and corrective measures to avert toxicity. *Cancer Treat Rep* 61:779–783, 1977.

19. Sadoff L, Rittmann A: The use of acetazolamide (AC) to alkalinize the urine in high dose methotrexate therapy in patients with advanced cancer. *Proc AACR* 17:304, 1976, (abstract C-272.)

20. Chan H, Evans WE, Pratt CB: Recovery from toxicity associated with high dose methotrexate: Prognostic factors. *Cancer Treat Rep* 61:797–804, 1977.

21. Von Hoff DD, Penta JS, Helman LJ, et al: Incidence of drug related deaths secondary to high dose methotrexate and citrovorum factor administration. *Cancer Treat Rep* 61:745–748, 1977.

22. Penta JS, Von Hoff DD, Louie A, et al: Drug related fatalities following methotreate and citrovorum factor administration, in *High Dose Methotrexate Pharmacology Toxicology and Chemotherapy.* (P Periti, ed) Firenze, Editrice Giuntina, pp 245–252.

23. Wang Y, Lantin E, Sutow WW: Methotrexate in blood, urine, and cerebrospinal fluid of children receiving high doses by infusion. *Clin Chem* 22(7):1053–1056, 1976.

24. Rosen G, Ghavimi F, Allen J, et al: Response of intracranial neoplasms to high dose methotrexate with citrovorum factor rescue. *Proc AACR* 18:296, 1977.

25. Rosen G, Ghavimi F, Vanucci R, et al: Pontine glioma: High dose methotrexate and leucovorin rescue. *JAMA* 230:1149–1152, 1974.

26. Djerassi I, Kim JS, Shulman K: High dose methotrexate–citrovorum factor rescue in the management of brain tumors. *Cancer Treat Rep* 61:691–694, 1977.

27. Isacoff, et al: Phase II clinical trial with high dose methotrexate therapy and citrovorum factor rescue. *Cancer Treat Rep* 62:1295–1304, 1978.

28. Shapiro WR: High dose methotrexate in malignant gliomas. *Cancer Treat Rep* 61:753–756, 1977.

29. Burcheneal JH, Karnofsky DA, Kingsley-Pilliers EM, et al: The effects of the folic acid antagonists and 2,6 diaminopurine on neoplastic disease: With special reference to acute leukemia. *Cancer* 4:549–569, 1951.

30. Schoenbach EB, Colsky J, Greenspan EM: Observations on the effects of the folic acid antagonists, aminopterin and amethopterin, in patients with advanced neoplasms. *Cancer* 5:1201–1220, 1952.

31. Wright JC, Cobb JP, Golomb FM, et al: Chemotherapy of disseminated carcinoma of the breast. *Ann Surg* 150:221–240, 1959.

32. Greening W: Methotrexate in the treatment of advanced cancer of the breast, in *Methotrexate in the Treatment of Cancer.* (Porter and Wiltshaw, eds). pp 29–33, 1962.

33. Condit PT, Shnider BI, Owens AH: Studies on the folic acid vitamins: VII. The effects of large doses of amethopterin in patients with cancer. *Cancer Res* 22:706–712, 1962.

34. Wilson HE, Louis J: The use of low dosage drug regimens in the treatment of neoplastic disease. *Ann Intern Med* 63:918, 1965 (abstract).

35. Vogler WR, Huguley CM, Kerr W: Toxicity and antitumor effect of divided doses of methotrexate. *Arch Intern Med* 115:285–293, 1965.

36. Eastern Cooperative Group in Solid Tumor Chemotherapy: Comparison of antimetabolites in the treatment of breast and colon cancer. *JAMA* 200:770–778, 1967.

37. Sullivan RD, Miller E, Zurek WZ, et al: Re-evaluation of methotrexate as an anticancer drug. *Surg Gynecol Obstet* 125:819–824, 1967.

38. Andrews NC, Wilson WL: Phase II study of methotrexate (NSC-740) in solid tumors. *Cancer Chemother Rep* 51:471–474, 1967.

39. Vogler WR, Furtado VP, Huguley CM: Methotrexate for advanced cancer of the breast. *Cancer* 21:26–30, 1968.

40. Nevinny HB, Hall TC, Haines C, et al: Comparison of methotrexate (NSC-740) and testosterone propionate (NSC-9166) in the treatment of breast cancer. *J Clin Pharmacol* 8:126–129, 1968.

41. Vogler WR, Jacobs J: High divided dose methotrexate (MTX) with leucovorin (LCV) rescue vs low oral divided dose MTX vs single dose IV MTX in advanced carcinoma of head, neck, breast, and colon. *Proc Am Assoc Cancer Res* 16:266, 1975 (abstract).

42. Henderson IC, Canellos GP, Blum RH, et al: Prolonged disease-free survival in advanced breast cancer treated with "super-CMF" adriamycin: An alternating regimen employing high dose methotrexate (M) with citrovorum factor (CF) rescue. *Proc AACR* 20:327, 1979.

43. Yap HY, Blumenschein GR, Yap BS, et al: High dose methotrexate for advanced breast cancer. *Cancer Treat Rep* 63:757–761, 1979.

44. Pratt CB, Roberts D, Shanks EC, et al: Clinical trials and pharmacokinetics of intermittent high-dose methotrexate "leucovorin rescue" for children with malignant tumors. *Cancer Res* 34:3326–3331, 1974.

45. Pratt CB, Roberts D, Shanks E, et al: Response, toxicity and pharmacokinetics of high dose methotrexate with citrovorum factor rescue for children with osteosarcoma and other malignant tumors. *Cancer Chemother Rep* Part 3 6:13–18, 1975.

46. Pitman SW, et al: Clinical trial of high-dose methotrexate (NSC-740) with citrovorum factor rescue (NSC-3590): Toxicologic and therapeutic observations. *Cancer Chemother Rep* Part 3 6:43–49, 1975.

47. Ablin AR, Bleyer WA, Finklestein JZ, et al: Failure of moderate-dose prolonged infusion methotrexate and citrovorum factor rescue in patients with previously treated metastatic neuroblastoma: A phase II study. *Cancer Treat Rep* 62:1097–1099, 1978.

48. Moertel CG, Reitemeier RJ, Hahn RG: Oral methotrexate therapy of gastrointestinal carcinoma. *Surg Gynecol Obstet* 130:292–294, 1970.

49. Cheng E, Magill GB, Golbey RB: High dose methotrexate therapy in carcinoma of the pancreas. *Proc AACR* 17:295, 1976.

50. Isacoff WH, Tisman G, Block JB: Treatment of advanced colorectal carcinoma with high dose methotrexate (HDMTX) given alone and in combination with 5-Fluorouracil (5-FU). *Proc AACR* 20:381, 1979.

51. Gad-el-Mawla N, Hamsa B, Cairns J, et al: Phase II trial of methotrexate in carcinoma of the bilharzial bladder. *Cancer Treat Rep* 62:1075–1076, 1978.

52. Altman CC, McCague NJ, Ripepi AC, et al: The use of methotrexate in advanced carcinoma of the bladder. *J Urol* 108:271–273, 1972.

53. Turner AG, Hendry WF, Williams GB, et al: The treatment of advanced bladder cancer with methotrexate. *Br J Urol* 49:673–678, 1977.

54. Wyatt JK, McAninch LN: A chemotherapeutic approach to advanced testicular carcinoma. *Can J Surg* 10:421–426, 1967.

55. Garnick MB, Skarin AT, Steele GD: Metastatic carcinoma of the penis: Complete remission after high dose methotrexate chemotherapy. *J Urol* 122:265–266, 1979.

56. Barlow JJ, Piver MS: Methotrexate with citrovorum factor rescue alone and in combination with cyclophosphamide in ovarian cancer. *Cancer Treat Rep* 60:527–533, 1976.

57. Parker LM, Griffiths CT, Yankee RA, et al: High dose methotrexate with leucovorin rescue in ovarian cancer: A phase II study. *Cancer Treat Rep* 63:275–279, 1979.

58. Roy D: Treatment of advanced or recurrent carcinoma of the cervix by cytotoxic drugs. *Indian J Cancer* 4:32, 1967.

59. Haffner WHJ, Frick HC: Intermittent intravenous methotrexate in the treatment of advanced epidermoid carcinoma of the cervix and vulvovagina. *Cancer* 26:812–815, 1970.

60. Mills EED: Intermittent intravenous methotrexate in the treatment of advanced epidermoid carcinoma. *S Afr Med J* 46:398–401, 1972.

61. Nikrui N, Magill GB, Ochoa M, et al: High dose methotrexate (HDMTX) therapy in carcinoma of the cervix. *Proc AACR* 17:173, 1976.

62. Hakes T, Nikrui M, Magill G, et al: Cervix cancer: Treatment with combination vincristine and high doses of methotrexate. *Cancer* 43:459–464, 1979.

63. Ross GT, Goldstein DP, Hertz R, et al: Sequential use of methotrexate and actinomycin D in the treatment of metastatic choriocarcinoma and related trophoblastic disease in women. *Am J Obstet Gynecol* 93:223–229, 1965.

64. Hreschchyshyn MM, Graham JB, Holland JF: Treatment of malignant trophoblastic growth in women, with special reference to amethopterin. *Am J Obstet Gynecol* 81:688–705, 1961.

65. Constantino PM, Benitez I, Estrella F: Amethopterin in the treatment of trophoblastic tumors. *Am J Obstet Gynecol* 82:641–645, 1961.

66. Hertz R, Lewis J, Lipsett MB: Five years experience with the chemotherapy of metastatic tumors in women. *Am J Obstet Gynecol* 82:631–640, 1961.

67. Hertz R, Ross GT, Lipsett MB: Primary chemotherapy of non-metastatic trophoblastic disease in women. *Am J Obstet Gynecol* 86:808–814, 1963.

68. Lamb EJ, Morton DG, Byron RC: Methotrexate therapy of choriocarcinoma and allied tumors. *Am J Obstet Gynecol* 90:317–327, 1964.

69. Brewer JI, Gerbie AB, Dolkart RE, et al: Chemotherapy in trophoblastic diseases. *Am J Obstet Gynecol* 90:566–578, 1964.

70. Dietzel HA, Schwarz RH: Primary treatment of choriocarcinoma with methotrexate. *Arch Surg* 92:301–303, 1966.

71. Hammond CB, Hertz R, Ross GT, et al: Primary chemotherapy for nonmetastatic gestational trophoblastic neoplasms. *Am J Obstet Gynecol* 98:71–78, 1967.

72. Wei PY, Ouyang PC: The use of methotrexate in the treatment of trophoblastic diseases, especially choriocarcinoma. *Am J Obstet Gynecol* 98:79–84, 1967.

73. Johnson FD, Jacobs EM, Silliphant WM: Trophoblastic tumors of the uterus problems of methotrexate therapy. *California Med* 108:1–13, 1968.

74. Hsu CT, Cheng YS: Methotrexate therapy in trophoblastic disease at the Provincial Taipei Hospital. *Am J Obstet Gynecol* 103:60–67, 1969.

75. Goldstein DP, Saracco P, Osathanondh R, et al: Methotrexate with citrovorum factor rescue for gestational trophoblastic neoplasms. *Obstet Gynecol* 51:93–96, 1978.

76. Huseby RA, Downing V: The use of methotrexate orally in treatment of squamous cancer of the head and neck. *Cancer Chemother Rep* 16:511–514, 1962.

77. Papac RJ, Jacobs EM, Foye LV, et al for the Western Cooperative Cancer Chemotherapy Group: Systemic Therapy with amethopterin in squamous carcinoma of the head and neck. *Cancer Chemother Rep* 32:47–54, 1963.

78. Condit PT, Ridings GR, Coin JW, et al: Methotrexate and radiation in the treatment of patients with cancer. *Cancer Res* 24:1524–1533, 1964.

79. Hellman S, Iannotti AT, Bertino JR: Determinations of the levels of serum folate in patients with carcinoma of the head and neck treated with methotrexate. *Cancer Res* 24:105–113, 1964.

80. Papac R, Lefkowitz E, Bertino JR: Methotrexate (NSC-740) in squamous cell carcinoma of the head and neck: II. Intermittent intravenous therapy. *Cancer Chemother Rep* 51:69–72, 1967.

81. Lefkowitz E, Papac RJ, Bertino JR: Head and neck Cancer: III. Toxicity of 24 hour infusions of methotrexate (NSC-740) and protection by leucovorin (NSC-3590) in patients with epidermoid carcinomas. *Cancer Chemother Rep* 51:305–311, 1967.

82. Lane M, Moore JE, Levin H, et al: Methotrexate therapy for squamous cell carcinomas of the head and neck. *J Am Med Assoc* 204:561–564, 1968.

83. Leone LA, Albala MM, Rege VB: Treatment of carcinoma of the head and neck with intravenous methotrexate. *Cancer* 21:828–837, 1968.

84. Adler GF, Hagan B, Indyk JS, et al: Methotrexate in the treatment of squamous cell carcinomas of the head and neck. *Med J Aust* 1:747–748, 1973.

85. Mitchell MS, Wawro NW, DeConti RC, et al: Effectiveness of high dose infusions of methotrexate followed by leucovorin in carcinoma of the head and neck. *Cancer Res* 28:1088–1094, 1968.

86. Buechler M, Mukherji B, Chasin W, et al: High dose methotrexate (MTX) with and without BCG therapy in advanced head and neck malignancy. *Proc AACR* 18:329, 1977.

87. Buechler M, Mukherji B, Chasin W, et al: High dose methotrexate with and without BCG therapy in advanced head and neck malignancy. *Cancer* 43:1095–1100, 1979.

88. Capizzi RL, DeConti RC, Marsh JC, et al: Methotrexate therapy of head and neck cancer: Improvement in therapeutic index by the use of leucovorin "rescue." *Cancer Res* 30:1782–1788, 1970.

89. Bertino JR, Levitt M, McCullough JL, et al: New approaches to chemotherapy with folate antagonists: Use of leucovorin "rescue" and enzymic folate depletion. *Ann NY Acad Sci* 186:486–495, 1971.

90. Levitt M, Mosher MB, DeConti RC, et al: High dose methotrexate - leucovorin (N^5-formyl tetrahydro folate) in epidermoid carcinomas of the head and neck. *Proc AACR* 13:20, 1972.

91. Levitt M, Mosher MB, DeConti RC, et al: Improved therapeutic index of methotrexate with "leucovorin rescue." *Cancer Res* 33:1729–1734, 1973.

92. Woods RL, Tattersall MHN, Sullivan J: A randomized study of three doses of methotrexate (MTX) in patients with advanced squamous cell cancer of the head and neck. *Proc AACR* 20:262, 1979. Abstract 1063.

93. Goldberg NH, Chretien PB, Elias EG, et al: Preoperative high dose methotrexate (MTX): A well tolerated regimen in head and neck cancer. *Proc AACR* 18:292, 1977.

94. Khandekar JD, Wolff A: Clinical trial of high dose methotrexate with leucovorin "rescue" (HDMTX) in advanced epidermoid carcinoma of the head and neck. *Proc AACR* 18:281, 1977.

95. Frei E III, et al: In press.

96. Weichselbaum RR, Miller D, Pitman SW, et al: Initial adjuvant weekly high dose methotrexate with leucovorin rescue in advanced squamous carcinoma of the head and neck. *Int J Radiat Oncol Biol Phys* 4:671–674, 1978.

97. Ambinder EP, Perloff M, Ohnuma T, et al: High dose methotrexate followed by citrovorum factor reversal in patients with advanced cancer. *Cancer* 43:1177–1182, 1979.

98. Kirkwood JM, Miller D, Weichselbaum R, et al: Symposium: Adjuvant cancer therapy of head and neck tumors. Predefinitive and postdefinitive chemotherapy for locally advanced squamous carcinoma of the head and neck. *Laryngoscope* 89:573–581, 1979.

99. Wang JJ, Freeman AI, Sinks LF: Treatment of acute lymphocytic leukemia by high dose intravenous methotrexate. *Cancer Res* 36:1441–1444, 1976.

100. Holland JF: CALGB data, unpublished.

101. Perrin JCS, Mauer AM, Sterling TD: Intravenous methotrexate (amethopterin) therapy in the treatment of acute leukemia. *Pediatrics* 31:833–839, 1963.

102. Huguley CM, Vogler WR, Lea JW, et al: Acute leukemia treated with divided doses of methotrexate. *Arch Intern Med* 115:23–28, 1965.

103. Frei E III, Freireich EJ, Gehan E, et al: From the acute leukemia group B: Studies of sequential and combination antimetabolite therapy in acute leukemia: 6-Mercaptopurine and methotrexate. *Blood* 18:431–454, 1961.

104. Sweet DJ, Ultmann JE, et al: Symposium on chemotherapy of non-Hodgkin's lymphoma, in *Proc. International Congress of Chemotherapy,* 1977.

105. Vogler WR, Huguley CM, Kerr W: Toxicity and antitumor effect of divided doses of methotrexate. *Arch Intern Med* 115:285–293, 1965.

106. Frei E III, Spurr Cl, Brindley CO, et al: Clinical studies of dichloromethotrexate. *Clin Pharmacol Ther* 6:160–171, 1965.

107. Burkitt D, Hutt MSR, Wright DH: The African lymphoma. *Cancer* 18:399–410, 1965.

108. Tejada F, Radomsky JL, Greenhawt M, et al: Methotrexate (MTX) CSF levels during high dose MTX-leucovorin (LCV) rescue. *Proc AACR* 18:91, 1977.

109. Pitman S, Frei E III: Weekly methotrexate citrovorum (MTX-CF) with alkalinization: Tumor response in a phase II study. *Proc AACR* 18:124, 1977.

110. Skarin AT, Zuckerman KS, Pitman SW, et al: High dose methotrexate with folinic acid in the treatment of advanced non-Hodgkin's lymphoma including CNS involvement. *Blood* 50:1039–1047, 1977.

111. Pitman SW, Frei E III: Weekly methotrexate calcium leucovorin rescue: Effect of alkalinization on nephrotoxicity; Pharmacokinetics in the CNS; and use in CNS non-Hodgkin's lymphoma. *Cancer Treat Rep* 61:695–701, 1977.

112. Djerassi I, Kim JS: Methotrexate and citrovorum factor rescue in the management of childhood lymphosarcoma and reticulum cell sarcoma (non-Hodgkin's lymphoma). Prolonged unmaintained remissions. *Cancer* 38:1043–1051, 1976.

113. Turman S, Coleman M, Silver RT: Treatment of resistant phase lymphoma with "high dose" methotrexate and folinic acid rescue. *Proc AACR* 17:302, 1976.

114. Ross CA, Selawry OS: Comparison of three dose schedules of methotrexate in lung cancer. *Proc AACR* 6:54, 1965.

115. Reed LJ, Muggia FM, Klipstein FA, et al: Intermittent parenteral methotrexate (NSC-740) therapy for carcinoma of the lung. *Cancer Chemother Rep* 51:475–481, 1967.

116. Selawry OS, Krant M, Scotto J, et al: Methotrexate compared with placebo in lung cancer. *Cancer* 40:4–8, 1977.

117. Djerassi I, Rominger CJ, Kim SJ, et al: Phase I study of high doses of methotrexate with citrovorum factor in patients with lung cancer. *Cancer* 30:22–30, 1972.

118. Minna J, Pelsor F, Ihde D, et al: High dose methotrexate - citrovorum factor rescue: Treatment of adeno and large cell carcinoma of the lung. *Proc AACR* 18:289, 1977.

119. Jacobs SA, Dilettuso BA, Santicky MA: Rescue from high dose methotrexate: Correlation between 30 hour MTX concentration and dose of leucovorin. *Proc AACR* 18:322, 1977.

120. Minna J, Pelsor F, Ihde D, et al: High dose methotrexate therapy by 6 or 30 hour infusion with leucovorin rescue in non-small cell lung cancer. *Proc AACR* 19:135, 1978.

121. Tornyos K, Faust H: Oral high dose methotrexate with citrovorum factor rescue in metastatic squamous cell carcinoma of the lung. *Cancer* 41:400–402, 1978.

122. Greco FA, Fer MF, Richardson RL, et al: High dose methotrexate with citrovorum factor rescue in non-small cell lung cancer. *Cancer Chemother Pharmacol* 1:255–257, 1978.

123. Ettinger DS, Stanley KE, Nystrom JS: High dose methotrexate (HDMTX) with citrovorum factor (CF) rescue in inoperable non-oat cell bronchogenic carcinoma. *Proc AACR* 20:347, 1979.

124. Eilber FR, Isacoff W: High dose methotrexate therapy for disseminated malignant melanoma. *Proc AACR* 17:262, 1976.

125. Fisher RI, Chabner BA, Myers CE: Phase II study of high dose methotrexate in patients with advanced malignant melanoma. *Cancer Treat Rep* 63:147–148, 1979.

126. Karakovsis CP, Carlson M: High dose methotrexate in malignant melanoma. *Cancer Treat Rep* 63:1405–1407, 1979.

127. Jaffe N: Recent advances in the chemotherapy of metastatic osteogenic sarcoma. *Cancer* 30:1627–1631, 1972.

128. Jaffe N: High dose methotrexate therapy in osteogenic sarcoma, in *High Dose Methotrexate Pharmacology Toxicology and Chemotherapy*, P Periti (ed). *Chemioterapia Oncologica*, vol 2, no 4, December 1978, pp 183–190.

129. Ambinder EP, Perloff M, Ohnuma T, et al: High dose methotrexate followed by citrovorum factor reversal in patients with advanced cancer. *Cancer* 43:1177–1182, 1979.

130. Wiltshaw E: Methotrexate in treatment of sarcomata. *Br Med J* 2:142–145, 1967.

131. Berenzweig M, Muggia FM, Kaplan BH: Chemotherapy of alveolar soft part sarcoma: A case report. *Cancer Treat Rep* 61:77–79, 1977.

132. Woods RL, Fox RM, Tattersall MHN: Treatment of advanced head and neck cancers: A randomized study of three methotrexate doses (to be published).

133. Osteosarcoma Panel Discussion, (JF Holland) Chairman, in *Therapeutic Progress in Ovarian and Testicular Cancers and the Sarcomas*. A Van Oosterom, F Muggia, F Cleton (eds). Martinus Nijhoff, The Hague, 1980.

134. Rosen G, Nirenberg A, Caparros B: Evaluation of high dose methotrexate with citrovorum factor rescue single agent chemotherapy in osteogenic sarcoma. *Proc AACR ASCO* 21:122, 1980.

135. Muggia FM, Catane R, Lee YJ, Rozencweig M: Factors responsible for therapeutic success in osteosarcoma: A critical analysis of adjuvant trial results, in *Adjuvant Therapy of Cancer II*. Salmon SE, Jones SE (eds). Grune and Stratton, Inc, New York, 1977, pp 383–390.

136. Edmonson JH, Green SJ, Ivins JC, et al: Post-surgical treatment of primary osteosarcoma of bone: Comparison of high dose methotrexate vs observation: Preliminary report. *Proc AACR ASCO* 21:476, 1980.

137. Natale R, Yagoda A, Molander D: In vitro and in vivo sensitivity of human bladder carcinoma: Correlation with phase II trials of AMSA, PALA and Methotrexate (MTX). *Proc AACR ASCO* 21:297, 1980.

25

The Cooperative Group Method of Cancer Research

John R. Durant

The advantages of cooperative group studies in oncology and other specialties dealing with therapeutic research have become increasingly obvious in the 25 years since the cooperative cancer study groups were first formed by the National Cancer Institute in 1955. A variety of important reasons have led several other National Institutes of Health to adopt this approach, particularly when it was deemed advisable to answer important questions about proposed strategies for improving the management of a wide variety of diseases. It is in circumstances such as rheumatoid arthritis, chronic infectious diseases such as cryptococcal meningitis, diabetes, and cancer where nonprogression, a variable natural history, and uncertain prognosis make the evaluation of the effect of treatment difficult. It is these same circumstances which invite quack remedies and anecdotes about miracle treatments that do not stand rigorous, but seldom used, skeptical analysis. The history of clinical medicine is replete with brilliant, insightful, but incorrect observations. Further, a new therapy is rarely such an advance that it is obvious by inspection. The story of the development of successful treatments is coexistent with the development of techniques for reducing the chances of coming to the wrong conclusion from the data available. In order to advance as rapidly as possible, there must be as few false starts as possible. The inclusion of a chapter on the advantages of cooperative group studies in a book concerning controversies in oncology therefore seems almost a statement of a dilemma rather than a controversy. How can we make rapid studies that are not in the wrong direction? We must push forward, but, to do so, we must not make unwarranted conclusions. Simultaneously, we must conserve our resources and not ask trivial questions. Implicitly, it seems our conclusions should be based on a sufficient but not excessive number of observations. With many variables, however, a large number of observations is usually necessary in order to make few conclusions with great certainty.

Various questions of scientific and medical importance have been subjected so often to the multi-institutional, cooperative approach that one wonders why the approach is controversial. Examples include the MRC studies of acute leukemia (1), the University Group Diabetes Project (2), the antiviral chemotherapy studies of the NIAID (3), the prophylactic granulocyte transfusion study of the NIHLB (4), as well as the cooperative group studies of the National Cancer Institute. Although expensive and often negative, these studies frequently serve a very useful function both of debunking fervently held beliefs and documenting solid advances. The negative studies are sometimes criticized as having been done incorrectly; however, good science with negative results is not popular, especially if it is expensive and the results at variance with those of vocal proponents. Thus, the controversy appears to center on a complex interplay of science, politics, and economics, This is so because the federal government plays the essential role as the provider of funds for research. With a limited budget there is competition among investigators with a wide variety of research styles. Some believe in the orderliness of nature so much that if a phenomenon can be established in a model or an animal, they do not wish to do research in humans, where it is both more expensive and more uncertain. Furthermore, a relatively large budget such as that of NCI attracts attention and generates controversy. In FY 1980, the National Cancer Institute's budget was $1 billion, that of the American Cancer Society of America was $149,171,000, and that of the Leukemia Society was $11,700,000. These add up to $1,149,182,700. Although this once seemed a tremendous amount of money, inflation has reduced the work it will do, and the public is more than ever concerned with economy. Further, we are torn by conflicting ideas regarding where increasingly scarce research dollars should be spent, that is, on fundamental research that generates new scientific ideas or on establishing whether certain implications of fundamental research already done are now of value to humans. With an unlimited amount of funds, we would peacefully pursue both. Such is no longer the case, and the problem is compounded more recently by still other competitors for the investment of funds. Is that great research development, that is, the establishment of a successful strategy or strategies for the treatment of human cancer, documented so clearly under carefully controlled circumstances, really applicable to everyday medicine? What is the best way to convert a great idea to a socially useful program? The taxpayer does not care about style; he wants the cheapest strategy available. Since treatment is proving increasingly expensive, there is now also growing support for the conventional wisdom that holds prevention as the best investment of scarce resources. Each type of approach has its advocates, creating an important dilemma with both scientific and social implications. Depending on our own value systems, we may be more or less concerned with developing great ideas, proving their therapeutic relevance, inserting them in the proper place in our society, or abolishing the need for therapy altogether. It seems unlikely that one is more important than another. Rather the issue is: how important is the question being asked and is the method being applied suitable to answer the question with precision? It is the contention of this chapter that for establishing new therapies as effective there is no more reliable approach than collaborative, cooperative studies. That there is controversy about such research arises out of confusion over goals, different styles of research, diverse value systems, and competing funding priorities.

Some seem to believe that their insights and those of their colleagues are unique and so profound that they can with the resources available make the most progress if funds are preferentially granted or all patients referred to them. It is my prejudice that this is an arrogant, elitist view that as often leads to setbacks as to progress. Although we would all, no doubt, like to find a simple, nontoxic, universally effective treatment for cancer, we have learned enough fundamental cancer biology to doubt that such will ever be the case. Today's clinical research is based on the expectation that it is unlikely that there will be a development equivalent to penicillin for pneumococcal pneumonia. There is not, I believe, a single example in oncology of a situation in which a hopeless malignancy was suddenly rendered almost invariably curable as the result of the application of some new insight tested in a single small series of patients. Instead, we have learned, as stated recently by Aisenberg when writing about Hodgkin's disease, "It is paradoxic that the dramatic improvement in survival in Hodgkin's disease of the past two decades has made the choice of optimum management more difficult" (5). Stated another way, our understanding of disease leads us to recognize an increasing number of differing factors that may influence the outcome. A recent example of this is illustrated by the apparently better prognosis for patients with stage IIIA Hodgkin's disease when its abdominal involvement is confined to areas above the chysterna chyli when compared with the same stage of disease involving the lower abdomen (6).

The wise investigator knows the wisdom of making haste slowly. The experience of the cooperative groups supports their important role in making haste slowly. In 1955, no one expected chemotherapy to do very much or do it very rapidly. Indeed, the excitement of the times was that some drugs seemed to have a dramatic, although temporary, effect on some patients with some kinds of cancers. At that time, the emphasis was almost solely on looking for drugs with anticancer activity, not for developing treatment strategies. The search quickly concentrated on analogues of nitrogen mustard and the folic acid antagonists that had in small numbers of cases shown interesting activity. New classes of agents were also investigated. Protocols were simple and usually of short duration. As new drugs emerged from screening and other preclinical testing, it was increasingly obvious that large numbers of cases were needed in order to identify drugs with valuable new characteristics. It was quickly learned that such drugs had activity only in a fraction of certain malignancies. Thus, at the very outset, it was apparent that statistical advice, consultation, and then partnership were essential parts of the search for active cancer chemotherapeutic agents. At first, since the emphasis was almost exclusively on therapeutic and toxic effects, it was necessary to define and quantify these so that they could be reported and compared. All clinical research has benefited from these initial efforts in oncology. Probably more than in any other single area of clinical research, oncology has led the way by introducing discipline and careful definition into clinical research. It was the early clinical trial statisticians who insisted on defining terms, removing bias, and including controls. The progress made in the past 25 years is a tribute to the wisdom of discipline in clinical trials. Not a single disseminated malignancy was curable in 1955. Indeed, the natural history of most malignancies was rarely altered significantly by drugs. Twenty-five years later, 10% of all patients who have disseminated disease can be cured (7). We can confidently discuss reproducible response rates and survival. This has created the circumstance in which success is documented by studies to determine reasons for failure. Indeed, by the early 1970s, barely 15 years after a serious organized attack on the treatment of cancer with drugs had begun, increasingly sophisticated and complex technologies to analyze and compare results had been developed. These statistical techniques, along with the computers required to apply them, permitted studies of the value of new biologic tests and attempts to determine in advance whether an effective treatment was likely to be successful or not in different groups of patients with the same disease. This technology, capable of identifying important prognostic factors, led to the very important notion of stratification in clinical trials. The importance of this is indicated by the realization that if there are 20 important characteristics that might influence an outcome, at least one will be misallocated in a study with two arms that seeks a difference significant at $P = .05$. If an important but previously unrecognized factor is not accounted for, it can, therefore, reduce or exaggerate differences if not equally distributed among experimental groups. This led to the recognition that it is not reasonable to expect randomization to divide patients into equivalent groups without accounting for important prognostic factors in advance. The importance of the unexpected important prognostic factor is, however, diminished if the numbers of cases entered is increased or the significant difference desired is enlarged. As a consequence, staging, long recognized as important for prognosis, is gradually being replaced by substaging, as reflected in staging systems for invariably widely disseminated diseases such as chronic lymphocytic leukemia (8) or substaging Hodgkin's disease (6). These developments help to explain many otherwise inexplicable differences among studies, differences due, not to therapeutic regimens used, but to differences in the prognostic characteristics of patients comprising experimental groups in different studies. Even when these are taken into account, however, many other factors in the same stage influence prognosis.

Some recognized factors not related primarily to stage of disease but which influence results include the following:

1. Whether staging is clinical or pathologic (9,10)
2. Performance status (11,12)
3. Immune competence (13)
4. Nutritional status (14)
5. Age (15,16)

The following list includes a sample of some confounding variables that apply to individual diseases:

Breast Cancer

1. Number of involved axillary nodes (17)
2. Menopausal status (18,19)
3. Presence and quantity of receptors for estrogen and progesterone (20,21)
4. Predominant metastatic site for advanced disease (22)

Melanoma

1. Depth of invasion for stage I (23)
2. Location of the primary for stage I (23)
3. Number of positive nodes for stage II (24)

CLL

1. Activity of the disease (25)
2. Organomegaly (8)
3. Marrow failure (8)

ALL

1. Age (16)
2. Initial white count (26)
3. Origin of the leukemic lymphocyte (26,27)

Myeloma

1. Performance status (11)
2. Initial hemoglobin (28)
3. Uremia (28,29)
4. Immunoglobulin type (28,29)
5. Cell mass (30)
6. Initial marrow labeling index (28)

These many factors have the effect of increasing the number of patients required to achieve an adequate sample.

Recently, Zelen (31) reviewed the general effect of sample size on clinical trials for the Board of Scientific Counselors of the NCI's Division of Cancer Treatment. For reasons previously stated, he assumed that no new treatment was going to be so much better than a previous one as to be obvious from inspection. He stressed that the overall goal of clinical therapeutic research was to maximize the possibility of true positive results and minimize false positives. He then examined the effect of sample size on achieving this goal for a variety of differences in response rate and increase in survival. In order to calculate the current ratio of probable true versus false positives, he reviewed 54 prospective therapeutic trials appearing in 12 issues of *Cancer* from 1977 to 1979. The median sample size was 50 with a range from 10 to more than 400. His calculations showed that if the usual $P = .05$ two-sided test of significance was used and if 58 patients were studied, there was only a 40% probability of finding a true positive if the experimental arm increased the response rate from 20% to 40%. In other words, even with randomization and an impressive statistically significant difference, it is more likely than not that the new treatment is not better than the old. Similarly, there is only a 30% probability of a true positive if a median life span increase of 50% is produced in a two-armed study with only 50 patients. The need for more patients is reduced if one looks for larger differences, but obviously the risk of missing an improved treatment rises proportionately. A 95% probability of detecting a true positive for a treatment that doubles the response rate from 20% to 40% requires 308 patients, and 256 patients are necessary for a 90% probability of detecting a true increase of 50% in the median life span. He argues from his experience with clinical trials that about 1 out of 10 produces a significant difference. Adopting the standard P = .05 for a significant positive result and an average 50-patient study, he then calculates that for each positive study there are 1.5 false positive studies. This requires 22 or 23 studies to produce one true positive. In order to improve the efficiency of this process, he argues that we must reduce the chance of a false positive by designing comparative clinical trials that have between 100 and 200 patients per treatment arm.

The following example illustrates the problem. In June of 1977, the SECSG began to study whether *C. parvum* would improve the disease-free interval and survival of clinical stage I melanoma. Figure 1 shows that for all such patients there is no significant effect of *C. parvum* when compared with no therapy. Figure 2 shows further that for patients with lesions less than 4 mm thick there is also no effect. Since relatively few patients of this type relapse within the first few years, the follow-up may, however, be too short to detect a real difference. This possibility is increased if only those patients with lesions greater than 4 cm thick are examined. In this group, there is a marked early difference (Fig. 3). The results are blinded so that if the results hold up, *C. parvum* could have either a marked therapeutic advantage or disadvantage. Note, however, that almost all patients (122 out of 135) had lesions less than 4 cm thick (32). Thus, if this

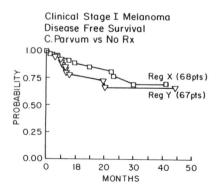

Figure 1. Interim analysis of Southeastern Cancer Study Group surgical adjuvant study of clinical stage I melanoma comparing no therapy with *C. parvum*. Results are blinded, but there is no evident difference.

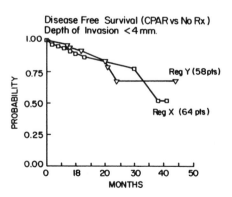

Figure 2. Interim analysis of Southeastern Cancer Study Group adjuvant study of clinical stage I melanoma comparing no therapy with *C. parvum* only in patients with primary lesions less than 4 mm thick. Results are blinded, but there is no evident difference.

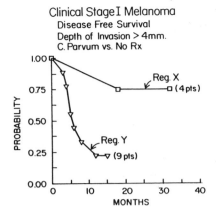

Clinical Stage I Melanoma
Disease Free Survival
Depth of Invasion > 4mm.
C. Parvum vs. No Rx

Figure 3. Same as Figure 2 only in patients with primary lesions thicker than 4 cm. One arm is statistically superior to the other, but confidence limits are very broad. Results are blinded.

difference is real, more than 500 patients with clinical stage I will be needed to provide 25 patients for each arm where an initial difference has been noted. Further, if there is a therapeutic effect, it should also be seen among these with thinner lesions, but their better prognosis will require many more years of follow-up to be documented. Thus, studies of new strategies for this disease should perhaps accept only patients with thick, stage I lesions. Results that include patients with both thick and thin lesions will likely be initially negative because of a preponderance of thin lesions. If rapid answers are desired, it is unlikely that a sufficient number of patients with thick stage I lesions can be found in any single institution. The solution is a multi-institutional study (a cooperative group).

Another example of this problem is illustrated by multiple myeloma. Figure 4 shows the predicted and actual survival of a group of 103 patients treated according to a current SECSG protocol. Figure 5 shows the differences in survival when these patients are divided into groups of good and poor risk patients (33). Since such poor risk patients comprise a small minority of the whole population studied, the effect of a very potent new therapy could easily be obscured by the favorable natural history of the large good risk group randomly distributed between the control and experimental arms. On the other hand, a new therapy applied only to good risk patients may look very promising when all that has been done is to exclude likely failures. Such may be the explanation for the remarkable results produced with the M-2 protocol from Memorial (34). A solution to this problem is to conduct phase II types of studies only on poor risk patients and determine whether you can beat the formula, much as a golfer may play a course of a given difficulty and try to better his score rather than beat an opponent. This, however, requires historical controls and assumes that no new nonspecific supportive measures will be introduced that will improve results. This assumption is generally believed to be dangerous and argues strongly for concurrent controls.

The problem with historical controls is that they often lead to mistaken conclusions. Carbone (35) recently reviewed the case for concurrent controlled trials. He cites two examples of instances in which the absence of concurrent controls

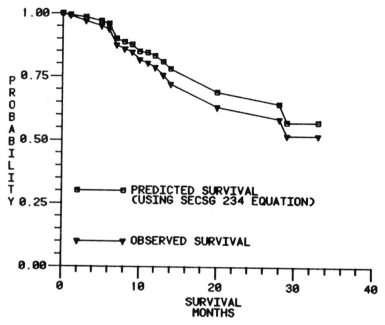

Figure 4. Comparison of predicted survival in multiple myeloma using formula derived for an old Southeastern Cancer Study Group study and actual observed survival in a new study. There is no difference.

resulted in the adoption of a falsely positive trial as standard, accepted treatment. The first was the use of urethane for multiple myeloma. The second was DES for prostatic cancer. In order to reduce the large number of patients required for comparative trials, Freireich has championed the use of historical controls using carefully matched pairs of patients (36). This use of historical controls has not, however, as stated above, gained wide acceptance. This is in part because of a recurrent problem with false positives resulting when such controls were used for trials of nonspecific immunotherapy, a treatment vigorously pursued by advocates of the historical control solution. BCG for stage I and II melanoma was found to be superior in two trials without concurrent controls (37,38); but when concurrent controls were used, the benefits are less obvious or confined to a small subset of patients (39). This is also generally true of the initially encouraging reports of the value of BCG in acute leukemia (40,41). In general, investigators agree with Carbone in insisting on concurrent controls and believing that historical controls are not sufficiently reliable to be a solution to the requirement for the large numbers of patients needed for comparative trials.

The need for large sample size and concurrent controls is compounded by the effects of prognostic variables previously discussed. To illustrate this, consider the sample size needs for adjuvant trials in stage II breast cancer. For the

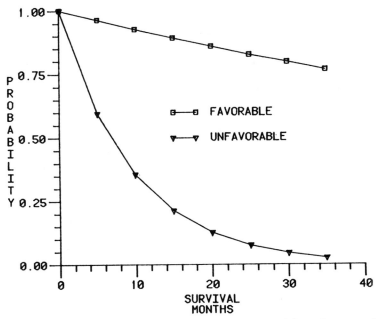

Figure 5. Difference between survival of good and poor risk patients as defined by Southeastern Cancer Study Group.

purpose of this discussion, the number of important variables affecting prognosis significantly is limited to three: the number of positive nodes, menopausal status, and whether or not the tumor has demonstrable estrogen receptors. If the effect of an experimental treatment were equal for each of these, no stratification would be necessary. Unfortunately, this has proved not to be the case. Thus, it is important to have enough patients in each subgroup to make independent comparisons. Eight groups of patients with stage II breast cancer are thus created:

1. 1–3 + nodes, premenopausal, ER+
2. 1–3 + nodes, postmenopausal, ER−
3. ≥ 4 + nodes, premenopausal, ER+
4. ≥ 4 + nodes, premenopausal, ER−
5. 1–3 + nodes, postmenopausal, ER+
6. 1–3 + nodes, premenopausal, ER−
7. ≥ 4 + nodes, postmenopausal, ER
8. ≥ 4 + nodes, postmenopausal, ER−

Assuming an equal distribution into each group, a two-armed study, a concurrent control, and using Zelen's minimal estimate of 100 patients per arm, 1,600 patients would be required. However, it is likely even more patients will be needed to complete the study. There are many more women with breast cancer who are postmenopausal and ER^+ than who are premenopausal or ER^-. Thus, the trial may go on much longer for some groups of patients than for others so as to achieve the requisite numbers to examine the effects of treatment in each subgroup. Furthermore, if for more confidence 200 patients in each group are desired, 3,200 patients are needed. Since not all patients will be evaluable, the requirement for more cases is increased still further. These estimates ignore the possibility that some additional important variable that influences prognosis exists and is unequally allocated in at least one of the subsets of patients. Such variables might include, for instance, unequal sensitivity to the chemotherapeutic agents used (42), socioeconomic status (43), the actual dose administered (44), or unequal toxicity (45). Were any of these misallocated in one or another of the treatment groups, the true result might either be obscured or magnified, leading to a false positive or negative, depending on the circumstances.

It thus seems self-evident that until a true single magic bullet is found, therapeutic trials will require large numbers of patients even if well designed and not subject to unexpected variables. We have recently had such an experience (45). We compared one schedule of Melphalan with one schedule of CMF in node positive stage II breast cancer (46). Early analysis indicated that Melphalan was significantly superior to CMF in preventing relapse and prolonging survival (Fig. 6). A multivariate analysis including six variables indicated that the only factors favorably influencing prognosis were having three or fewer positive nodes and receiving Melphalan. Melphalan, however, produced significantly greater numbers of patients with leucopenia and significantly fewer with nausea and vomiting. When the nadir white blood count achieved during treatment, a factor not originally included in the analysis, was entered in the multivariate analysis, Melphalan was no longer superior to CMF. It was found that leucopenia, produced primarily with Melphalan, was the important factor. It was among patients treated with Melphalan that leucopenia was most frequent, but it was among all

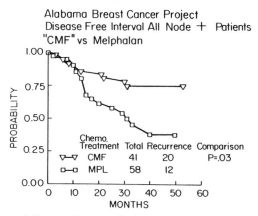

Figure 6. Comparison of disease free survival of node-positive breast cancer patients in Alabama. Melphalan appears to be superior to Cytoxan, Methotrexate, and 5-FU but is probably not (see text.)

those who achieved leucopenia that disease-free survival was the best. Further analysis showed that, as the nadir white blood count of patients treated with Melphan increased, there was a progressively greater chance for recurrence. Indeed, for the group of 26 patients with 1 to 3 positive nodes who received at least 9 months of therapy, none treated with Melphalan who had a nadir WBC <3,000 has relapsed with a median follow-up of greater than 40 months, whereas for the 28 whose white blood count never fell below 3,000, 18% have relapsed. The probability of selecting a characteristic that would identify 26 consecutive nonrelapsing patients by chance alone is $< 5.6 \times 10^{-4}$. The purpose of this illustration is not to argue the merits of one treatment over another but rather to note what may happen when two treatments are not given to the equivalent important biologic toxicity and when that factor is not included in the original analysis. Because of nausea and vomiting more patients considered CMF intolerable and withdrew, so that it was considered the more toxic arm. On the other hand, the real measure of an adequate dose was leucopenia, not nausea and vomiting. The conclusion from this trial, which required 623 patients with operable breast cancer to find enough to compare two adjuvant chemotherapies, is not that Melphalan is superior to CMF but rather that regimens must be given to the appropriate equivalent toxicity before valid comparisons can be drawn. In other words, this study did not really compare Melphalan with CMF, but that was not realized until after the study was over.

This discussion is intended to emphasize the notion that the more we learn about prognostic factors and the more sophisticated our analytic techniques become, the more patients it will require to compare any partially effective treatment with any other partially effective treatment. If learning whether one treatment is really better than another is the goal of a study, there is no solution except to enter adequate numbers of patients in every subgroup. Three thousand two hundred patients with node-positive breast cancer cannot, in my opinion, be accessioned in a reasonable time by any method but by a cooperative arrangement between collaborating institutions. Even then, it may be difficult as illustrated by the recent B06 protocol of the NSABP, a study of stage I and II breast cancer with three treatment arms.

This discussion is not intended to denigrate the role of single-institution studies where ideas can be tested quickly for feasibility using small numbers. It is not to deny that retrospective analyses of a single institution's experience cannot lead to valuable insights. It is meant to indicate that, if it is important to prove you have found a better treatment, there is a need for large numbers of cases or there will be a great risk of either promulgating a false positive result or missing a true positive.

The ability to acquire adequate numbers of cases in a reasonable period is not, however, the only advantage of the cooperative study approach.

It is often stated that only in single institutions can complex laboratory tests be satisfactorily studied as to their interaction with a new treatment. Indeed, it was in a single institution that the adverse effect of a mediastinal mass in older boys with acute lymphocytic leukemia was noticed and correlated with E rosetting of leukemic cells (27). That cooperative groups can rapidly and prospectively apply a complicated laboratory test in a study of the natural history of a disease is illustrated by the SWOG study of acute lymphocytic leukemia and the effect of having a leukemia whose cells were arrested at the pre-B cell stage of development. The observation that such a subcategory of disease existed was first made by Vogler et al. at the University of Alabama in 22 patients studied over 13 months (47). Quickly a reference laboratory was established, and in May of 1978 all SWOG pediatric institutions began to enter patients. In 18 months, 118 patients had technically satisfactory immunologic testing so as to identify one of four phenotypes in all patients. To date, it appears that the pre-B characteristic adversely affects prognosis for disease-free survival in a fashion almost equivalent to that of the T cell (48). Small numbers and a short follow-up, however, result in insignificant statistical differences at this time. Similarly, the SECSG is collecting data about the following factors in adult acute lymphocyticleukemia: E rosettes, surface immunoglobulins, terminal transferase, and glucocorticoid receptors. The requisite immunologic expertise to develop specific antisera, provides proper quality control for a host of laboratory parameters, and managing the data usually overwhelm the resources of a single institution. A collaborative arrangement between institutions can increase both available expertise and the probability that quality control will be effectively carried out. The combination of diverse expertise, adequate data management, effective quality control, and adequate sample size can usually be obtained only in a multi-institutional setting.

Another advantage of cooperative studies is the ability to collect data on the importance of low-frequency complications. In the SECSG, for instance, we noted that severe pulmonary failure occurred in a few patients treated with BCNU combinations. Because of the large number of studies, good follow-up, and good data management, we were able to determine that the frequency was between 1% and 2% in over 700 patients (49). Similarly, the resources of the cooperative groups have been invaluable in determining the frequency and importance of cardiotoxicity with Adriamycin (50). To illustrate the value of such studies further both the CALGB (51) and the SECSG (52) have noted that leukemia following Hodgkin's disease is much less frequent in patients whose complete remission is induced with nitrosourea combinations than it is with MOPP. Although 1,020 patients who achieved complete remission in the two groups provide the denominator for this observation, the statistical significance of the difference is not yet convincing. If the observation that nitrosourea combinations result in less leukemia is correct, it will have obviously enormous impact on therapeutic recommendations. Once again, no single institution could address this question. On the other hand, model system studies to examine whether nitrosourea cyclophosphamide combinations are antagonistic as regards carcinogenesis and teratogenesis can be done in one institution. This is currently being done at the UAB Cancer Center using the Ames assay, mitochondrial mutagenesis in fungi, the 10 T½ cell system, and mouse models for induction of lung cancer and retinal defects. Clinical observations derived from large multi-institutional studies thus can provide leads for single-institution studies examining biologic phenomena. In turn, confirmation of a biologic effect can lead to an important search for molecular explanations for such phenomena with subsequent far-reaching implications.

Finally, the impact of disciplined studies, properly stratified and quality-controlled, on the education of countless medical students, house officers, fellows, and faculty cannot be overstated. For instance, the current composition of the

Medical Oncology Subcommittee of the American Board of Internal Medicine includes a majority (5 out of 9) who are members of cooperative groups. The opportunity for the use of data regarding therapeutic options, the importance of staging, the role of prognostic factors, and the value of careful and sophisticated analysis that is provided by cooperative groups are unparalleled as an educational experience. It is the exposure to this process that provides the majority of American students and house officers an opportunity to learn that cancer is not only a curable disease but one that offers exciting opportunities both for research and for personal satisfaction. The cooperative groups have played an essential role in this process while documenting many of the therapeutic advances of the past quarter century. They will, no doubt, continue to do so.

REFERENCES

1. Comstock GW, Livesay VT, Webster RG: Leukemia and BCG. A controlled trial. *Lancet* 2:1062, 1971.
2. Klimt CR, Knatterud GL, Meinert CL, et al for the University Group Diabetes Program: A study of the effects of hypoglycemic agents on vascular complications in patients with adult onset diabetes: I. Design methods and baseline results. *Diabetes* 19:747–783, 1970.
3. Whitley RJ, Chien LT, Dolin R, et al (eds) and the Collaborative Study Group: Adenine arabinoside therapy of herpes zoster in the immunosuppressed: NIAID collaborative antiviral study. *N Engl J Med* 294:1193–1199, 1976.
4. National Heart, Lung and Blood Institute Prophylactic Granulocyte Toxicity Study: Unpublished data.
5. Aisenberg AC, Linggood RM, Lew RA: The changing face of Hodgkin's disease. *Am J Med* 67:921–928, 1979.
6. Stein RS, Golomb HM, Diggs CH, et al: Anatomic substages of stage III-A Hodgkin's disease. *Ann Intern Med* 92:159–165, 1980.
7. DeVita VT Jr: Personal communication.
8. Rai KR, Sawitsky A, Cronkite EP, et al: Clinical staging of chronic lymphocytic leukemic. *Blood* 46:219–234, 1975.
9. Donegan WL, Lewis JD: Clinical diagnosis and staging of breast cancer. *Semin Oncol* 5:373–384, 1978.
10. Glatstein E, Trueblood HW, Enright LP, et al: Surgical staging of abdominal involvement in unselected patients with Hodgkin's disease. *Radiology* 97:425–432, 1970.
11. Hammack WJ, Huguley CM Jr, Chan YK: Treatment of myeloma: Comparison of melphalan, chlorambucil, and arathioprine. *Arch Intern Med* 135:157–162, 1975.
12. Hansen HH, Dombernowsky P, Hirsch FR: Staging procedures and prognostic features in small cell anaplastic bronchogenic carcinoma. *Semin Oncol* 5:280–287, 1978.
13. Eilber FR, Nizze JA, Morton DL: Sequential evaluation of general immune competance in cancer patients: Correlation with clinical course. *Cancer* 35:660–665, 1975.
14. Lanzotti VJ, Copeland EM, George SL, et al: Cancer chemotherapeutic response and intravenous hyperalimentation. *Cancer Chemother Rep* 59:437–439, 1975.
15. Rosenberg SA: Hodgkin's disease, in *Cancer Medicine* (eds) Holland JF, Frei E III. Lea & Febiger, 1973, Philadelphia, pp 1276–1302.
16. Ortega JA, Nesbit ME, Donaldson MH, et al: L-Asparaginase, vincristine and prednisone for induction of first remission in acute lymphocytic leukemia. *Cancer Res* 37:535–540, 1977.
17. Fisher ER, Gregorio RM, Fisher B: The pathology of invasive breast cancer. *Cancer* 36:1–85, 1975.

18. Fisher B, Carbone P, Economou SG, et al: L-Phenylalanine mustard (L-PAM) in the management of primary breast cancer: A report of early findings. *N Engl J Med* 292:117–122, 1975.

19. Bonadonna G, Valagussa P, Rossi A, et al: Are surgical adjuvant trials altering the course of breast cancer? *Semin Oncol* 5:450–464, 1978.

20. McGuire WL, Horwitz KB, Pearson DH, et al: Current status of estrogen and progesterone receptors in breast cancer. *Cancer* 39:2934–2947, 1977.

21. Wittliff J: Steroid-binding proteins in normal and neoplastic mammary cells. *Methods Cancer Res* 11:293–254, 1975.

22. Smalley RV, Bartolucci AA: Variation in responsiveness and survival of clinical subsets of patients with metastatic breast cancer to two chemotherapy combinations (abstract). *EORTC Second Breast Cancer Working Conference,* Copenhagen, Denmark, June, 1979.

23. Balch CM, Murad TM, Soong S-J, et al: A multifactoral analysis of melanoma: I. Prognostic histopathological features comparing Clark's and Breslow's staging methods. *Ann Surg* 188:732–742, 1978.

24. Eilber FR, Morton DL, Holmes EC, Adjuvant immunotherapy with BCG: Results of treatment in patients with regional lymph node metastases of malignant melanoma. *N Engl J Med* 294:237, 1976.

25. Huguley CM Jr: Survey of current therapy and of problems in chronic leukemia, in *Leukemia-Lymphoma* (A Collection of Papers Presented at the Fourteenth Annual Clinical Conference on Cancer, 1969, at the University of Texas M. D. Anderson Hospital and Tumor Institute at Houston), 1970, pp 317–331.

26. Chessells JM, Hardisty RM, Rapson NT, et al: Acute lymphoblastic leukemia in children: Classification and prognosis. *Lancet* 2:1307–1309, 1977.

27. Borella L, Sen L: T cell surface markers on lymphoblasts from acute lymphocytic leukemia. *J Immunol* 111:1257–1260, 1973.

28. Durie BGM, Salmon SE, Moon TE: Pretreatment tumor mass, cell kinetics, and prognosis in multiple myeloma. *Blood* 55:364–372, 1980.

29. Cohen HJ, Silberman HR, Larsen WE, et al: Combination chemotherapy with intermittent 1,3-bis(2-chloroethyl)1-nitrosourea (BCNU), cyclophosphamide, and prednisone for multiple myeloma. *Blood* 54:824–836, 1979.

30. Durie BGM, Salmon SE: A clinical staging system for multiple myeloma. *Cancer* 36:842–854, 1975.

31. Zelen M: Personal communication.

32. Southeastern Cancer Study Group: Unpublished data.

33. Southeastern Cancer Study Group: Unpublished data.

34. Case DC Jr, Lee BJ III, Clarkson BD: Improved survival times in multiple myeloma treated with melphalan, prednisone, cyclophosphamide, vincristine, and BCNU: M-2 protocol. *Am J Medicine* 63:897–903, 1977.

35. Carbone PP: The case for clinical trials. *Ca-A Cancer J Clinicians* 30:53–54, 1980.

36. Freireich EJ: Who took the clinical out of clinical research: Mouse or man? Seventh Annual David A. Karnofsky Memorial Lecture, American Society of Clinical Oncology, May 5, 1976, Toronto, Ontario.

37. Morton DL, Eilber FR, Holmes EC, et al: BCG immunotherapy of malignant melanoma: Summary of a seven-year experience. *Ann Surg* 180:635–643, 1974.

38. Holmes EC, Eilber FR, Morton DL: Immunotherapy of malignancy in humans: Current status. *JAMA* 232:1052–1055, 1975.

39. Eilber FR: Personal communication.

40. Vogler WR, Bartolucci AA, Omura GA, et al: A randomized clinical trial of remission induction, consolidation and chemoimmunotherapy maintenance in adult acute myeloblastic leukemia. *Cancer Immunol Immunother* 3:153–170, 1978.

41. Omura GA, Vogler WR, Lynn MJ: A controlled clinical trial of chemotherapy vs. BCG immunotherapy vs. no further therapy in remission maintenance of acute myelogenous leukemia (AML). *Proc ASCO/AACR* 18:C–23, 1977 (abstract).

42. Salmon SE, Hamburger AW, Soehnlen B, et al: Quantitation of differential sensitivity of human-tumor stem cells to anti-cancer drugs. *N Engl J Med* 298:1321–1327, 1978.

43. Berg, JW, Ross R, Latourette HB: Economic status and survival of cancer patients. *Cancer* 39:467–477, 1977.

44. Bonadonna G, Valagussa P: Dose-response effect of CMF in breast cancer. *Proc AACR/ASCO* 21:C–374, 1980 (abstract).

45. Alabama Breast Cancer Project: Unpublished data.

46. Wirtschafter D, Carpenter JT Jr, Mesel E: A consultant-extender system for breast cancer adjuvant chemotherapy. *Ann Intern Med* 90:396–401, 1979.

47. Vogler LB, Crist WM, Bockman DE, et al: Pre-B-Cell leukemia: A new phenotype of childhood lymphoblastic leukemia. *N Engl J Med* 298:872–878, 1978.

48. Pullen DJ, Metzgar RS, Falletta JM, et al: Southwest Oncology Group experience with immunologic phenotyping in acute lymphoblastic leukemia of childhood. *Cancer Treat Rep* (in press).

49. Durant JR, Norgard MJ, Murad TM, et al: Pulmonary toxicity associated with bischloroethyl-nitrosourea (BCNU). *Ann Intern Med* 90:191–194, 1979.

50. Von Hoff DD, Layard MW, Basa P, et al: Risk factors for adriamycin induced congestive heart failure. *Ann Intern Med* 91:710–717, 1979.

51. Holland JF: Personal communication.

52. Southeastern Cancer Study Group: Unpublished data.

26

Are Single-Institution Studies More Innovative than Group Studies?

Clara D. Bloomfield

INTRODUCTION

Significant advances in cancer therapy have occurred in the last 25 years that have resulted in a reduction of national mortality from cancer below the age of 45 (1). Although basic and applied laboratory research (e.g., the development of new drugs) are responsible in part for these advances, major contributions have been made by clinical treatment research.

Clinical treatment research has been defined by the National Cancer Institute (NCI) (2) as research on human subjects encompassing any or all aspects of treatment involving individuals or groups of cancer patients, including validation of preclinical findings in a clinical setting. It includes all clinical trials. Clinical treatment research is particularly concerned with efforts to determine the best possible treatment of each type of human cancer. This type of research is generally performed either by single institutions or cooperative clinical trial groups. It appears that the ultimate goal of the research—the cure of cancer—will be most rapidly and effectively achieved if both participate.

The key steps in the development of new treatments or therapeutic modalities have been identified by the Division of Cancer Treatment (DCT) subcommittee for Clinical Trials Review (3) as (*1*) the availability of adequate resources (including new drugs, new instrumentation, and adequate local, regional, and national resources), (*2*) the innovative input of new ideas by individual investigators or small groups of investigators at one or more institutions or cancer centers, (*3*) scale-up and confirmation or refutation of results of pilot studies, and (*4*) comparison of promising new treatments as confirmed via this process to existing standard treatments so that the superior treatment can be translated into the control of cancer of specific types in patients throughout the nation. In general, the first and second steps have been performed primarily by single institutions and the third and fourth steps have been performed primarily by cooperative clinical trial groups.

Controlled experimentation, in particular the prospective controlled clinical trial, is now regarded as the principal way to generate scientific data on the value of medical treatments. The controlled clinical trial represents an important methodologic advance in the science of therapeutics, but, even with the best methodology, the outcome of a trial will be disappointing if promising treatments are not selected for study. Thus, the need for innovative and well-run pilot studies, carried out by skilled investigators, is as important as ever (4). In cancer clinical treatment research single institutions have in most instances been responsible for the development of new ideas and the formulation of hypotheses and their preliminary testing. In general, confirmation of the usefulness of a new treatment has been performed by cooperative clinical trial groups.

The purpose of this essay is to explore and document the contribution of research in single institutions to cancer clinical therapeutic research. In a time of increasingly scarce resources, there is a tendency to consider such a discussion a challenge to cooperative groups. Such is not the case; single institutions and cooperative group participation in clinical treatment research are clearly complementary. The purpose of this chapter is neither to impugn cooperative group trials nor to diminish their importance, which has been repeatedly emphasized of late (5–8) and is amply described by Dr. John Durant in this volume. However, the importance of single-institution clinical research is often not appreciated, and funding mechanisms have clearly been inadequate (2). It is for these reasons that this chapter is written.

In this chapter the advantages of single institutions for certain types of clinical treatment research are first discussed. Some of the major accomplishments of cancer research and how single institutions have contributed to them are then considered. Finally, the inadequacies of current funding mechanisms for single-institution clinical treatment research is discussed.

ADVANTAGES OF SINGLE-INSTITUTION CLINICAL TREATMENT RESEARCH

In a single institution it would appear to be easier (1) to conduct innovative studies, (2) to modify a study, (3) to initiate a study rapidly, (4) to perform a complex study, (5) to ensure uniformity of high-quality data, and (6) to perform ancillary studies. Each of these is considered in turn. However, it is important to realize that scientific study of the advantages of single-institution clinical research as compared with multicenter cooperative research has not been undertaken and is clearly indicated.

Conduct of Innovative Studies

There has been little study of the methodology of discovery and none that I could find relative to cancer clinical treatment research. However, almost all investigators would agree with Thomas (9) that "hunches and intuitive impressions are essential in getting the work started." Hunches and intuitive impressions are difficult to test in cooperative group trials for at least two reasons.

First the group process of generating a study is basically incompatible with a highly innovative study. Creativity has been defined by Ebashi (10) as "the result of the interaction, or rather, 'friction' between the contemporary scientific concept or understanding and the way of thinking of a particular individual. If (the individual's) thinking coincides perfectly with the current concept or understanding, he cannot be creative even if he is very bright." This definition of creativity or innovativeness explains in part why cooperative group studies cannot be truly innovative.

The generation of cooperative group studies, especially with the advent of multimodality input, is extremely complicated. A study idea is usually presented to a disease committee by an individual investigator. It is reviewed in its early draft form by the disease and modality committees. There are generally two to three cycles of reviews taking a minimum of from 6 to 12 months (11). The difficulties of initiating an innovative study under these conditions are obvious. Convincing one other like-minded individual of the soundness of a new idea without preliminary data is generally difficult; convincing 20 to 100 disease and modality committee members and as many as 1,000 investigators in 15 to 30 institutions with various training backgrounds and biases is probably impossible. Moreover, if a promising, highly innovative protocol is activated but almost all the participating investigators are not convinced of the soundness of the study, adequate numbers of patients may not be entered, and the study will fail.

Carter (12) has described this intrinsic problem of cooperative group studies as the compromise phenomenon. "The compromise phenomenon involves the reality that as multiple groups debate a study design compromises of the original proposed design will be required in order for all to agree to participate. The larger the number that are involved the greater the compromises that will probably have to be made. If these compromises are too great, then a least-common-denominator protocol will result which may no longer be innovative or worth undertaking."

The analogy between the innovative clinical research investigator and the cooperative group and the description by Morris (13) of the creative child and his playmates is of interest:

> One has to remember that when a child is trying out new patterns of play in a social context, it will be subject to conformist pressures from other members of its group. The child can be creative only when those pressures are ignored and it says: "I'm going to try this new thing anyway. I know the rest of the group don't want to do this, they all want to play that same game we played yesterday, but I want to try a new game now," and . . . is prepared to ignore the fact that there may be some nice rules that have been invented and will make a nice repetitive game that everybody knows how to do in a . . . comfortable way.

A second reason that cooperative groups cannot mount truly innovative studies is less well appreciated. Cooperative groups cannot afford to do highly innovative studies because almost all new ideas are wrong. The well-known philosopher of science, Karl Popper, has written (14):

> To get new and good ideas, what one must do is first to produce new ideas, and secondly to criticise them. This is also the way in which one gets a grip on a problem. That is to say, it is only after you have produced a hundred bad solutions to a problem—or a couple of hundred— that you see where the real difficulty lies. . . .

Einstein wrote somewhere . . . that in the 2 years before 1916—before his General Theory of Relativity—he may have had, on the average, an idea every two minutes: almost always, of course, an idea that he rejected. A similar point is implicit in John Archibald Wheeler's remark that "our whole problem is to make our mistakes as fast as possible."

Morris (15) has stated it in a somewhat different way:

The creative act is not linked inevitably with excellence, because the creative act is one that by virtue of its suddenness, by virtue of the fact that it is a dramatic shift in thinking, a change of direction, it is often full of errors and flaws. The most original thinkers often made the most terrible mistakes and when we look back at people who have changed the course of thinking we now say "Oh yes, he found a way to see things differently, but he was wrong on this, and this, and this. . . ."

Cooperative clinical trial groups can simply not afford the testing of multiple wrong ideas. The time involved to generate a study and the group resources invested in it (financial, statistical, and patient) preclude the undertaking of many studies that do not provide useful new information. It is difficult in cooperative groups to modify or stop studies that have been initiated, even when they develop problems or look as if they were not going to be productive. In the single institution, however, it is easy for the single investigator or small group of investigators to test a new idea on a few patients and if it does not seem to be correct to drop or modify the study.

There would undoubtedly be disagreement regarding what constitutes a truly innovative study in cancer clinical treatment research. Clinical treatment research studies can, however, reasonably easily be divided into exploratory, confirmatory, and explanatory studies (12). An exploratory study is one that explores a new idea or a new regimen, a confirmatory study is one that attempts to reproduce a positive result that has been previously reported, and an explanatory study is one that takes an established active regimen and attempts to dissect it or to modulate it in some way so as to improve its therapeutic index. It is obvious that truly innovative studies are exploratory, but exploratory studies are not necessarily highly innovative. Carter (12) has listed as examples of important exploratory studies in cancer clinical treatment research the MOPP study of DeVita et al. (16), the five-drug study on breast cancer of Cooper (17), the VAMP study of Freireich et al. (18), the initial evaluation of total nodal irradiation for Hodgkin's disease by Kaplan (19), and the Hexa-CAF study in advanced ovarian cancer by Young et al. (20). All these have been performed at single institutions. This is not to say that important innovative studies cannot occur in cooperative groups, but the majority of cooperative group studies are confirmatory or explanatory (12), and almost all important innovative or exploratory studies have been performed in single institutions (see the next section).

Ease of Modification of Studies

The study design in almost all exploratory or innovative studies will require modification from that initially proposed. It is for this reason that it is almost universal in clinical research to do a preliminary or trial experiment before one starts a major study. The importance of the preliminary trial is well described by Hamilton in his excellent book *Lectures on the Methodology of Clinical Research* (21):

> Before an experiment is started it is well to do a preliminary or trial experiment. It is only in this way that one has an opportunity of seeing the practical difficulties that can appear. In clinical research, the preliminary trial is largely a test of what one might call the administrative procedures, but sometimes one will be involved in more than plain observation of patients, one will be using apparatus. In such case, a preliminary trial is absolutely necessary to see that all is going well. I am not referring to the tests to see if apparatus is working, but a trial of the actual procedures to be used in the experiment.

> During the preliminary trial, the data should be collected as if it were a full trial. . . . In this way one has an opportunity of seeing whether the material is amenable to analysis. . . .

> The preliminary run may also show you that your hypothesis is inadequate and may need to be revised. Some of the first findings may even suggest big changes in the experimental design, as well as in the hypothesis.

In a single-institution study, difficulties in experimental design are rapidly recognized and can be rectified immediately. In cooperative group studies identification of problems are often delayed because no one person sees all the patients. Even once the problem is brought to the attention of the study chairman, he must be convinced of its validity and confirm it by checking with all the other investigators. Any modifications must then be discussed and agreed on by all participants. Finally, an official addendum modifying the study must be written and distributed. When the change is major, the data collected previously may no longer be of use. In the cooperative group setting, as discussed earlier, this may constitute a major wasting of group resources.

Rapid Initiation of Studies

In a single institution, investigators can usually rapidly initiate a study. Indeed, initially new ideas are generally tested on a few patients in the absence of a formally designed study. If the results look promising, a formal protocol is written and submitted to the institution's committee on the use of human subjects in research. The single-institution protocol generally does not require the kind of detail needed in a multicenter trial protocol (22). In a single institution the initiation of a complex study may take several months but almost never requires the 6 to 12 months indicated by the cooperative groups as being the usual time course of generation of a study (11). Indeed, the 6- to 12-month period is a conservative estimate, as can be seen in Table 1, which describes the time course for generation of the lymphoma studies in Cancer and Leukemia Group B initiated since I became Vice-Chairman of the Lymphoma Committee. Similarly, the EORTC—gnotobiotic project group has stated that, even with its experience, it needs one to two years to develop a new protocol (22).

Table 2 lists clinical treatment research in lymphoma initiated at the University of Minnesota during approximately the same period as the CALGB studies listed in Table 1. All were initiated within three months of formulating the idea. Three (MN 5, MN 6, MN 8) served as prepilots for CALGB studies; all these were

Table 1. Time from Initial Discussion of Idea to Activation of Protocol for Lymphoma Studies Activated in CALGB 11/77–4/80

Protocol Number	Type of Study and Description	Month of Initial Discussion	Month Activated	Time (mo)
7751	*Phase III*. Comparison of combination chemotherapy alone and with radiation therapy by involved field in poor risk patients with stage I and II Hodgkin's disease	4/75	12/77	32
7772	*Phase II* study of Chlorozotocin	7/77	7/78	12
7804	*Pilot*. CHOP in combination with low-dose 5-day IV infusion bleomycin in the treatment of poor histology lymphomas and nodular PDL	11/77	10/78	11
7851	*Phase III*. Treatment of advanced diffuse histiocytic lymphoma; CHOP versus CHOP-infusion bleo followed by high-dose methotrexate versus conventional dose methotrexate	8/77	4/79	20
7902	*Pilot*. Methotrexate, Leucovorin rescue, VM-26, Procarbazine, Dexamethasone in the treatment of poor histology lymphoma or nodular poorly differentiated lymphocytic lymphoma refractory to prior therapy	12/77	9/79	21
7903	*Pilot*. The treatment of advanced Hodgkin's disease with induction chemotherapy followed by late intensification	11/77	10/79	23
7951	*Phase III*. The management of stage III and stage IV nodular poorly differentiated lymphocytic lymphoma and nodular mixed lymphocytic histiocytic lymphoma CHOP-bleo versus Cytoxan	7/78	1/80	18
7972	*Phase II* trial of AMSA	11/78	8/79	9

activated within one month of return from the CALGB meeting where the idea was initially discussed and basically as soon as the first eligible patient was seen.

Performance of Complex Studies

The complexity of a study may be defined in a number of ways. Cancer clinical treatment studies may be complex because they combine numerous modalities in treatment, they contain multiple drugs, the drugs are administered in unusual ways in terms of route of administration or timing, unusual measurements are required, resources of limited availability are needed (e.g., unusual equipment, clinical tests, clinical facilities, or support mechanisms), or excessive personnel (e.g., physician, clerical, or nursing) time is required. It is obviously easier to

Table 2. Lymphoma Studies at University of Minnesota Initiated Between 1975 and 1980

MN 1 — *Pilot.* Whole lung irradiation for stage I and II Hodgkin's disease with large mediastinal masses

MN 2 — *Pilot.* Glucocorticoid receptors in lymphomas and response to treatment with glucocorticoid alone

MN 3 — *Pilot.* Restaging including laparotomy following chemotherapy for advanced Hodgkin's disease

MN 4 — *Pilot.* CRAB followed by allogeneic bone marrow transplantation for Burkitt's and T-cell lymphoma

MN 5 — *Pilot.* C-HOPE in advanced lymphoma

MN 6 — *Pilot.* CALGB 7804 pretest

MN 7 — *Phase II.* Vindescine in lymphoma

MN 8 — *Pilot.* Tolerance of extended field radiotherapy followed by combination chemotherapy in Hodgkin's disease; pretest for CALGB 7751

Table 3. Comparison of Complexity of Lymphoma Treatment Studies of CALGB and the University of Minnesota

Study Number[b]	Modalities Involved[c]	Complexity Rating of Study According to:[a]				
		Number of Drugs	Drug Route/ Timing	Required Measure- ments	Required Resources	equired Personnel Time
7751	MO/RO/SO	R	R	R	R	R
7772	MO	R	R	R	R	R
7804	MO	R	I	I	I	R
7851	MO	R	I	R	I	R
7902	MO	R	R	R	R	R
7903	MO	R	I	R	R	R
7951	MO	R	R	R	R	R
7952	MO	R	R	R	R	R
MN 1	MO/PO/RO/SO	. . .	. . .	I	R	R
MN 2	MO/SO	R	R	C	C	C
MN 3	MO/SO	R	R	I	R	R
MN 4	PO/MO/RO	I	I	C	C	C
MN 5	MO	R	R	R	R	R
MN 6	MO	R	I	I	I	R
MN 7	MO	R	I	R	R	R
MN 8	MO/RO	R	R	R	R	R

[a]R = routine (compatible with standard treatment for the disease); I = intermediate complexity; C = unusually complex (much different from what is required in standard treatment).

[b]See Tables 1 and 2.

[c]MO = medical oncology; RO = radiation oncology; SO = surgical oncology; PO = pediatric oncology.

execute a complex study, which has been designed to suit the unique capabilities of a single institution, in that institution. Circumstances and resources are rarely the same in multiple institutions.

I know of no study comparing the complexity of single-institution with cooperative group trials. Such a study might be useful. For interest I compared the complexity of the CALGB lymphoma studies described previously (Table 1) with our local studies in lymphoma performed during the same period (Table 2). As illustrated in Table 3, our local protocols were more likely to involve several therapeutic modalities and tended to be more complex in terms of the measurements, resources, and personnel time required. Bonadonna has suggested that one of the problems with cancer treatment research occurring in single institutions is the resulting development of highly sophisticated treatments that cannot be easily administered in general hospitals (5). Obviously, however, if such treatments substantially improve survival, this is a minor consideration.

Uniformity of High Quality Data

The relative ease of monitoring a protocol so that all criteria are adhered to and all eligible patients entered and the uniformity in type of patient studied and how the protocol is executed are considered by most clinical trial methodologists as among the most important advantages of the single-institution clinical trial compared with multicenter trials (6,12,22–25). These advantages of single-center studies and disadvantages of multicenter trials have been stated in a number of ways, but I think one of the clearest statements is that of Gaus (22):

> The problems in cooperative and multicenter trials are in principle the same problems as in single-center studies, but they are more difficult to handle and control. It is especially more difficult to:
>
> 1. Get samples of the same statistical population of patients in all participating hospitals
> 2. Observe the same points and use the same laboratory methods in all participating hospitals
> 3. Ensure the same treatment, the same standard of nursing care, and the same environmental conditions in all participating hospitals
> 4. Get a small "variance within treatments" due to the differences among hospitals, their organization and structure, the language barrier, and the different attitudes of the patients.

The uniformity of protocol execution when a small number of experienced investigators make the measurements and take care of all patients in a single institution using a single set of laboratories and the same nursing and support facilities can obviously not be duplicated in multicenter trials. Moreover, in single institutions when problems in uniformity or interpretation of measurements occur, these can readily be solved. Missing data are also more readily retrieved.

An additional aspect of nonuniformity in multicenter trials that has not been extensively considered has been pointed out by Israel (24):

> Eligibility and exclusion criteria vary considerably from one institution to another owing to dissimilarity in the accuracy of available diagnostic procedures, the equipment available and the energy put into obtaining these diagnostic investigations.

The practical importance of uniformity in protocol evaluation has been questioned. It has been argued that if only one group can effectively use a treatment, it obviously has limitations. The problem with this argument is that cancer treatment research is done to test a hypothesis, not administer therapy. If an effective treatment is discovered, subsequent studies can modify the treatment to make it more widely applicable.

These differences in both patient population and ability to execute a study can cause serious problems in interpretation of results in multicenter trials. The variable quality of data coming from differing institutions may result in what Carter (12) calls the dilution phenomenon. Poor-quality data or poor execution of the protocol regimens lessen (dilute) the import of high-quality data. If a great deal of poor-quality data come into a study, the dilution may be so great that a false negative may result. That differing results will be achieved by different centers in a cooperative group trial has been demonstrated repeatedly and described for SWOG by Freireich (5).

Performance of Ancillary Studies

A major advantage of single-institution clinical treatment research is that ancillary or adjunct studies are readily performed. Adjunct studies are important not only because they result in advances in clinical cancer treatment but also because they often increase our understanding of basic biology (26). Of the major contributions to cancer clinical treatment research of single institutions identified at the conference on Clinical Research in Cancer Centers many related to this area (see Table 4) (27).

Ancillary studies may be of a number of types. One type of adjunct study involves associated laboratory or basic research such as study of malignant cells for immunologic, cytogenetic, cytokinetic, or other features both to learn about basic biology and to correlate these features with clinical course and response to various treatment modalities. Another type of adjunct study relates to the development of treatment support techniques (e.g., control of opportunistic infection, the use of platelets and white cells during chemotherapy, the use of hyperalimentation, the use of indwelling venous catheters for administration of intravenous products over prolonged periods, the use of Ommaya reservoirs, pain control, etc.).

Other examples of ancillary studies that have been important in cancer treatment advances and done in single institutions are measurements of drug blood levels and pharmacology in general, assessment of various baseline host conditions for response to treatment (e.g., immune status), and the use of various tumor markers such as carcinoembryonic antigen for screening and prognosis. An additional type of ancillary study involves long-term follow-up of the patient for the development of late complications of treatment. A single institution, with its stability of personnel and record keeping, is particularly suitable for such studies.

Such ancillary studies have resulted in important advances in our ability to treat patients. Ancillary studies have almost always been done in single institutions for a number of reasons. First, ideas for such adjunct studies are more likely to be recognized when a single investigator evaluates a series of patients

Table 4. Contributions of Single Institutions (Cancer Centers) to Clinical Research; Concensus of the Conference on Clinical Research in Cancer Centers (27)

The primary role of (cancer centers is) in the area of innovative ideas and pilot studies. Confirmatory studies (are) possible in some cases as well and, certainly, the cancer center has a responsibility to contribute to the improved care of the cancer patient in practice. The cancer center seems uniquely suited, however, to the development of therapeutic hypotheses and preliminary testing through well designed pilot studies. In addition:

1. The single institution, with its stability of personnel and record keeping, is particularly suitable to long-term studies. With improved treatment regimens, survival for patients with some cancers is now measured in years rather than months. Final assessment of the results of a specific treatment protocol may require from five to ten years of follow-up. Particularly important in this long-term evaluation are such additional features as late consequences of cancer and its treatment and the possibility of such clinical problems as secondary neoplasms.

2. Clinical research in cancer centers allows for the formulation of hypotheses, design of clinical trials to test the hypothesis and, upon review of the resulting data, formulation of new hypotheses for further testing. Thus, the series of clinical trials in cancer centers is characterized by sequential development of protocol study approaches. The pool of accumulating clinical data also allows for repeated analysis to further our understanding of the biology of human cancer.

3. Implementation of protocol studies within a cancer center allows for close monitoring for quality and consistency of data.

4. Treatment regimens under study are often associated with a variety of ancillary studies dealing with related clinical care problems or laboratory investigation involving human cancer.

5. The accumulation of well controlled observations on patients with cancer expands the knowledge concerning clinical characteristics of human cancer, observations about etiology and both short and long-term treatment complications.

6. A cancer center provides the opportunity for multidisciplinary or multimodal approaches to the treatment and investigation of human cancer. Within a center, a variety of specialists and subspecialists are available who can be involved in the care and study of the patient with cancer.

7. After failure of an initial protocol study, it is characteristic for patients to be entered into second and third line studies with the objective to provide the patient with additional opportunity for treatment as well as for investigators to learn further about the efficacy of other drugs and drug combinations.

8. The environment in a cancer center is usually such that a variety of related and unrelated scientific disciplines are present and thus investigators involved in clinical research can seek out advice and even collaborative research opportunities when it is appropriate.

9. Since there is this mix of scientific disciplines in the environment of a cancer center, it is also conducive to the clinical studies being reviewed and reported locally in a critical environment usually involving people in basic cancer research as well as other related clinical disciplines.

10. Most cancer centers have strong laboratory and clinical training programs. The clinical research is an important part of the educational opportunities available to trainees.

---

being treated under similar circumstances. Flexibility in study design and the following of new leads such as can be done in a single institution are important in the development of newer techniques. Finally, such studies are often too complex to involve multiple institutions, either for technical reasons or because of the quality and consistency of clinical data required.

CONTRIBUTIONS OF SINGLE INSTITUTIONS TO THE CURE OF SELECTED ADVANCED CANCERS

Significant advances have resulted from clinical cancer treatment research. It has been estimated that using surgery, radiotherapy, and chemotherapy, alone or in combination, approximately 41% of cancer patients are now cured (28). There are currently at least 12 cancers in which drugs have been responsible for a fraction of patients with advanced disease achieving a normal life span (Table 5) (1). Study of the contributions of single institution and cooperative group research to the ability to cure these cancers might be useful in order to help make rational decisions regarding funding and the structuring of environmental conditions to accelerate our ability to cure cancer. An interesting analysis of the studies that resulted in 10 major clinical advances in cardiovascular and pulmonary medicine and surgery has been done by Comroe and Dripps (29); a similar study in cancer treatment advances would be of interest.

Since no such study has been performed, I have tabulated for three of the cured cancers some of the key clinical studies contributing to these cures. A rigorous analysis is beyond the scope of this article. I have simply selected some recent review articles describing the development of curative therapies for various tumors and listed the studies that the authors felt were the key ones. Then I have determined if they were cooperative group or single-institution studies. The methodologic inadequacies of this approach are obvious; this is not meant to be definitive analysis. However, the results tend to support the process de-

Table 5. Advanced Cancers in Which Drugs Have Been Responsible for a Fraction of Patients Achieving a Normal Life Span (1)

Choriocarcinoma
Testicular cancer
Acute lymphoblastic leukemia, pediatric
Acute myelogenous leukemia, adult
Burkitt's lymphoma
Hodgkin's disease
Diffuse histiocytic lymphoma
Nodular mixed lymphoma
Ewing's sarcoma
Rhabdomyosarcoma
Wilms' tumor
Ovarian cancer

scribed earlier, that initial studies usually come from single institutions and confirmatory studies from cooperative groups.

The first proof that chemotherapy could cure metastatic disease came from the work of Li, Hertz, and Spencer in choriocarcinoma in 1956 (30). The key studies resulting in the cure of metastatic choriocarcinoma have been identified by Zubrod in his article on "Historic Milestones in Curative Chemotherapy" (28). All the studies he references (see Table 6), except the last one, were performed in single institutions. The last study, which basically confirms the earlier work done at the National Cancer Institute, was done by a group of cooperating hospitals organized by Duke University. It is worth noting that none of these studies is a comparative trial, not even the study of the cooperative group.

A more complete list of the first studies reporting cures in gestational trophoblastic tumors has been compiled by Li (31). Six of these were performed in single institutions and two by cooperative groups. The earlier reports all came from single institutions.

Table 6. Cure of Metastatic Choriocarcinoma—Key Articles from Zubrod CG (28)

I. *Observation.* A short course of methotrexate in a hypophysectomized woman with metastatic melanoma resulted in a reduction of a previously high titre of gonadotropin.
   A. Min Chin Li, Sloan-Kettering Institute (unpublished).

II. *Pilot Study* in two patients with choriocarcinoma
   A. Li et al, National Cancer Institute: Effect of methotrexate therapy upon choriocarcinoma and chorioadenoma. *Proc Soc Exp Biol Med* 93:361, 1956.
   Dosage schedule based on work of:
      1. Goldin et al, National Cancer Institute: Modification of treatment schedules in the management of advanced mouse leukemia with amethopterin. *J Natl Cancer Inst* 17:203, 1956.
      2. Paul T. Condit, National Cancer Institute: Duration of the effects of the folic acid antagonists in man. *Proc AACR* 2:194, 1957.
   B. Hertz et al, National Cancer Institute: Five years' experience with the chemotherapy of metastatic choriocarcinoma and related trophoblastic tumors in women. *Am J Obstet Gynecol* 82:631, 1961.

III. *Pilot Studies* on other agents in patients resistant to methotrexate
   A. Hertz et al, National Cancer Institute: Effect of vincaleukoblastine on metastatic choriocarcinoma and related trophoblastic tumors in women. *Cancer Res* 20:1052, 1960.
   B. Ross et al, National Cancer Institute: Actinomycin D in the treatment of methotrexate-resistant trophoblastic disease in women. *Cancer Res* 22:1016, 1962.

IV. *Confirmatory Studies*
   A. Hammond CB, et al, Southeastern Regional Trophoblastic Disease Center: Treatment of metastatic trophoblastic disease: Good and poor prognosis. *Am J Obstet Gynecol* 115:451, 1973.

Table 7. Cure of Metastatic Testicular Cancer—Key Articles from Fraley et al (32)

I. Demonstration that combination chemotherapy with actinomycin D, chlorambucil, and methotrexate could cause complete remissions in disseminated testicular cancer
  Li et al, Sloan-Kettering Institute:
  Effects of combined drug therapy on metastatic cancer of the testis. *JAMA* 174:1291, 1960.
   A. *Confirmatory Studies*
    1. Mackenzie, James Ewing and Memorial Hospitals: *Cancer* 19:1369, 1966.
    2. Moore, Letterman General Hospital: *J Urol* 100:527, 1968.
II. Identification of other active agents
   A. Mithramycin
    1. Curreri and Ansfield, University of Wisconsin: *Cancer Chemother Rep* 8:18, 1960.
    2. Kofman et al, Presbyterian-St. Luke's Hospital: *Cancer* 17:938, 1964.
    3. Brown and Kennedy, University of Minnesota: *N Eng J Med* 272:111, 1965.
   B. Vinblastine
    1. *Samuels and Howe*, M. D. Anderson: *Cancer* 25:1009, 1970.
   C. Bleomycin
    1. EORTC: Study of clinical efficiency of bleomycin. *Br Med J* ii:643, 1970.
    2. Samuels, M. D. Anderson: Personal communication of data to Kenneth Agre, M.D., PhD., Bristol Labs, Syracuse, New York, 1970.
III. Development of more active combination chemotherapy regimens
   A. Samuels et al, M. D. Anderson: *Cancer* 36:318, 1975. *Cancer Chemother Rep* 59:563, 1975.
   B. Wittes et al, Memorial Sloan-Kettering Cancer Center: *Cancer* 37:637, 1976.
IV. Identification of the activity of *cis*-diamminedichloroplatinum in testicular cancer
   A. Rossof et al, Rush Medical College: *Cancer* 30:1451, 1972.
   B. Higby et al, Roswell Park Memorial Institute: *Cancer* 33:1219, 1974.
V. Development of curative combination chemotherapy regimens in a substantial fraction of patients: the addition of platinum
   A. Cvitkovic et al, Memorial Sloan-Kettering Cancer Center: *Proc AACR* 16:174, 1975.
   B. Einhorn et al, Indiana University: *Proc ASCO* 17:240, 1976. *Ann Intern Med* 87:293, 1977.
VI. Confirmation and exploration of role of maintenance
   A. Bosl et al, University of Minnesota: *Am J Med* 68:492, 1980.

Table 8. Early Clinical Cancer Treatment Research Contribution to the Cure of Childhood Acute Lymphoblastic Leukemia (28,33–35)

I. Elucidation of active drugs
   A. Folate antagonists
      1948–1952 series of reports from single institutions demonstrating activity of aminopterin and amethopterin (methotrexate) in ALL
         [*Farber et al., N Engl J Med 238:787, 1948; Farber et al., Arch J Dis Child 77:129, 1949; Domeshek, Blood 4:168, 1949; Sacks et al., Ann Intern Med 32:80, 1950; Burchenal et al., Cancer 4:549, 1951; Schoenbach et al., Cancer 5:1201, 1952*]
   B. Glucocorticoids
      1950–1954 series of reports from single institutions demonstrating activity of ACTH and cortisone in ALL
         [*Farber in Mote (ed) Proc of the First Clinical ACTH Conf. NY Blakiston, 1950 p. 338; Stickney et al., Proc Staff Meeting Mayo Clinic 25:488, 1950; Schulman et al., Pediatr 8:34, 1951; Fessas et al., Arch Intern Med 94:384, 1954*]
      1956 first study using prednisone (from single institution)
         [*Hyman and Sturgeon, Cancer 9:2, 1956*]
   C. 6-Mercaptopurine
      1953–1954 series of reports from single institutions demonstrating activity in ALL
         [*Burchenal et al., Blood 8:965, 1953; Hall et al., Ann NY Acad Sci 60:374, 1954; Bernard and Seligmann, Ann NY Acad Sci 60:385, 1954; Farber, Ann NY Acad Sci 60:412, 1954; Pierce, Ann NY Acad Sci 60:415, 1954; Rundles and Crago, Ann NY Acad Sci 60:425, 1954; Hyman et al., Ann NY Acad Sci 60:430, 1954; Bethell and Thompson, Ann NY Acad Sci 60:436, 1954; Fountain, Ann NY Acad Sci 60:439, 1954; Rosenthal et al., Ann NY Acad Sci 60:448, 1954; Gaffney and Cooper, Ann NY Acad Sci 60:478, 1954; Wilson, Ann NY Acad Sci 60:499, 1954*]
   D. Vincristine
      1962–1964 series of reports from single institutions demonstrating activity in ALL
         [*Karon et al., Pediatr 30:791, 1962: Rohn and Hodes, Proc AACR 3:355, 1962; Selawry and Delta, Proc AACR 3:360, 1962; Tan and Aduna, Proc AACR 3:367, 1962; Evans et al., Cancer 16:1302, 1963; Selawry, JAMA 183:741, 1963; Shaw and Brunner, Cancer Chemother Rep 42:45, 1964*]

II. Combining of drugs to achieve high complete remission rates and remissions of longer duration
   1960–1968 series of reports from single institutions and cooperative groups demonstrating efficacy or superiority of drug combinations
   1. Single institutions:
      [*Zeulzer and Flatz, Am J Dis Child 100:886, 1960; Evans et al, Cancer 16:1302, 1963; Perrin et al., Pediatr 31:833, 1963; Freireich et al., Proc AACR 5:20, 1964, Freireich et al., Proc AACR 6:20, 1965; Henderson et al., Proc AACR 7:30, 1966; George et al., Proc AACR 7:23, 1966*]
   2. Cooperative groups:
      [*Frei et al., Blood 18:431, 1961; Sullivan et al., Cancer Chemother Rep 16:161, 1962; Frei and Taylor, Proc AACR 4:20, 1963; Selawry and Frei, Clin Res 12:231, 1964; Frei et al., Blood*

26:642, 1965; Krivit et al., J Pediatr 68:965, 1966; Fernbach et
al., N Engl J Med 275:451, 1966]

III. Development of maintenance therapy approaches
    1. 1957–1963 series of reports from single institutions
       suggesting superiority of maintained remissions in ALL
       [Hyman et al., Cancer Res 17:851, 1957; Zeulzer and Flatz, Am J
       Dis Child 100:886, 1960; Condit and Eliel, JAMA 172:451,
       1960; Bernard et al., Nouv Rev France Hematol 2:195, 1962;
       Boggs et al., Medicine 41:163, 1962; Perrin et al., Pediatr
       31:833, 1963]
    2. 1961–1970 series of reports primarily from cooperative
       groups, the NCI and St. Judes exploring the use of various
       drugs and the best ways to administer them for maintenance
       (see 33 & 35 for summaries)

IV. Development of the concept of prophylactic treatment of the
central nervous system to prevent relapse in this area
    A. Development of effective treatment of CNS leukemia and
       recognition of its increasing incidence (including during
       remission) with prolongation of survival in childhood ALL
       1. 1954–1959 series of reports from single institutions on the
          use of intrathecal amethopterin
          [Sansone, Ann Paediatr 183:33, 1954; Whiteside et al., Arch
          Intern Med 101:279, 1958; Murphy, Pediatr Clin N Am
          6:611, 1959; Hyman et al., Proc AACR 3:29, 1959]
       2. 1957–1960 series of reports from single institutions on the
          use of radiotherapy
          [Sullivan, Pediatr 20:757, 1957; D'Angio et al., Am J
          Roentgen Rad Therapy Nuclear Med 82:541, 1959; Shaw et
          al., Neurology 10:823, 1960]
    B. 1963–1966 series of reports on the use of prophylactic
       therapy to the CNS. First published report from a
       cooperative group; the remaining studies are from single
       institutions
       [Frei and Taylor, Proc AACR 4:20, 1963; Spevak, Iowa Med
       Soc 54:238, 1964; George and Pinkel, Proc AACR 6:22, 1965;
       Mathé, Bull int Un Cancer 3:4, 1965; Sharp and Nesbit, Proc
       AACR 7:64, 1966; George et al, Proc AACR 7:23, 1966]

One of the most recent advanced cancers to be cured in a sizable number of patients by chemotherapy alone is nonseminomatous testicular cancer. The key studies resulting in the cure of this tumor have recently been reviewed by Fraley et al (32) and are listed in Table 7. As can be seen, only one of the key studies (EORTC study of bleomycin) was performed by a cooperative group. A few confirmatory studies relative to the treatment of advanced testicular cancer have been published or recently undertaken by cooperative groups (7).

Among the 12 advanced cancers currently cured by chemotherapy, the major contributions toward cure from cooperative group studies have occurred in acute leukemia. Thus, I have evaluated how single institutions have contributed to the cure of acute lymphoblastic leukemia (ALL). The early studies (before 1970) contributing to the cure of ALL are indicated in Table 8. These studies represent a fairly complete list of the earliest studies for each major step toward the cure of ALL. The studies have been selected from four articles (28,33–35).

The first step in the cure of ALL was the discovery that a number of drugs were highly active. The effectiveness of the first three major classes of drugs (folate antagonists, glucocorticoids, and 6-mercaptopurine) was demonstrated in single institutions before 1954–1955, when the major cooperative groups for study of leukemia were formed. Even in the case of the more recent drugs, however, initial activity has been demonstrated in single institutions. Controlled trials, primarily performed by cooperative groups, have subsequently defined the optimal dosage and scheduling of these drugs (33–35). The subsequent steps towards cure (Table 8, II,III) have resulted from both single-institution and cooperative group research. In general, the major innovations have come from single institutions, and the cooperative group studies have been confirmatory or explanatory, although this has not invariably been the case.

FUNDING MECHANISMS FOR SINGLE-INSTITUTION CANCER CLINICAL TREATMENT RESEARCH

It is clear from the preceding discussion that single institutions have made important contributions to cancer treatment research. As indicated in the report of the DCT Subcommittee for Clinical Trials Review (3), the first step toward the development of new treatments is the availability of adequate research resources. Funding for clinical treatment research in single institutions has been difficult to obtain. Funding for clinical treatment research in cancer comes primarily from four sources: the government (primarily the NCI), industry (primarily drug companies), other charitable organizations (e.g., the American Cancer Society), and donations from relatives and friends of patients and other interested individuals to specific institutions. The relative contributions of these various sources to cancer clinical treatment research has not been evaluated, but presumably a major portion of the support comes from the NCI.

Eight funding mechanisms for support of clinical therapeutic research from the NCI have been identified (27). They are as follows:

1. Cancer center core grants
2. Cooperative group grants (R10)
3. Program project grants (P01)
4. Contract support
5. Cancer research emphasis grants
6. Organ site programs (R26)
7. Cancer control
8. Individual investigator applications (R01)

Of these funding mechanisms, only the program project grants and the individual investigator grants allow the investigator the opportunity for development of self-initiated research programs.

Clinical treatment research consumes only 10.5% of the NCI budget, even though human subjects research is generally more expensive than preclinical research. In fiscal year 1978, $19.3 million in direct costs were awarded to 135 grants for clinical treatment research (2). Forty-five percent, or 8.6 million, was awarded to the clinical cooperative groups (R10). R10s constituted 62% ($n =$ 84) of the total clinical treatment grants awarded. The remaining clinical treatment grants awarded consisted of 20 P01s, 19 R01s, and 12 R26s. Of the grants submitted for each group, this represented funding of 63% of the R10s requested, 60% of the R26s, 53% of P01s, and only 23% of R01's. Funding awarded for clinical treatment research in each category was for P01s 9.2 million, for R10s 8.6 million, for R01s 0.9 million, and for R26s 0.6 million.

Most single-institution grant research is funded via R01s and P01s; thus only $10.1 million was awarded for single-institution clinical treatment research, even though such research has made a major contribution to the cure of cancer. Moreover, the current grant review mechanism awarded only 32% of requested single-institution grants and only 23% of those were individual-investigator-instigated rather than cancer center grants. More than twice the percentage of clinical research R01 grants were disapproved in FY78 as compared with all other competing NCI R01 grants. This problem of insufficient monies available for single-institution research and an inadequate review mechanism has recently been acknowledged by the NCI. It has recently solicited more cancer clinical treatment research grants from single institutions and has set up a separate study section for reviewing these grants (36).

SUMMARY

The past 25 years have witnessed significant progress in our ability to cure advanced cancers. Much of this progress can be attributed to cancer clinical treatment research. Although important clinical treatment research has been done both in single institutions and by cooperative clinical trial groups, the development of therapeutic hypotheses and their preliminary testing have usually been done in single institutions. This is primarily because in the single institution it is easier (1) to conduct innovative studies, (2) to modify a study, (3) to initiate a study rapidly, (4) to perform a complex study, (5) to ensure uniformity of high-quality data, and (6) to perform ancillary studies. Although clinical treatment research in single institutions has all the advantages above and has made significant contributions to the cure of advanced cancer, current funding is inadequate, and more resources need to be directed, in particular, to individual-initiated clinical treatment cancer research.

REFERENCES

1. DeVita VT, Oliverio VT, Muggia FM, et al: The drug development and clinical trials programs of the division of cancer treatment, National Cancer Institute. *Cancer Clin Trials* 2:195, 1979.
2. *Division of Cancer Treatment Analysis of FY78 NCI Supported Treatment Research Grants.* Feb. 23, 1979.
3. Salmon SE: Draft Proposal—September 1, 1979. Subcommittee Report for Clinical Trials Review. DCT Board of Scientific Counselors.

4. Biostatistics and the Clinical Cancer Cooperative Group Program. Document prepared for DCT Board of Scientific Counselors Review of Clinical Trials, March 26–27, 1979.

5. Carter SK, Mathé G: An overview of the 1978 international meeting on comparative therapeutic trials. *Biomedicine Special Issue* 28:6, 1978.

6. Machin D, Staquet MJ, Sylvester RJ: Advantages and defects of single-center and multicenter clinical trials, in Tagnon HJ, Staquet MJ (eds): *Controversies in Cancer. Design of Trials and Treatment.* New York, Masson Publishing USA, Inc, 1979, p 7.

7. Carbone PP: Cooperative Group Clinical Trials Review. Working Document prepared for DCT Board of Scientific Counselors Review of Clinical Trials, March 26–27, 1979.

8. Editorial: UK national cancer trials—unstarted business. *Lancet* ii:618, 1979.

9. Thomas L: Biostatistics in medicine. *Science* 198:676, 1977.

10. Ebashi S: in Krebs HA, Shelley JH (eds): *The Creative Process in Science and Medicine,* Proceedings of the C. H. Boehringer Sohn Symposium. Taunus, 1974, p 130.

11. Davis HL, Durant JR, Holland JF: An overview of the cooperative groups and their interrelationship with the National Cancer Institute and other governmental agencies, in Carbone PP (ed): *Cooperative Group Clinical Trials Review.* Working Document prepared for DCT Board of Scientific Counselors Review of Clinical Trials. March 26–27, 1979.

12. Carter SK: Some thoughts on collaborative clinical research and its review. *Cancer Clin Trials* 2:257, 1979.

13. Morris DJ: in Krebs HA, Shelley JH (eds): *The Creative Process in Science and Medicine,* Proceedings of the C. H. Boehringer Sohn Symposium. Taunus, 1974, p 14.

14. Popper K: in Krebs HA, Shelley JH (eds): *The Creative Process in Science and Medicine,* Proceedings of the C. H. Boehringer Sohn Symposium. Taunus, 1974, p 18.

15. Morris DJ: in Krebs HA, Shelley JH (eds): *The Creative Process in Science and Medicine,* Proceedings of the C. H. Boehringer Sohn Symposium. Taunus, 1974, p 24.

16. DeVita VT, Serpick AA, Carbone PP: Combination chemotherapy in the treatment of advanced Hodgkin's disease. *Ann Intern Med* 73:881, 1970.

17. Cooper R: Combination chemotherapy in hormone resistant breast cancer. *Proc Am Assoc Cancer Res* 10:15, 1969.

18. Freireich EJ, Frei E III: Recent advances in acute leukemia, in *Progress in Hematology.* New York, Grune & Sratton, 1964, p 187.

19. Kaplan HS: The radical radiotherapy of regionally localized Hodgkin's disease. *Radiology* 78:553, 1962.

20. Young RC, Chabner BA, Hubbard SP, et al: Advanced ovarian adenocarcinoma: A prospective clinical trial of melphelan (L-Pam) versus combination chemotherapy. *N Engl J Med* 229:1261, 1978.

21. Hamilton M: *Lectures on the Methodology of Clinical Research.* Edinburgh and London, E & S Livingstone Ltd, 1961, p 46.

22. Gaus W: The experience of the EORTC-gnotobiotic project group in planning, organizing, performing, and evaluating cooperative clinical trials, in Tagnon HJ, Staquet MJ (eds): *Controversies in Cancer: Design of Trials and Treatment.* New York, Masson Publishing USA, Inc, 1979, p 17.

23. Bonadonna G, Valagussa P: The logistics of clinical trials. *Biomedicine Special Issue* 28:43, 1978.

24. Israel L: Practical and conceptual limitations of best conceived randomized trials. *Biomedical Special Issue* 28:36, 1978.

25. Freireich EJ, Gehan EA: The limitations of the randomized clinical trial, in DeVita VT, Busch H (eds): *Methods in Cancer Research* XVII:277, 1979.

26. Swazey JP, Reeds K: *Today's Medicine, Tomorrow's Science: Essays on Paths of Discovery in the Biomedical Sciences.* Washington, DC, Government Printing Office, 1978.

27. Mauer AM, Carter SK: *Minutes of Meeting of Conference on Clinical Research in Cancer Centers.* National Institutes of Health, Nov. 30–Dec. 1, 1978.

28. Zubrod CG: Historic milestones in curative chemotherapy. *Semin Oncol* 6:490, 1979.

29. Comroe JH, Dripps RD: *The Top Ten Clinical Advances in Cardiovascular-Pulmonary Medicine and Surgery 1945–1975*. Washington, DC, Government Printing Office, 1978.

30. Li MC, Hertz R, Spencer DB: Effect of methotrexate upon choriocarcinoma and chorioadenoma. *Proc Soc Exp Biol Med* 93:361, 1956.

31. Li MC: Trophoblastic disease: Natural history, diagnosis and treatment, *Ann Intern Med* 74:102, 1971.

32. Fraley EE, Lang PH, Kennedy BJ: Germ-cell testicular cancer in adults. *N Engl J Med* 301:1420, 1979.

33. Carter SK: Acute lymphocytic leukemia, in Staquet MJ (ed): *Randomized Trials in Cancer: A Critical Review by Sites*. New York, Raven Press, 1978, p 1.

34. Livingston RB, Carter SK: *Single Agents in Cancer Chemotherapy*. New York, IFI/Plenum, 1970.

35. Goldin A, Sandberg JS, Henderson ES, et al: The chemotherapy of human and animal acute leukemia. *Cancer Chemother Rep* 55:309, 1971.

36. *NIH Guide for Grants and Contracts*, vol 9, no 3, Feb. 22, 1980.

Index